ENCYCLOPEDIA OF

Infectious Diseases

ENCYCLOPEDIA OF

Infectious Diseases

Carol Turkington and
Bonnie Ashby, M.D.

Facts On File, Inc.

Encyclopedia of Infectious Diseases

Copyright © 1998 by Carol Turkington and Bonnie Ashby, M.D.

Facts On File, Inc.
11 Penn Plaza
New York NY 10001

Library of Congress Cataloging-in-Publication Data

Turkington, Carol.
Encyclopedia of infectious diseases / Carol Turkington and Bonnie Ashby.
p.   cm.
Includes bibliographical references and index.
ISBN 0-8160-3512-1 (alk. paper)
1. Communicable diseases—Encyclopedias. I. Ashby, Bonnie. II. Title.
[DNLM: 1. Communicable Diseases—encyclopedias. WC 13 T939e 1998]
RC112.T87   1998
616.9'03—dc21
97-50440

Facts On File books are available at special discounts when purchased in bulk quantities for businesses,
associations, institutions or sales promotions. Please call our Special Sales
Department in New York at (212) 967-8800 or (800) 322-8755.

You can find Facts On File on the World Wide Web at http://www.factsonfile.com

Cover design by Semadar Megged

Printed in the United States of America

MP Hermitage 10 9 8 7 6 5 4 3 2

This book is printed on acid-free paper.

For

William M. Roulston
(1948–1997)

In loving memory

Far better it is to dare mighty things, to win glorious triumphs even
though checkered by failure, than to take rank with those poor
spirits who neither enjoy much nor suffer much because they live
in the grey twilight that knows not victory nor defeat.

—Theodore Roosevelt

CONTENTS

ACKNOWLEDGMENTS

This book would not have been possible without the cooperation of countless men and women whose generosity of spirit contributed to the massive task of keeping track of the ever-evolving global picture on infectious disease.

Thanks to everyone who gave time and effort at the National Institutes of Health, the medical libraries of the National Library of Medicine, the Hershey Medical Center, and the University of Pennsylvania Medical Center. Thanks to staffers at Pharmaceutical Research and Manufacturers of America, to Eli Lilly, Astra USA, Bristol-Myers, Ciba-Geigy, Hoffmann-LaRoche, Pfizer, Smith-Kline Beecham, and Solvay Pharmaceuticals. Thanks also to the staffs of the Centers for Disease Control and Prevention, the National Institute of Allergy and Infectious Diseases, the World Health Organization and its Collaborating Center on AIDS, the Food Safety and Inspection Service, the American Public Health Association, the International Research Foundation for Helicobacter and Intestinal Immunology, Allan Brownstein at the American Liver Foundation, the American Leprosy Missions, the National AIDS Clearinghouse, the National Vaccine Compensation Program, the Emerging Infections Information Network, the WHO Division of Control of Tropical Diseases, the WHO Emerging and Other Communicable Diseases Surveillance and Control, the National Center for Infectious Disease, the folks at the Bug Bytes web site, and the American Lyme Disease Foundation.

Finally, my thanks as ever to my agent Bert Holtje, to the very patient Anne Baxter at Facts On File, and to Michael and Kara.

INTRODUCTION

From birth until death, the human body is under relentless attack by hordes of living organisms that compete for survival in our environment. The air we breathe, the food we eat, the ground we walk on, the water we drink, the buildings we live in, the vegetation that surrounds us—all harbor infectious organisms.

These agents of infectious disease come in all shapes and sizes, from microscopic viruses, bacteria, and protozoans to foot-long parasitic worms. While these germs may vary wildly in appearance, they all share a dependence on human beings for at least part of their life cycle. They enter the body by hitching a ride in contaminated food or beverages, or by invading the genital tract or the eyes. They may attack even before birth, passing through the mother's placenta where they attack the developing cells of the fetus so that the baby may be diseased or deformed at birth.

Luckily, the human body is not defenseless against this ever-present danger. Because the human environment is biologically hostile, our bodies have developed exquisitely sensitive methods that react quickly in the presence of infectious organisms. The skin and the immune system are the body's primary methods of preventing infection, and when intact they can protect admirably well. But when these barriers break down or are affected by another disease, the body becomes vulnerable to invasion by a frightening array of microorganisms both mild and deadly.

Of all the dangers threatening life on the planet today, the threat of infectious disease is one of the most insidious. Most Americans are unaware of the danger that still exists from new and emerging infections throughout the world. The developed world has become complacent with the belief that modern science had triumphed over the deadly infectious diseases of our grandparents' generation—cholera, tuberculosis, malaria, diphtheria, smallpox, influenza, polio.

It is not so.

Diseases we thought we had conquered long ago have returned with new virulence. In Kentucky, a particularly nasty form of TB that spreads like wildfire appears to infect almost everyone who comes in contact with a carrier. In Texas, an especially virulent strain of group A strep killed 18 residents in 3 months, 6 of them children.

Modern transatlantic air travel is capable of transferring infections from one city to another and from one country to another in a matter of minutes to hours. What once took tens or hundreds of years can today be accomplished overnight.

Even as we struggle with the ancient infections, new viruses may still appear. The human immunodeficiency virus and AIDS showed us that previously unknown viruses can emerge at any time to threaten the world's health, even as the older diseases gain new strength. These new dangers are growing even as antibiotics are becoming less effective. In late 1997 a deadly new strain of influenza—the H5 "bird flu"—crossed from chickens to humans, killing a group of young and healthy Hong Kong citizens before the government took drastic measures to contain the disease by killing every chicken in Hong Kong. The flu was of enormous concern because scientists believed that no human anywhere in the world had immunity to this new virus. Had it continued to spread and mingled with more common influenza viruses, the flu could have developed into the next pandemic that scientists fully expect sometime in the future.

The fight between human and microbe is a struggle of epic proportions. It is not a fight that is won easily. Still, modern medicine has far more ability to combat new and emerging infections than did our ancestors long ago. Modern methods of tracking disease can pinpoint problem areas and move to contain them before the problem gets worse. At least in the developed world, better methods to control the spread of disease organisms, including better sanitation, water purification, clean housing, pest control, personal hygiene, and quarantine procedures have vastly improved the health of its people. Vaccines together with general better health and nutrition have boosted immunity.

This book is designed as a guide and reference to a wide range of infectious diseases and their causes, and to additional information and addresses of organizations that deal with infectious disease. *It is not a substitute for prompt medical attention from a medical profes-sional trained in the treatment of infectious dis-ease.* All cases of suspected infectious disease should immediately be reported to a physician for treatment.

Information in this book comes from the most up-to-date sources available and includes some of the most recent research in the field of infectious disease. Readers should keep in mind, however, that changes occur very rapidly in this field. Because space limitations made it impossible to include all of the information in this very large specialty, a detailed bibliography has been provided for readers who seek additional sources of information. To reduce the number of cross-references, all drugs used to treat infectious disease are included in a separate list at the back of the book. All other entries are cross-referenced, and appendices provide additional information.

—Carol Turkington
Lancaster, Pennsylvania

ENCYCLOPEDIA OF

Infectious Diseases

abscess An inflammatory pus-containing nodule that is usually caused by a bacterial infection. The pus is made up of dead and live microorganisms, and destroyed tissue from white blood cells carried to the area to fight the infection. An abscess may either grow larger or smaller depending on whether the white blood cells or the bacteria win the fight. Abscesses may be found in the soft tissue beneath the skin (such as the armpit or groin), where a large number of lymph glands are located.

Cause While bacteria (such as staphylococci) are the most common cause of abscesses, fungal infections sometimes cause abscesses as well.

Diagnosis Abscesses can usually be diagnosed by sight, although a scan (such as CAT or MRI) may be used to confirm the diagnosis.

Treatment Antibiotics are usually prescribed to treat a bacterial infection, and antifungal agents will treat fungal infections. However, the lining of the abscess cavity tends to cut down on the amount of the drug that can pass from the blood into the source of the infection. Therefore, the cavity itself needs to be drained by cutting through the lining. This allows the pus to escape through a drainage tube or by leaving the cavity open to the skin. Many abscesses heal after simple drainage; others require both drainage and drug treatment.

Acinetobacter A genus of aerobic bacteria, of the family Neisseriaceae. The genus do not produce spores or move of their own accord. Found everywhere in nature, some members of the family can cause illness in humans.

acquired immunodeficiency syndrome (AIDS) A usually fatal viral disease of the immune system for which there is no immunization and no cure as yet. The disease has a crippling effect on the human immune defense system, rendering the victim unable to fight off many types of other infections, and prone to certain cancers. Eventually, these infections or cancers in themselves may be fatal. First identified in 1980, AIDS was soon recognized as epidemic throughout the world. The dominant feature of late AIDS is an extreme wasting and weight loss, leading to its nickname of "slim disease" in Uganda, the heart of the epidemic.

The World Health Organization (WHO) estimates that 17 million people are infected with HIV (human immunodeficiency virus, the viral cause of AIDS) and 4 million have full-blown AIDS; more than 90 percent of all people with AIDS live in Third World countries. The largest number of AIDS cases (more than 2.5 million) is found in sub-Saharan Africa, where more than 10 million people with HIV live. In the United States, AIDS is still primarily a disease of homosexual and bisexual males (making up 47 percent of all reported cases in 1993), although IV drug users make up a large percentage of the total. The WHO estimates that by the year 2000, 40 million people around the world could be infected.

No one knows where the human virus originated. One theory is that the virus existed undetected for centuries in isolated African villages. Since a person can harbor the virus for years before developing AIDS, and because rural Africans often contract many diseases that kill them at an early age, it's possible that the virus could have been infecting people for a very long time without being identified. Other scientists believe the virus somehow "jumped" from infected African monkeys to humans fairly recently, since viruses in monkeys are genetically similar to the HIV. However, trying to place the origin of HIV infection in Africa angers many people who feel this is blaming Africa for the AIDS problem.

The earliest documented case of HIV infection was located in a 1959 blood sample from central Africa. Epidemiologists believe the virus may have traveled from Africa to the United States during the mid-1970s, where it was first transmitted via anal intercourse among gay men in New York and San Francisco. The Rwanda capital of Kigali and the capital of Zaire both reported epidemics in 1980, and by 1982 Uganda and Zambia reported similar epidemics.

Within 10 years, U.S. scientists began to notice among young gay men an outbreak of formerly rare diseases such as PNEUMOCYSTIS CARINII pneumonia and KAPOSI'S SARCOMA that had previously been found only in those with damaged immune systems. Next, IV-drug users began to come down with the disease, together with hemophiliacs and others who received blood transfusions or blood products.

By 1991, the cumulative number of cases from 52 African countries was almost 93,000, increasing to an estimated 7.5 million people in 1993 infected with HIV in sub-Saharan Africa. By 1994, scientists reported as many as 30 different strains of HIV that often escape conventional tests to detect their presence in blood. (The new strains, first isolated in Cameroon, had not yet been detected in the United States.)

AIDS is being diagnosed in more Americans than ever, according to new statistics from the U.S. Centers for Disease Control and Prevention, but it's claiming fewer lives. The greatest increase in new cases is showing up among certain groups of young people, especially heterosexuals, women, and African Americans. The incidence among young black heterosexual women rose almost 160 percent

from 1990 to 1995, the largest increase in all groups of young people. Incidence among all young women rose more than 70 percent; incidence among young men remained unchanged. The only significant decrease in AIDS incidence in the United States occurred among young white gay and bisexual men, with a 30 percent decrease in new cases from 1990 to 1995.

However, for the first time since the disease was reported, there was no increase in the rate of HIV-related deaths in 1995, according to the CDC. The death rate has leveled off and is expected to plummet with the spread of newer antiviral drug treatment. Health experts in New York said that HIV-related deaths in that city had dropped from a peak of 7,000 a year in 1994 and 1995 to 5,000 in 1996. Similar decreases have been seen in other cities. The drop in deaths coincided with the introduction of improved antiviral drugs.

Cause   AIDS is caused by the HUMAN IMMUNODEFICIENCY VIRUS (HIV, also called the AIDS virus) that is found in all body fluids of infected people. However, only blood, semen, vaginal discharge, and breast milk have enough of the virus to spread it readily to others. The virus attaches to and attacks the helper T cells in the white blood cells. White blood cells are a part of the immune system and help fight infection and disease. When the immune system is damaged, it can't keep the body healthy. In AIDS, T cells die slowly as the HIV invades and destroys them.

HIV is the third of five human RETROVIRUSES identified since 1980, although scientists believe there are more retroviruses in existence. (A retrovirus contains an enzyme—reverse transcriptase—that converts viral RNA into a DNA copy that becomes part of the host cell's DNA.) HIV is part of a class of retroviruses known as lentiviruses, ordinarily associated with arthritis and anemia. (Lentiviruses are retroviruses that cause slowly progressive, usually fatal diseases.)

In the case of the HIV, the virus attaches itself to the cells that control the immune system (the T lymphocytes). Once inside this T cell, the virus releases its RNA with a chemical that allows it to join the cell's own DNA. All offspring of this altered T cell therefore contains the virus's genetic code. The T cell produces new HIVs, which destroy the host cell as they are created.

HIV is spread by sexual contact with an infected person, by needle-sharing among injecting drug users, or (now rarely) through blood or blood-product transfusions. An infected mother may spread the virus to her unborn baby before or during birth or during breast-feeding. In the health care setting, workers have been infected with HIV after being stuck with a needle containing HIV-infected blood, or (rarely) when infected blood enters an open cut or splashes into a mucous membrane. There has been only one demonstrated case of patients being infected by a health care worker, which involved transmission from an infected dentist to five of his patients. In investigations of more than 15,000 patients of 32 HIV-infected doctors and dentists, not one other case of this type of transmission has been found.

A person cannot get AIDS from someone else by touching, sneezing or coughing, sharing eating or drinking utensils, or from a swimming pool or other public place. AIDS is not spread from tears, urine, sweat, or saliva. In thousands of households where families have cared for AIDS patients, AIDS has not been transmitted via sharing laundry, kitchen or bathroom facilities, meals, eating utensils, drinking cups or glasses.

There has been no known risk of HIV transmission to coworkers, clients, or consumers. Food service workers known to be HIV infected need not be restricted from work, unless they have other infections such as diarrhea or HEPATITIS A, which are readily contagious.

HIV has not been transmitted through closed-mouthed kissing, although open-mouthed kissing is not recommended by the Centers for Disease Control because of the slight risk of contact with blood. No case of AIDS has ever been reported to the CDC that occurred from any kind of kissing.

While a tiny amount of HIV has been found in saliva and tears, it is important to understand that this does not necessarily mean that it can be transmitted by contact with tears. No virus has been found in sweat.

While many people have been concerned about the possibility of transmission via insect bites, CDC studies have shown no evidence that insects can transmit HIV, even in areas where there are many cases of AIDS and large populations of insects. This could be because when an insect bites a person, it doesn't inject its own, or a previous person's, blood into the new victim; instead, it injects its own saliva. Some diseases (like MALARIA or YELLOW FEVER) are transmitted by saliva, but HIV lives for only a short time within an insect. Even if a mosquito carried the virus, it doesn't become infected and can't transmit the virus to the next person it bites.

Diagnosis The presence of HIV is determined by a blood test that shows antibodies to HIV. The disease is defined as a positive AIDS test and a T-cell count less than 200. (A healthy person's T-cell count should be more than 440.) In May 1996, the FDA approved the first HIV test system with a home-use blood collection kit to test for HIV infection. A second test kit was approved in July. Scientists hope that the reliable home test kits will make diagnosis easier and more accessible. In June 1996, the FDA approved a highly reliable new home test that does not require a blood sample, but instead uses a treated cotton pad to collect a tissue sample from between the gum and cheek. The sample is tested for antibodies to HIV.

Symptoms A person who has been infected with the AIDS virus may not have any symptoms for months or even years. Many patients remain relatively healthy from 8 to 11 years after being infected.

While symptoms are different from one person to the next, early signs often include lymph node swelling in neck, jaw, armpit, or groin. Other signs include night sweats, fatigue, weight loss, fever and cough, THRUSH, or diarrhea. After some time, many AIDS patients develop other infections and cancers, including Kaposi's sarcoma, non-Hodgkin's lymphoma, pneumocystis carinii, CYTOMEGA-LOVIRUS, TOXOPLASMOSIS, MYCOBACTERIUM AVIUM COMPLEX, or TUBERCULOSIS.

Treatment While at present there is no cure for AIDS, intensive research has produced new medications that can prolong life. There are three groups of medicines that currently treat AIDS: antiviral drugs, prophylactic medicines to protect against certain infections, and other drugs to fight infections and cancer.

An enormous number of new antiretroviral drugs for treating HIV infection have been introduced, including new nucleoside agents, the first generation of HIV protease inhibitors, and non-nucleoside reverse transcriptase inhibitors (NNRTIs). In addition, tests to evaluate how much virus is circulating in a patient's blood make it possible to monitor the effectiveness of these drugs. This combination of new agents for HIV infection, together with new ways to monitor the effectiveness of therapy, has significantly improved the prognosis for today's HIV-infected patients. Combination therapy, the use of more than one antiretroviral drug at a time, is often implemented. By combining several drugs, the likelihood that a patient will develop resistance is much lower.

Reverse transcriptase inhibitors are divided into two groups: the nucleoside and the non-nucleoside drugs. Nucleoside reverse transcriptase inhibitors (NRTIs) include zidovudine (ZDV), didanosine (ddI), zalcitabine (ddC), and lamivudine (3TC). They are used primarily in combination with NNR-TIs and protease inhibitors because of their potent effect. Non-nucleoside reverse tran-

scriptase inhibitors include nevirapine (NVP) and delavirdine (DLV).

A third category of drugs are the protease inhibitors. These compounds interfere with a viral enzyme, preventing the formation of new infectious virus. The FDA has approved for protease inhibitors: saquinavir (Invirase), indinavir (Crixivan), ritonavir (Norvir), and nelfinavir (Viracept), for use in combination with NRTIs like ZDV and 3TC. A number of other HIV protease inhibitors are currently under development.

Prevention Abstinence from sexual contact and not sharing needles is the only sure way to prevent AIDS. Other than that, using a latex (rubber) condom during sexual intercourse is the best protection against the sexual transmission of HIV. Latex condoms should always be used for oral, anal, and vaginal sex in any relationship or if there is a chance that either partner is infected. Condom manufacturers in the United States electronically test all condoms for holes and weak spots. In addition, the FDA requires that manufacturers use a water test to examine samples from each batch for leakage. Only water-based lubricants should be used with latex condoms because oil-based lubricants, such as petroleum jelly, weaken natural rubber.

For people allergic to latex, the FDA has approved several polyurethane condoms, which are comparable to latex as a barrier to sperm and HIV virus.

In the United States, blood and blood products have been tested since 1985 for the AIDS virus and are considered safe. In addition, the FDA inspects the more than 3,000 donor centers where blood and blood components are collected and processed. The risk of HIV infection from transfusions has dropped from 1 in 2,500 units of blood in 1985 to 1 in 440,000 to 640,000 units by the end of 1995.

Although 13 experimental AIDS vaccines have been tested on more than 1,500 U.S. volunteers since 1988, the federal government has rejected large-scale immunization.

Outside the body, the HIV is easily killed by common disinfectants such as alcohol or peroxide.

actinomycosis A bacterial infection caused by *Actinomyces israelii* or *Arachnia propionica,* bacteria normally present in the mouth and tonsils that can cause infection when introduced into broken tissue. It's possible to transmit the bacteria via a human bite.

Abdominal actinomycosis usually follows an acute inflammatory process in the stomach or intestines such as appendicitis. Generalized actinomycosis may involve the skin, brain, liver, and urogenital system. A pelvic form of abdominal actinomycosis may occur with the use of an intrauterine contraceptive device.

Symptoms The most common form of the disease affects the mouth and jaw, causing a painful swelling. Small openings later develop on the skin of the face, discharging pus and characteristic yellow granules. Poor oral hygiene may contribute to this particular manifestation.

Diagnosis A diagnosis is usually confirmed by the presence of the microorganism.

Treatment All forms of the disease can be treated with penicillin, which is usually successful, although treatment may be needed for several months in severe infections. Penicillin is the drug of choice, but other antibiotics are also effective. Adequate surgical drainage is important, together with bed rest and proper diet.

adenovirus A family of more than 40 DNA-containing viruses identified by sequential letters and numbers that cause infections of the eyes, upper respiratory tract, and gastrointestinal system. Whereas some adenoviruses attack only animals, the ones that inhabit humans account for 2 percent of all respiratory illness from mild flu to PNEUMONIA.

After the illness fades away, the virus persists in the tonsils, adenoids, and other lymph tissue. Adenoviruses do not become latent (like the HERPES viruses) but instead reproduce constantly and slowly.

The virus was first isolated in adenoids back in the 1950s, but the virus probably was causing respiratory illnesses long before that. Respiratory disease caused by adenoviruses has been a problem since the Civil War and was known as acute respiratory disease (ARD) during World War II. The viruses are still found among adults, usually as a cold or upper respiratory infection. There is no vaccine against this virus family.

Aedes A genus of mosquito found widely in tropical and subtropical areas. Several species are capable of transmitting to humans disease-causing organisms that cause a variety of illnesses, including DENGUE FEVER, EASTERN EQUINE ENCEPHALITIS, ST. LOUIS ENCEPHALITIS, and YELLOW FEVER.

Aedes albopictus **mosquito** Also called the Asian tiger, this type of mosquito can transport the dengue virus. This mosquito, now found in the United States, entered Houston, Texas, after hitching a ride with a used tire shipment from Japan in 1995. It is now established in 17 states.

Although this mosquito has not yet caused any known cases of DENGUE FEVER in the United States, it was found to carry another dangerous arbovirus—EASTERN EQUINE ENCEPHALITIS—in locations around a Florida tire dump.

AIDS See ACQUIRED IMMUNODEFICIENCY SYNDROME.

alveolar hydatid disease See ECHINOCOCCOSIS.

amebiasis (amoebiasis) Also known as amoebic dysentery, this infection of the liver or intestine is caused by the parasite *Entamoeba histolytica,* normally found in the human intestinal tract and feces. It is most serious in infants, the elderly, and those with impaired immune systems.

Anyone can get the disease, but it is found more often in homosexual males, and those arriving from tropical or subtropical areas and those in institutions. Some people carry the parasite for weeks to years, often without symptoms.

Cause Food can be tainted with the protozoa through fecal contamination, such as when infected food handlers don't wash their hands after using the bathroom. A person contracts the disease by swallowing the cyst stage of the parasite in contaminated food or water. The disease can also be spread by person-to-person contact, especially during anal intercourse.

Symptoms If there are symptoms, they may include tenderness over the abdomen and liver, abdominal pain, jaundice, loose morning stools, diarrhea, nervousness, anorexia, weight loss, and fatigue. Symptoms usually occur from a few days to a few months after exposure, but usually within two to four weeks. Most people exposed to the disease don't become seriously ill.

Rarely, the parasite will invade the body beyond the intestines, causing a more serious infection (such as a liver abscess).

Diagnosis The disease is diagnosed by examining stools under a microscope; multiple samples of fresh feces may have to be studied because the number of parasites changes from day to day, and they are hard to see.

Treatment Metronidazole is often effective in curing the infection. It is not usually necessary to isolate an infected person, since casual contact at work or school is not likely to transmit the disease. Special precautions may be needed by food handlers or children enrolled in day care.

Prevention Careful handwashing after going to the bathroom and proper disposal of sewage can help prevent the disease. Infected patients should refrain from intimate contact until effectively treated.

amebic abscess A collection of pus in the liver caused by the protozoan parasite *Entamoeba histolytica*. When the organism's cysts are ingested in contaminated food or water, they pass into the intestine and, from there, into the intestinal walls.

Symptoms Nausea and vomiting, abdominal pain, and severe diarrhea.

Treatment Oral metronidazole and chloroquine.

amebic carrier state A condition in which a patient may carry amebic organisms without showing symptoms of infection. A carrier appears to be healthy, but subsequently may develop the amebic infection. The carrier is always contagious if feces aren't disposed of carefully.

American Lyme Disease Foundation, Inc. A national nonprofit organization created to advance research, treatment, prevention, and public awareness of Lyme Disease throughout the United States. Public and professional education are a major focus of the foundation. The group offers a toll-free information number and an established national physician referral system. In addition, members produce educational videos for both the elementary and junior high school levels.

For more information, contact the American Lyme Disease Foundation, Inc., Mill Pond Offices, 293 Route 100, Suite 204, Somers, NY 10589; telephone (914) 277-6970 or (800) 876-LYME; fax (914) 277-6974.

aminoglycosides A family of antibiotics that include gentamicin, amikacin, kanamycin, neomycin, streptomycin, and tobramycin. These drugs may be toxic to the nerve involved in balance or hearing and can damage kidney function.

amoeba (ameba) A microscopic single-celled parasite that is a type of protozoan that takes different shapes as it moves through its watery world. When an amoeba senses food (such as bacteria), it heads in that direction by stretching out a "pseudopod" (false foot) until it is right beside the food. Then the pseudopods stretch out and around the food, trapping it.

Amoeba reproduce by cell division at an extremely fast rate—thousands of generations in one day. However, most of the cells die almost as quickly as they reproduce.

Several species prey on humans, including *Entamoeba coli* and *E. histolytica*.

anaerobic bacterial infections A bacterial infection that flourishes in complete or almost complete absence of oxygen, such as CLOSTRIDIUM BOTULINUM. These bacteria (called anaerobes) are found throughout nature and in the body. Infections are usually found in deep puncture wounds that are not exposed to air, or in damaged tissue as the result of trauma, tissue death (necrosis), or an overgrowth of bacteria. Anaerobic organisms can lead to GANGRENE, TETANUS, or BOTULISM.

ancylostomiasis See HOOKWORM DISEASE.

anisakiasis A type of food poisoning caused by the parasitic worm *Anasakis simplex* (herring worm) or related worms that are found in sushi, the Japanese dish made of raw fish.

Fewer than 10 cases are diagnosed in the United States every year; however, it is suspected that many cases go undiagnosed. Japan has the highest number of cases because of the large amounts of raw fish eaten there.

Anisakiasis can be misdiagnosed as acute appendicitis, Crohn's disease, peptic ulcer, or cancer of the intestine.

Cause The parasitic worm *Anisakis simplex* infests small crustaceans eaten by many kinds of fish, dolphins, and whales. Fertilized eggs from the female parasite are eliminated by the host fish, which develop into larvae that hatch in salt water.

The disease is transmitted by raw, undercooked, or insufficiently frozen fish and shellfish. Its incidence is expected to increase with the increasing popularity of sushi and sashimi bars. In addition to sushi, sashimi, and ceviche, the larvae can be found in raw herring and Pacific salmon and in cod, haddock, fluke, flounder, and monkfish.

Symptoms If the worm is not coughed up or passed into the bowels, it can penetrate the stomach and cause severe pain, nausea, and vomiting and require surgery. Removing the worm or worms is the only known method of reducing the pain and eliminating the infestation.

In North America, the disease is usually diagnosed when the patient begins to feel a tingling or tickling sensation in the throat, and coughs up a worm. In more severe cases, the pain is akin to acute appendicitis, accompanied by nausea.

Symptoms may appear from an hour to two weeks after consuming raw or uncooked seafood.

Diagnosis In cases where the patient coughs up the worm, the diagnosis may be made by examining the worm itself. Otherwise, the physician may need to examine the inside of the stomach and the small intestine.

Prevention The worm is killed by cooking or freezing the fish. Marinating raw fish in lemon or vinegar does *not* kill all the harmful bacteria or parasites that the fish could contain. Visual inspection of the raw fish, even by the most experienced Japanese chef, will not guarantee the absence of worms.

***Anopheles* mosquito** A genus of mosquito, many species of which transmit the MALARIA parasites to humans.

anthrax This bacterial infection primarily affects livestock, but it is occasionally spread to humans, causing a skin or lung infection. Bible experts believe the "very severe plague" on the Pharaoh's cattle described in Exodus 9 was almost certainly anthrax. Anthrax is one of the zoonotic diseases, which means that it resides mainly in animals, not in people.

In the 1800s, anthrax was known as "woolsorter's disease" in England and "ragpicker's disease" in Germany because workers caught it from spores in hides and fibers (respectively). By 1876, bacteriologist Robert Koch developed a way to grow pure anthrax cultures in a lab. Within a year, as anthrax raced through French sheep herds, Louis Pasteur began work on developing a vaccine. He was successful in 1881.

In the 1920s, the United States enacted laws to require testing of horsehair or pig bristle shaving brushes. The largest outbreak ever recorded in this country occurred in 1957, when nine employees of a goat hair processing plant got sick after touching a contaminated shipment from Pakistan; four of the five patients with the pulmonary form of the disease died. Other cases appeared in the 1970s when contaminated goatskin drumheads from Haiti were brought into the country as souvenirs.

Today, anthrax, even among cattle, is rare largely because a vaccine has been developed to protect against the disease. However, some serious epidemics still occur among herds and humans in developing countries because of ineffective control programs. A recent outbreak in Russia occurred when contaminated beef was inadvertently distributed to schools and workers; about 1,500 people were thought to have eaten the diseased meat or had contact with affected animals. Nine people were infected and one died. Infectious diseases, including anthrax, have been on the rise in Russia in the past few years as the state health care system has steadily deteriorated.

There has been some interest in the bacteria as a means of biological warfare; 50 percent of those who inhale between 8,000 and 10,000 spores will die, according to the U.S. Defense Department. Indeed, the largest documented outbreak ever of human inhalation anthrax

occurred in Russia in 1979. While officials at the time claimed that the 77 victims got anthrax after eating contaminated meat, in 1992 Russian president Boris Yeltsin said the KGB had admitted a military cause. Two years later, an independent team of American and Russian experts found that a windborne aerosol of anthrax spores from a military lab on April 2, 1979, produced the epidemic that killed 69 of the 77 victims. Why the release occurred has never been explained.

Cause Anthrax is caused by the bacterium BACILLUS ANTHRACIS, which produces spores that can remain dormant for years in soil and animal products such as hides, wool, hair, or bones. *B. anthracis* can live in pastures for a long time, multiplying rapidly during damp, warm weather. It is especially hardy in the alluvial soil of the Nile valley and the Mississippi River valley (the first North American cases were found among animals in Louisiana in the early 1700s). The disease is often fatal to cattle, sheep, and goats, and their hides, wool, and bones are often heavily contaminated. However, the bacillus is not highly infectious in humans and doesn't depend on multiplication within humans to survive.

If the bacteria are breathed in, they can cause a type of rare and fatal anthrax known as pulmonary anthrax, which attacks the lungs. Intestinal anthrax is a very rare, fatal form of the disease caused by eating the flesh of animals who have died of anthrax. Cutaneous anthrax is the milder form, caused when spores enter the body via a cut.

Symptoms The most common symptom of anthrax is a raised, itchy area at the site of the bacteria's entry, which progresses to a large blister. This is followed by a black scab surrounded by swollen tissue. In fact, the disease gets its name from the Greek word for coal because of this characteristic coal-black sore it causes. Patients also experience shivering and chills, but few other symptoms. In more than 90 percent of cases in humans, the bacteria remain within the sore.

Occasionally, the bacteria may spread to the nearest lymph node, or in rare cases it may escape into the bloodstream, causing rapidly fatal blood poisoning, internal bleeding, or anthrax meningitis.

Intestinal anthrax causes stomach and intestinal inflammation and ulcers, much like the sores that appear on the skin in cutaneous anthrax.

Pulmonary anthrax patients experience a suffocating bronchitis that is usually fatal.

Treatment   Anthrax is curable in the early stages with high doses of penicillin, but it can be fatal in advanced stages. A vaccine is available to protect against the disease.

Prognosis   One or 2 out of 10 patients will die from anthrax of the skin if it is not properly treated. A full 100 percent of patients will die of inhalation anthrax if untreated.

antibacterial drugs   A group of drugs used to treat infections caused by bacteria. These drugs share the same actions of antibiotic drugs but (unlike the antibiotics) have always been produced synthetically. The largest group of antibacterial agents are the sulfonamides. Medically, physicians do not differentiate antibacterials from antibiotics.

antibiotic drugs   A group of drugs used to treat infections caused by bacteria. Originally prepared from molds and fungi, antibiotic drugs are today produced synthetically. Antibiotics fight infection when the body has been invaded by harmful bacteria, or when the bacteria in the body begin to multiply uncontrollably.

Some drugs, known as broad-spectrum antibiotics, are effective against a wide range of bacteria, whereas others are useful only in treating a specific bacterium. Some of the best-known antibiotics include the macrolides (erythromycin and clarithromycin); the penicillins (amoxicillin, penicillin V, and oxacillin); the aminoglycosides (gentamicin and streptomycin); the cephalosporins (cefaclor and cephalexin); the quinolones (ciprofloxacin and ofloxacin); and the tetracyclines (doxycycline and oxytetracycline).

Still, these drugs can cause some side effects. Antibiotics kill bacteria, but they can also reduce the "good" bacteria naturally present in the body. When this happens, different bacteria or fungi can grow in their place, causing oral, intestinal, or vaginal candidiasis (THRUSH).

Some patients are allergic to antibiotics and can develop swelling, itching, or breathing problems if they take these drugs. A severe allergic reaction to antibiotics (especially PENICILLIN) can be fatal.

When penicillin was first introduced in the 1940s, doctors finally had a good way to treat infections that had previously claimed thousands of lives. Penicillin and its cousin, ampicillin, were called "wonder drugs" and were soon among the most widely prescribed drugs in the world. Unfortunately, even the best of these drugs can't kill every single bacterium. When an antibiotic was used against a bacterial infection, it destroyed only those bacteria that were susceptible to the drug; resistant strains were left behind, to survive and spread. Over time, this occurred often enough so that today there are many bacteria resistant to the most-prescribed antibiotics. Resistance occurs when a bacterium is able to evolve so that it is no longer harmed by the specific antibiotic.

The problem is worse in other parts of the world (Europe, the Far East, and South America), where antibiotics are widely available without a prescription. This has led even more quickly to drug-resistant strains in other parts of the world, which are now circulating the globe. See also ANTIBACTERIAL DRUGS.

Resistance   Resistance is likely to develop if a person doesn't take antibiotics long enough; this leaves a few super-strong germs behind. Drugs kill the vulnerable strains of germs, but the tough survive and flourish. Indeed, half of all antibiotics prescribed in the

United States today are either misused or unneeded, according to medical experts.

Resistance also occurs when doctors over-prescribe antibiotics instead of saving them for specific infections that really require such a drug. Too often, doctors prescribe antibiotics for viral infections (which antibiotics cannot treat). Some doctors defend this practice by saying the cost of a culture to identify the source of the infection is more expensive than the antibiotic. Patients also pressure physicians to prescribe antibiotics. For this reason, the U.S. Centers for Disease Control and Prevention (CDC) has issued guidelines urging hospitals and doctors to use antibiotics more sparingly to slow the development of drug-resistant strains of germs.

Among bacteria that have concerned public health officials are certain types of "flesh eating" strep, and bacteria that cause EAR INFECTION, TUBERCULOSIS, PNEUMONIA, MENINGITIS, and sepsis (an often-fatal blood infection). Some hospitals cannot treat enterococci that can infect kidneys, bladders, wounds, and blood because they have become resistant even to vancomycin, the drug of last resort. (See VANCOMYCIN-RESISTANT ENTEROCOCCI.) According to one CDC study, about 13,300 Americans died in 1992 alone from infections that were no longer sensitive to antibiotics. Every year, another 60,000 to 70,000 patients die from hospital-acquired infections, half of which are caused by drug resistant super-bugs. Scientists believe that antibiotic resistance is a major threat to the nation's health, since many diseases are no longer treatable by antibiotics that were effective against them even a few years ago.

Scientists are racing against time to develop new types of drugs that will be effective against some of the most deadly infections. Because scientists had mistakenly thought the world had enough antibiotics, drug companies began moving away from antibiotic research in the 1980s. Drug development is also expensive: It costs about $237

million to bring one new drug to the market. For every drug that does make it that far, many others are abandoned along the way.

New Drugs　A new class of experimental antibiotics may prove to be such a weapon against bacteria showing resistance to standard drugs. The new drugs would attack the lipid coating of the cell wall in resistant bacteria. The coating is needed by the bacteria; without it, the microbes die. The new drugs (L-573,655 and L-161,240) were able to cure mice infected with normally lethal doses of *E. coli* bacteria. Much more work must be done in the lab and on animals, however, before the new medicine can be tested on humans.

In other research, scientists are turning to DNA to find a weapon against resistant bacte-

---

WHO'S AT RISK FOR RESISTANT BACTERIA?

Certain groups of people are considered more vulnerable to drug-resistant infections. They include the following:

- anyone who takes small amounts of antibiotics to ward off frequent infections
- health care workers
- child care workers
- anyone with impaired immune function
- people with prolonged hospital stays

ANTIBIOTIC CAUTIONS

It's possible to cut down on resistant bacterial infections if patients change the way they use antibiotics. Patients should

- not self-medicate with antibiotics
- not put pressure on the physician to prescribe antibiotics
- try not to use antibiotics for minor infections
- complete the full course of medicine, as prescribed
- never share antibiotics
- never save leftover pills for future use

ria. North Carolina State University researchers have modified a small strand of DNA to interfere with a vital protein-making mechanism used by bacteria and yeasts. Scientists hope this altered molecule will be the forerunner of a new type of antibiotic drug. If they can program these DNA fragments to shut down protein construction only in fungi or bacteria and NOT human cells, the molecules could then be used in the development of an effective antibiotic that would be immune to resistance.

antidiarrheal drugs A type of medicine used to relieve the symptoms of diarrhea. They work by several means: absorbing water from the digestive tract, changing the action of the intestines, altering electrolyte transport, or adsorbing toxins or microorganisms. See also TRAVELER'S DIARRHEA.

antifungal/antiyeast drugs A group of drugs prescribed to treat infections caused by either fungi or yeasts (and sometimes both) and that can be administered directly to the skin, taken orally, or by injection. They are commonly used to treat different types of TINEA, including ATHLETE'S FOOT, JOCK ITCH, and scalp ringworm. They are also used to treat THRUSH and fungal infections such as CRYPTOCOCCUS.

Side effects Agents applied to the skin, scalp, mouth, or vagina may sometimes increase irritation. Systemic antifungal agents that are given by mouth or injection may cause more serious side effects, damaging the kidney or liver.

Types Antifungal agents are available as creams, injections, tablets, lozenges, suspensions, and vaginal suppositories. The most common antifungals include terbinafine, amphotericin B, cyclopirox, clotrimazole, econazole, griseofulvin (by mouth only), itraconazole (by mouth and IV only), fluconazole (by mouth and IV only), ketoconazole, miconazole, and tolnaftate. While amphotericin B is the standard drug for treating serious systemic fungal infections, it is usually given in the hospital because of the danger of side effects. On the other hand, itraconazole and fluconazole are the two most recently approved drugs to enter the antifungal arsenal. These two cause fewer side effects and can be taken orally on an outpatient basis.

Nonprescription creams may help treat usual candidal vaginal yeast infections. They are of no use in treating candidal infections affecting the brain, kidney, or other organs, which do occur in immunocompromised patients.

Antiyeast agents such as mycostatin do not kill most fungi. Most antifungals inhibit yeasts as well—except for griseofulvin. Drugs that are used for both systemic fungal and yeast infections include fluconazole, ketoconazole, amphotericin B, and itraconazole.

Most yeast infections are superficial. Systemic, life-threatening yeast infections do NOT occur in healthy people.

antihelmintic drugs A group of drugs used to treat worm infestations. A large proportion of the world's adult population harbor many worms in their intestines. The amount of parasites is described as their "worm burden."

Because the body's immune system does not fight worms well, persistent infestations are not uncommon. The antihelmintic drugs eliminate the worms from the body, preventing the potential complications.

Different types of antihelmintic drugs—including niclosamide, niridazole, piperazine, praziquantel, thiabendazole, albendazole, and mabendazole—are used to treat infestation by different types of worms.

In the case of intestinal worms, the drugs work by either killing or paralyzing the worms, thus preventing them from gripping onto the intestinal walls. They are then eliminated from the body in the feces. To speed up this process, laxatives may be used at the same time.

In other tissues, antihelmintics kill worms by boosting their vulnerability to the immune system; once these worms have died, they may need to be surgically removed along with any cysts that they have caused.

Adverse effects of antihelmintics include nausea and vomiting, stomach pain, headache, dizziness, and rash.

antimalarial drugs   A type of medicine used to destroy or prevent the development of plasmodia (protozoa that cause MALARIA). Chloroquine hydrochloride and hydroxychloroquine sulfate are effective against *Plasmodium vivax, P. malariae,* and certain strains of *P. falciparum.* Anyone with drug-resistant strains of *P. falciparum* may be treated with a combination of different antimalarial drugs. Resistance by the malarial organism to usual forms of therapy is becoming a worldwide problem.

antimicrobial drugs   Drugs that destroy or inhibit the growth of microorganisms. See ANTIBACTERIAL DRUGS and ANTIBIOTIC DRUGS.

antipyretic drugs   A type of medicine designed to lower fever by reducing the body temperature. Most popular types of antipyretics include acetaminophen, aspirin, and other nonsteroidal antiinflammatory drugs (NSAIDs), such as ibuprofen.

antiseptic   A germicide that slows down the growth and reproduction of germs on human skin or tissue (not inanimate objects). They weaken microbes but don't usually kill them. Health care antiseptics in soaps or other products help prevent the spread of infection in medical facilities. Antiseptics include alcohol (ethanol or isopropanol), iodine (iodophor), povidone-iodine (Betadine), hydrogen peroxide, chlorhexidine, or hexachlorophene (pHisoHex).

Experts advise against using hydrogen peroxide as an antiseptic, since it does NOT kill bacteria and interferes with capillary blood flow and wound healing. Other experts note that ethyl alcohol is not a good wound antiseptic because it irritates already damaged tissue and causes a scab to form, which may in fact protect bacteria.

The FDA is considering a ban on some ingredients in antiseptics, which the government believes may not be generally recognized as safe and effective. These include mercury, cloflucarban, fluorosalan, and tribromsalan.

Over-the-counter antiseptics applied to the skin can help prevent infection in minor cuts, scrapes, or burns. They can be kept in the first-aid kit to pour on a dirty cut after clean-

---

FDA LISTS SAFE ACTIVE INGREDIENTS IN ANTISEPTICS

- ethyl alcohol (48 to 95 percent)
- isopropyl alcohol
- benzalkonium chloride
- benzethonium chloride
- camphorated metacresol
- camphorated phenol
- phenol
- hexylresorcinol
- hydrogen peroxide solution
- iodine tincture
- iodine topical solution
- povidone-iodine
- methylbenzethonium

ing it with soap and water. If an injury is extensive, it should be taken care of by a doctor. Antiseptics should not be used for cuts that are deep, that keep bleeding, or that require stitches. Antiseptics should not be used for scrapes with imbedded particles that can't be flushed away, large wounds, or serious burns.

Over-the-counter antiseptics should not be used for more than one week on an injury; if it persists or gets worse, consumers should seek medical care.

antiserum   A preparation containing antibodies to a specific germ that combine with specific foreign invaders (antigens). Antiserum usually includes components of living things such as viruses or bacteria, and is usually used as an emergency treatment when an unvaccinated person has been exposed to a dangerous infection. Treatment includes immunization as well.

Antiserum is prepared from the blood of animals or humans who have already been immunized against the organism.

The antiserum helps to provide some immediate protection against the microorganisms while full immunity develops. However, these measures are not as effective in preventing disease as is immunization before exposure.

antitoxin   An antibody produced by the body to fight off a toxin formed by invading bacteria or a biological poison such as botulism or snakebite. Antitoxins are also produced commercially to contain an antibody that can neutralize the effect of a specific toxin released into the blood by bacteria (such as those that cause TETANUS or DIPHTHERIA). They are often life saving, especially in the case of food poisoning from botulism.

Antitoxins are prepared by injecting animals (usually horses) with specific toxins that provoke the animal's immune system into producing antibodies that neutralize the

toxin. The extracts are taken from the animal's blood to be used as an antitoxin.

Antitoxins are usually injected into the muscle of the victim. Once in a while, it may cause an allergic reaction or, more rarely, anaphylactic shock.

Antivenin is an antitoxin specifically made to combat snakebite poison. Antivenins are specific for each poisonous snake.

antitussive drugs   A type of medicine used to suppress coughing, possibly by reducing the activity of the cough center of the brain and by depressing breathing. These drugs include both narcotics and nonnarcotics that act on the central and peripheral nervous systems to suppress the cough reflex. Because the cough reflex is important in clearing the upper respiratory tract of secretions, antitussives should not be used with a productive cough (one that produces mucus). Codeine and hydrocodone are strong narcotic antitussives. Dextromethorphan is equally effective but does not carry the danger of inducing patient dependence. Antitussives are given by mouth (usually in a syrup with an expectorant and alcohol). They may also be given as a capsule with an antihistamine and mild painkiller.

antiviral agents   A group of drugs used to treat viral infections. To date, there is no drug that completely eradicates viruses and cures the illnesses they cause. This is because viruses live only within cells; a drug capable of killing a virus would also kill its healthy host cell.

However, scientists are making exciting discoveries in the race to discover a drug that will fight viruses. New antiviral agents that interfere with viral replication or that otherwise disrupt chemical processes of viral metabolism have been developed. Some of these new agents prevent viruses from penetrating into healthy cells. One of the most well known of the new antivirals (AZT) works in one of these new ways, by interrupting the replication cycle of the HIV virus; it has been demonstrated to delay the progression of HIV infection.

They are not without problems, however; some useful antivirals have a wide variety of side effects and patients receiving these drugs must be monitored carefully. Some resistant virus strains have developed in patients receiving initially effective therapy. Some of the better-known antivirals include amantadine, rimantadine, ribavirin, idoxuridine, vidarabine, trifluridine (trifluorothymidine), acyclovir, ganciclovir, zidovudine (ZDU, formerly called AZT, or azidothymidine), foscarnet, and interferons.

arboviral infections Arboviral (short for *ar*thropod-*bo*rne) infections are caused by any of a number of viruses transmitted by arthropods such as mosquitoes and ticks. The infections, which include ENCEPHALITIS, EASTERN EQUINE ENCEPHALITIS, ENCEPHALOMYELITIS, RIFT VALLEY FEVER, hemorrhagic fever, ST. LOUIS ENCEPHALITIS and CALIFORNIA ENCEPHALITIS, usually occur during warm weather months when insects are active. There are more than 520 known arboviruses; about 100 of these can cause human disease.

Cause Anyone can get an arboviral infection, although youngsters and the elderly are most susceptible. Most of these type of infections are spread by infected mosquitoes, but only a few types of mosquitoes are capable of transmitting disease—and only a few of these actually carry a virus. Infection with one arbovirus can provide immunity to reinfection by that specific virus and may also protect against other related viruses.

Symptoms Symptoms of the different types of arboviruses are usually similar, although they differ in severity. Most infections don't cause any symptoms at all; mild cases may involve a slight fever or headache. Severe infections quickly cause an intense headache, high fever, disorientation, coma, tremor, convulsions, paralysis, or death.

Symptoms usually occur between 5 and 15 days after exposure.

Treatment There are no specific treatments for these kinds of infections. Treatment is typically aimed at relieving symptoms.

Prevention The arboviral diseases can be prevented by using insect repellents when outdoors in mosquito-infested areas, screening, and community control programs. Epidemics are not likely to occur wherever insects that carry the diseases are kept under control.

arenavirus A family of viruses named for the Latin word for sand, a reference to the virus's granular outer appearance. The arenaviruses were first identified during a 1933 ENCEPHALITIS outbreak in St. Louis. The various viruses include Ampari, Junin, Lassa, Latino, Machupo, Parana, Pichinde, Tacaribe, Tamiami; they may cause MENINGITIS or hemorrhagic fevers when humans encounter these viruses in excrement from bats, rats, or mice.

These unusual viruses can be deadly. Argentinian hemorrhagic fever, which is caused by the Junin virus, was identified in 1953 near the Junin River; the disease kills 20 percent of those infected by causing fatal hemorrhaging. The mortality rate for the Bolivian variety (Machupo, named for another river) is 30 percent; this disease was first called the black typhus. LASSA FEVER may kill as many as 60 percent of its victims.

Most of these viruses have been limited to certain geographic areas, and since direct person to person contagion is unusual, worldwide pandemics are not expected to occur.

arthritis, septic Also known as infective arthritis or pyogenic arthritis, this joint disease is caused by the invasion of bacteria into the joint from a nearby infected wound or from a blood infection.

Cause In addition to a nearby infection, septic arthritis also may occur as a complication of an infection elsewhere in the body, such as with GONORRHEA or STAPHYLOCOCCAL INFECTION.

Symptoms The infected joint usually becomes hot, painful, and swollen.

Diagnosis Diagnosis is made from the appearance of the joint and the joint fluid, which may be withdrawn through a needle from the affected joint and examined for the presence of microorganisms; a culture may be made from this fluid as well.

Treatment Antibiotic drugs are used to treat septic arthritis. Occasionally, surgical cleansing of the joint space is necessary.

ascariasis See ROUNDWORMS.

Asian flu See INFLUENZA.

Asian tiger mosquito See *AEDES ALBOPICTUS* MOSQUITO.

aspergillosis A rare infection in which the fungus *Aspergillus fumigatus* (found in old buildings or decaying plants) affects the ear or any other organ; sometimes it attacks the mucous membranes of the nose or urethra, or internal organs such as the lungs, liver, and kidneys. It is an occasionally fatal opportunistic infection among those with impaired immune systems, especially if the infection has spread throughout the body.

Allergic aspergillosis usually occurs as asthma; it can occur if susceptible people inhale spores of aspergillus.

Treatment Amphotericin B is used to treat systemic aspergillosis (especially if it has spread to the lungs). Steroids are used to treat acute allergic reactions to *ASPERGILLUS*. Itraconazole (Sporonox) has been recently successful in some cases in treating systemic aspergillosis.

Aspergillus A genus of fungi (including many common molds), some of which cause respiratory infections in humans. It is a common contaminant in the laboratory and is a rare cause of hospital-acquired infection. The fungus is found everywhere in soil and proliferates rapidly. The species *A. fumigatus* causes ASPERGILLOSIS. *A. niger* is commonly found in the external ear. Inhalation of *A. fumigatus* and *A. flatus* is common, but infection is rare. More commonly, an allergic reaction ensues.

athlete's foot A common fungal condition causing the skin between the toes (usually the fourth and fifth toes) to itch, peel, and crack with diffuse scaling and redness of the soles and sides of the foot. Associated with wearing shoes and sweating, the condition is rare in young children and in places of the world where people do not wear shoes. It is primarily found in adolescents and men, especially those who wear sneakers without socks. A person with athlete's foot is infectious for as long as the lesions exist.

Itchy skin on the foot is probably not athlete's foot if it occurs on the top of the toes. If the foot is red, swollen, sore, blistered, and oozing, it is more likely some form of contact dermatitis, although inflammatory fungal infections can sometimes look like this. Secondary bacterial infections of the eroded skin can also look like this.

Cause The fungi that are responsible for athlete's foot are called DERMATOPHYTES; they live only on dead body tissue (hair, the outer layer of skin, and nails). The two main dermatophytes responsible for athlete's foot are *TRICHOPHYTON rubrum* and *T. mentagrophytes*. The condition occurs both by direct and indirect contact; it can be passed in locker rooms, showers, or shared towels and shoes.

Symptoms Symptoms may include scaling and cracking of the skin between the toes and the sides of the feet; the skin may itch and peel. There may be small water blisters between the toes; it can spread to the instep or the hands. There is often an odor.

Diagnosis Scrapings from the affected area will be examined under a microscope for certain fungal characteristics.

Treatment The condition may clear up without any attention, but it usually requires treatment. An untreated fungal infection can lead to bacteria invading cracks in the skin. The affected area should be kept dry, clad in dry cotton socks or in sandals, or kept uncovered. A number of nonprescription fungicide sprays will cure athlete's foot, including clotrimazole, ketoconazole, miconazole-nitrate, sulconazole, or tolnaftate. Before applying, the feet should be bathed well with soap and water, then well dried (especially between the toes). The sprays should be applied to all sides of the feet twice a day for up to four weeks. After the spray has been applied, the feet should be covered in clean, white cotton socks.

For cases that don't respond to the sprays, a physician may prescribe one of several oral medicines.

When the acute phase of the infection passes, the dead skin should be removed with a bristle brush in order to remove the living fungi. All bits of the skin should be washed away. In addition, the skin underneath toenails should be scraped every two or three days with an orange stick or toothpick.

Prevention Good hygiene is the best way to prevent athlete's foot. Disinfecting the floors of showers and locker rooms can help control the spread of infection.

Once an infection has cleared up, the patient should continue using antifungal cream now and then—especially during warm weather. Avoid plastic or too-tight shoes or any type of footwear treated to keep out water. Natural materials (cotton and leather) and sandals are the best choices, whereas wool and rubber can make a fungal problem worse by trapping moisture.

Shoes should be aired out regularly in the sun and wiped inside with a disinfectant-treated cloth to remove fungi-carrying dead skin. The insides of shoes should then be dusted with antifungal powder or spray. Those individuals who perspire heavily should change socks three or four times daily. Only natural white cotton socks should be worn, and they should be rinsed thoroughly during washing.

Feet should be air dried after bathing and then powdered. To reduce the risk of infection, it is important to wear sandals or flip-flops in public bathing areas.

avian flu A deadly type of influenza normally affecting chickens that abruptly jumped to humans in Hong Kong in 1997, infecting 18 people and killing six.

Avian flu, or "bird flu," is caused by the avian-flu virus, a rod-shaped virus that can cut through protective mucus and attach to cells that line the nose and throat. For reasons that are not clear, it travels more efficiently from chickens to humans than from humans to humans. Unlike the more traditional flu viruses that cause little more than chills, fever, and aches, this version attacks not just the respiratory system but every tissue in the body, including the brain, leading to severe hemorrhaging throughout the system.

No new cases have been diagnosed since December 1997, but virologists consider the emergence of this new virus to be one of the most troubling medical events of the century. The danger with this purely avian virus is that unlike the common flu, humans would have no immunity against it. High-speed travel linking countries around the world means that a pandemic of this unusually deadly influenza virus could circle the globe in a matter of months.

The virus is termed "H5 flu," because it carries the H5 variation of the H gene, a variation that is notoriously lethal in chickens. In the Hong Kong epidemic, the many outdoor markets held the key to why the confirmed cases of H5 avian flu were sprinkled throughout the city. Some people had had direct contact with poultry, and then others appeared to have caught the disease from contact so casual that the people weren't aware of it.

It is believed that the epidemic was halted when the city government decided to kill every chicken in Hong Kong. The decision, which was widely ridiculed at the time, apparently prevented a more widespread disaster. However, scientists are convinced that the avian virus is still circulating in the environment.

Although there have been no new cases since the end of 1997, scientists fear that the virus could exchange genetic material with the common flu virus. If someone were to be infected with both viruses at once, the RNA from one virus could combine with the RNA from the other, producing a new virus that is both highly contagious and deadly. This is exactly what happened in the deadly flu epidemic of 1918 that killed more than 20 million people, many of them young and healthy.

B

babesiosis (babesiasis) A rare, occasionally fatal, disease caused by a tick-borne microorganism similar to both LYME DISEASE and human granulocytic ehrlichiosis (HGE). Also known as Nantucket Fever, it is most often seen in the elderly and those with impaired immune systems. Severe cases have been diagnosed in those who have had their spleen removed prior to exposure.

Most cases of babesiosis have been reported in summer and fall in the northeastern United States, especially Nantucket, Shelter Island in New York, and other offshore islands in New England. However, cases have recently been identified in the upper Midwest, the Pacific Coast states, and Europe. A related species has caused a babesiosis-like illness in Washington and California.

Cause Babesiosis is caused by protozoa similar to those that cause MALARIA (the species *Babesia microti*); it is passed via the bite of ticks; the most common is the species *Ixodes dammini*. The tick is carried by meadow voles, mice, and deer. The disease can also be transmitted via contaminated blood transfusions. The protozoa causing babesiosis was first identified by Roman bacteriologist Victor Babes, for whom the organism and the disease was named.

Symptoms Babesiosis typically causes mild illness in otherwise healthy people, but it can be overwhelming to those with impaired immune systems. Symptoms appear within 1 to 12 months after infection and include fever, fatigue, and hemolytic anemia lasting from several days to several months. A person may also have the disease with no symptoms at all. It is not known if a past infection renders a patient immune.

Diagnosis Molecular tests are being developed, but currently the disease is diagnosed by microscopic examination of blood smears.

Treatment Standardized treatments have not been developed; however, a combination of antimalarial drugs as quinine and an antibiotic (clindamycin) are usually the drugs of choice.

Prevention The spread of babesiosis can be curtailed with the control of rodents around houses and the use of tick repellents.

bacillary angiomatosis An infectious disease that causes blood vessels to grow out of control in bone, liver, and skin, forming tumorlike masses that look like those of KAPOSI'S SARCOMA.

bacillary dysentery See SHIGELLOSIS.

***Bacillus* (pl. bacilli)** A large genus of gram-positive, spore-bearing bacteria (in the family Bacillaceae) that includes 33 species, three of which cause disease. They are found in soil and air and are responsible for many diseases, including ANTHRAX and FOOD POISONING. Most feed on dead matter and are responsible for food spoilage. The genus includes *BACILLUS ANTHRACIS, BACILLUS POLYMYXA* and *BACILLUS SUBTILIS*.

Bacillus anthracis A species of gram-positive bacteria that causes ANTHRAX, a disease mostly affecting cattle and sheep. If inhaled, the spores of this organism can cause a pulmonary form of anthrax. Spores live for many years in hides and wool.

Bacillus pestis See *PASTEURELLA PESTIS*.

Bacillus polymyxa A species of *Bacillus* that is commonly found in soil and is the source of the polymyxin group of antibiotics.

Bacillus subtilis A species of *Bacillus* that may cause CONJUNCTIVITIS in humans; it is also used to produce the antibiotic bacitracin.

bacteremia An invasion of bacteria into the bloodstream. This is an uncommon complication of STREP THROAT, TONSILLITIS, or streptococcal skin infection; it may also occur a few hours after minor surgery. Infection can spread via the bloodstream to other parts of the body, producing abscesses, peritonitis (inflammation of the abdomen), inflammation of the heart, or MENINGITIS. Bacteremia may also lead to shock, causing a generalized illness with high fever, circulatory collapse, and eventually, organ failure.

Those at greatest risk include patients with an impaired immune system, children with CHICKEN POX, burn victims, elderly patients with CELLULITIS, diabetes, blood vessel disease, cancer, or anyone taking steroids or chemotherapy. IV-drug users are also at risk.

Bacteremia may occur as well in healthy young adults with no known risk factors.

bacteria Bacteria are microbes whose genetic material is not organized into a cell nucleus, like plants or animals. Some bacteria feed on other organisms, some make their own food (like plants do) and some bacteria do both. Some need air to survive, and others exist without air (anaerobic). Some move by themselves, and others can't move at all. Bacteria also come in a variety of shapes, colors, and sizes.

It's important to remember that not all bacteria are harmful; most are helpful, such as those that break down dead plant and animal matter in the soil. Some (like the actinomycetes) produce antibiotics such as streptomycin. Plants can't grow without nitrogen, and bacteria help nitrogen to form in the soil. Bacteria are also used to make cheese out of milk and leather out of animal hide. Grazing animals use bacteria to digest the grass they eat.

Bacteria can be found in the air, the water, food, and everything we touch. Since few of these are harmful, humans are seldom bothered by them. When harmful bacteria do enter the body, the immune system usually can kill the invading microbes.

They are of incredible importance because of their extreme flexibility, capacity for rapid growth and reproduction, and their ancient age—the oldest known fossils are those of bacteria-like organisms that lived nearly 3.5 billion years ago.

Bacteria in humans are essential to digestion. More than 400 different kinds help digest food and fill niches in the intestine that might otherwise be colonized by harmful bacteria.

At least one type of bacteria (*Bacteroides thetaiotaomicron*) interacts with cells lining the intestine, benefitting both the human host and the bacteria. Without this type of bacteria, cells in the intestines may fail to produce a sugar found in human milk that is used as food by the bacteria and other beneficial intestinal organisms. When these naturally occurring bacteria are killed (because of ANTIBIOTIC use or other illnesses) harmful bacteria can take over. Diarrhea is one result.

As scientists understand more about the interaction between helpful bacteria and intestines, they may be able to use these bacteria to protect a patient with an impaired immune system or who is taking antibiotics. See also DIARRHEA AND INFECTIOUS DISEASE; ANTIDIARRHEAL DRUGS; TRAVELER'S DIARRHEA.

Unfortunately, some disease-causing bacteria are beginning to become resistant to many of the antibiotics doctors use to treat the infections. A 1996 World Health Organization report found that drug-resistant strains of microbes causing MALARIA, TUBERCULOSIS, PNEUMONIA, CHOLERA, and traveler's diarrhea are on the rise. Certain drug-resistant microbes in the United States cause up to 60 percent of hospital-acquired infections, the report adds.

bacterial infections   One of the most important types of infectious disease. These include GONORRHEA, bacterial MENINGITIS, WHOOPING COUGH, bacterial PNEUMONIA, TUBERCULOSIS, TYPHOID FEVER, and many others.

bacterial pneumonia   See PNEUMONIA, BACTERIAL.

bactericide   Any substance that kills bacteria.

Bang's disease   The common name for BRUCELLOSIS.

Bartonella   A genus of small, gram-negative coccobacilli that infect red blood cells and cells of the lymph nodes, liver, and spleen. Named for the 18th-century Peruvian bacteriologist who discovered them (Alberto Barton), they are transmitted at night by the bite of a sandfly of the genus *Phlebotomus*. The only known species of *Bartonella* is *B. bacilliformis*, the organism that causes BARTONELLOSIS.

bartonellosis   An acute or chronic bacterial infection transmitted to humans by the bite of the sandfly. The risk of this disease exists in the mountain valleys of southwest Colombia, Ecuador, and Peru, at altitudes between 2,500 and 8,000 feet.
   Cause   The *Phlebotomus* sandfly carries the disease-producing bacterium *Bartonella bacilliformis*. Transmission occurs between dusk and dawn (which is sandfly feeding time).
   Symptoms   Bartonellosis has two distinct types: Oroya fever and Veruga peruana. Symptoms of Oroya fever begin between two to three weeks after being bitten, with fever, weakness, headache, and bone or joint pain followed by severe anemia and swollen lymph nodes. The disease lasts between two and six weeks and then subsides, but it is occasionally fatal. Death is usually associated with secondary and overwhelming *Salmonella* infection.

Veruga peruana is characterized by the appearance of nodules on the face and limbs that bleed easily and last for up to a year. They finally heal without scarring.
   Treatment   Chloramphenicol or ampicillin is the preferred treatment, although tetracycline, penicillin, or streptomycin also are effective. More recently, doctors may combine two or more antibiotics because of the frequent presence of *Salmonella*.
   Prevention   This disease can be prevented by avoiding high-risk areas between sundown and sunup, together with the use of insect repellents.

BDV   See BORNA DISEASE VIRUS.

bird flu   See AVIAN FLU.

black death   See PLAGUE.

bladder infection   See URINARY TRACT INFECTION.

blastomycosis   A mild, often self-limiting yeast infection that usually begins in the lungs and spreads to other sites in the body, especially skin and bone. The disease is found most often in children and in men between the ages of 40 and 60.
   The disease is also known as Chicago disease, Gilchrist's disease, and North American blastomycosis.
   Cause   The disease is caused by the yeast *Blastomyces dermatiidis;* it can be confused with *Coccidioides immitis* or *Cryptococcus neoformans*.
   Symptoms   The amount and type of inflammation may vary from one site on the body to another and from one patient to another. There is usually widespread inflammation in the lungs, with small areas of abscesses.
   Treatment   Amphotericin B is the drug of choice; hydroxystilbamidine has been successful in treating the form of the disease that affects the skin, but it is less helpful with

other forms. Both ketaconazole and itraconazole have been used successfully.

blepharitis A chronic or long-term inflammation of the eyelids and eyelashes affecting people of all ages. It is characterized by red, irritated scaly skin at the edges of the lids.

Cause Among the most common causes are poor eyelid hygiene, excess oil produced by the glands in the eyelids, a bacterial infection, or an allergic reaction. Seborrheic blepharitis is the most common form. It is often associated with dandruff of the scalp or skin conditions such as acne.

Symptoms Blepharitis usually appears as greasy flakes or scales around the base of the eyelashes and as a mild redness of the eyelid. Sometimes, seborrheic blepharitis may result in a roughness of the tissue that lines the inside of the eyelids or in nodules on the eyelids. Styes can also result from an acute infection of the eyelids.

A less common form of blepharitis is ulcerative blepharitis. It is characterized my matted, hard crusts around the eyelashes which, when removed, leave small sores that may bleed or ooze.

Treatment Blepharitis is usually not serious. In many cases, good eyelid hygiene and a regular cleaning routine can control it. Scales can be removed with cotton moistened with warm water. The inflammation often recurs, which requires more treatment. Ulcerated eyelids must be treated by a physician, since severe cases can lead to problems with the cornea.

blood-borne infectious disease See INFECTIOUS DISEASES.

blood fluke See FLUKE.

blood poisoning See SEPTICEMIA.

boil An inflamed, pus-filled section of skin (usually an infected hair follicle) found often on the back of the neck or moist areas such as the armpits and groin. Very large boils are called a CARBUNCLE.

Cause Boils are usually caused by infection with the bacterium *Staphylococcus aureus*, which invades the body through a break in the skin, where it infects a blocked oil gland or hair follicle. When the body's immune system sends in white blood cells to kill the germs, the resulting inflammation produces pus.

Symptoms A boil begins with a red, painful lump that swells as it fills with pus, until it becomes rounded with a yellowish tip. It may either continue to grow until it erupts, drains, and fades away or is reabsorbed by the body. Recurrent boils may occur in people with known or unrecognized diabetes mellitus or other diseases involving lowered body resistance.

Treatment Putting pressure on a boil might spread the infection into surrounding tissue. Instead, apply a hot compress for 20 minutes every two hours to relieve discomfort and hasten drainage and healing. After treating a boil, wash hands thoroughly before cooking to guard against staph infection getting into food or breaks in the skin.

It may take up to a week for the boil to break on its own. To further reduce chance of infection, take showers, not baths. If the boil is large and painful, a physician may prescribe an antibiotic or open the boil with a sterile needle to drain the pus. Occasionally, large boils must be lanced with a surgical knife; this is usually done using a local anesthetic.

Complications More seriously, bacteria from a boil may find its way into the blood, causing blood poisoning; for this reason, doctors advise against squeezing boils that appear around the lips or nose, since the infection can be carried to the brain. (Other danger areas include the groin, the armpit, and the breast of a nursing woman.) Signs of a spreading infection include generalized symptoms of fever and chills, swelling lymph nodes, or red lines radiating from the boil.

Prevention Some experts note that boils are usually infected cysts and recommend leaving cysts untouched or having them lanced by a physician. For patients prone to boils, some experts recommend washing the skin with an antiseptic soap.

Keep skin around a boil clean while drainage is occurring, and take showers to lessen the chance of spreading the infection.

Bordetella A genus of gram-negative bacteria discovered by Belgium bacteriologist Jules J. B. V. Bordet. Some species cause respiratory disease in humans involving the bacteria *Bordetella bronchiseptica, B. parapertussis,* and *B. pertussis.* See WHOOPING COUGH.

Bordetella pertussis A species of tiny gram-negative anaerobic bacterium (in the genus *Bordetella*) that causes WHOOPING COUGH, one of the most common infections on earth. All the other species of the *Bordetella* genus cause diseases that resemble whooping cough.

It is extremely virulent, infecting more than 90 percent of susceptible victims after close contact. It usually strikes during childhood; before the advent of modern medicine it was a major cause of infant death around the world. It is still a significant health problem in underdeveloped areas, causing about 40 million cases worldwide and about 400,000 deaths. A vaccine against the bacteria was developed in the mid-1940s, although local outbreaks still occur among unvaccinated individuals.

The disease was named *pertussis* (from the Latin word for "intense cough") and was known popularly as "whooping cough" in the 17th century; earlier, it was called "chin cough." French physicians called it *quinta* because of the five-hour respites between coughing spasms, or "coqueluche." Since 1940, the vaccine against *Bordetella pertussis* (a combination of DIPHTHERIA, TETANUS, and pertussis), or "DPT," has cut the incidence of whooping cough by 99 percent, but the shot

was linked to rare but serious side effects, including high fever, convulsions, and rarely, brain damage and death. In 1988, the United States established an $80 million fund to compensate children who were injured by the vaccine, which initiated 4,700 claims. Since then, the National Institutes of Health spent $16 million to develop a safer vaccine—the acellular vaccine, so named because it was derived from only part of a *B. pertussis* cell.

Borna disease virus (BDV) A type of virus known to cause behavior disruptions and neurological disease in several animal species, and recently found in humans as well. Infection with this virus may trigger depressive episodes in humans who are already vulnerable to major depression or manic-depression.

Borna disease virus is a single-stranded RNA virus that establishes a persistent infection without directly damaging host cells. BDV infection may contribute to depressive illness by altering neuronal cells in the limbic system. The leading hypothesis is that BDV, as it inserts itself into neurons, may disrupt the function of those cells by binding to neurotransmitter receptors.

It causes neurological symptoms in domestic animals, which is where it gets its nickname, "crazy virus." The neurological symptoms resemble those seen in humans with manic-depression. This virus is entirely separate from MAD COW DISEASE, although the neurological symptoms are what led researchers to study BDV more closely.

The virus infects cells of the limbic system implicated in many psychiatric disorders, including bipolar depression and schizophrenia. BDV infects cells in the nervous system just as its distant viral relative, rabies, does, causing brain damage in animals and humans. Previous studies have shown that a large proportion of psychiatric patients with certain affective disorders, such as depression and manic-depressive disorder, have antibodies specific to proteins of BDV. Since Borna viral material tends to appear during episodes of depression, scientists suspect that the virus brings on depressive episodes in people predisposed to mood disorders by their genes or other factors (perhaps by disrupting communication between brain cells). In most people, however, the infection appears to cause no problems.

It's too soon to say how big a factor Borna virus might be in depression or manic-depression, and it's not clear whether Borna virus can jump from animals to people, nor how it might spread between people. However, scientists do know that humans can't get Borna virus from eating meat or other products of infected animals.

BDV was first reported more than a century ago as a cause of neurological disease in horses in Borna, Germany. Since then, outbreaks of the virus have been documented in cattle, sheep, and cats. Rats injected with BDV exhibit damage to brain cells in the limbic system, the part of the brain that governs mood and emotions. Interestingly, the virus affects various animal species differently. While rats' brains are destroyed, the virus causes only subtle abnormal social patterns in tree shrews. Further animal studies as well as larger studies of psychiatric patients may help scientists better understand how the virus causes disease and how to develop a way to diagnose and treat it.

The cause of most of the common psychiatric disorders, including depression, manic-depression, anxiety, and schizophrenia, remains a mystery. In some cases, symptoms appear suddenly and the disease follows a catastrophic course, while in other cases the disease may be intermittent. Despite a large amount of research, and a lot of familial association evidence, the search for causative genes has produced mixed results. This has helped fuel the search for other factors, such as viral infection.

One group of investigators at the National Institute of Mental Health is pursuing the hypothesis that schizophrenia might be caused by viruses transmitted from household pets to pregnant women or young children. Another group of researchers at the University of Southern California is looking for a link between chronic fatigue syndrome and "stealth viruses" (viruses that have been incorporated into the host DNA and are no longer recognized by the immune system). These viruses cannot be detected by standard immunological methods or standard culture techniques. However, they can be detected with PCR based techniques, matching DNA sequences with known viral DNA.

borrelia   See RELAPSING FEVER.

Borrelia burgdorferi   A species of large parasitic spirochete bacteria (in the genus *Borrelia*) that cause LYME DISEASE. The species *B. duttonii, B. persica,* and *B. recurrentis* cause RELAPSING FEVER.

botulism   The most common type of the infectious disease known as botulism is a food-borne illness involving the toxin produced by the bacteria *Clostridium botulinum,* which is both rare and very deadly (two thirds of those afflicted die). Another type is known as "infant botulism," an uncommon illness that strikes infants under the age of one. Because botulism is technically a poisoning, not an infection, the patient cannot infect others even though the bacteria will be excreted in feces for months after the illness.

Botulism is more common in the United States than anywhere else in the world, owing to the popularity of home canning; there are about 20 cases of food-borne botulism poisoning each year. Botulism got its name during the 1800s from *botulus,* the Latin word for "sausage," because of a wave of poisoning from contaminated sausages.

Cause   Botulism toxins are a type of neurotoxin that attaches to the nerves, blocking the messages that are sent to the muscles. The

C. botulinum spores (latent form of the bacteria) are found in air, water, and food; they are harmless until deprived of oxygen (such as inside a sealed can or jar). If conditions are favorable, the spores will start to generate and multiply, producing one of the most deadly toxins known—7 million times more deadly than cobra venom.

Cases of botulism from commercially canned food are rare because of strict health standards enforced by the U.S. Food and Drug Administration, although some people have gotten botulism from eating improperly handled commercial pot pies. In Canada, cases have been reported from seal meat, smoked salmon, and fermented salmon eggs. *Most cases occur during home canning.*

Canned foods that are highly susceptible to contamination include green beans, beets, peppers, corn, and meat. Although the spores can survive boiling, the ideal temperature for their growth is between 78 degrees F and 96 degrees F. They can also survive freezing.

Botulism can also occur if the *C. botulinum* bacteria in the soil enters the body through an open wound, although this is extremely rare.

Symptoms   Onset of symptoms may be as soon as three hours or as late as 14 days after ingestion, although most symptoms usually appear between 12 and 26 hours. The first sign is usually muscle weakness beginning with the head, often leading to double vision. This is followed by problems in swallowing or speaking, followed by the paralysis of the muscles needed to breathe. Other symptoms can include nausea, vomiting, diarrhea, and stomach cramps. The earlier the onset of symptoms, the more severe the reaction. Symptoms generally last between three to six days; death occurs in about 70 percent of untreated cases, usually from suffocation as a result of respiratory muscle paralysis. In infants, symptoms may go unrecognized by parents for some time until the poisoning has reached a critical stage.

Diagnosis   Large commercial labs or state health labs can test for the toxin in food, blood, or stool; it's also possible to grow the bacteria from food or stool in a special culture. The diagnosis is most often made by an astute health care practitioner who recognizes the signs and symptoms. In an outbreak, the first victim to become sick usually dies.

Treatment   Prompt administration of the antitoxin (type ABE botulinus) lowers the risk of death to 10 percent. Most untreated victims will die. The Centers for Disease Control is the only agency with the antitoxin, and it makes the decision to treat. Local health departments should be called first for this information. While induced vomiting may help following ingestion of food known to contain botulism toxin, it may not be complete. Because the disease can occur with only a small amount of toxin, botulism may still develop.

Patients are usually put on a respirator to ease breathing. In infant botulism, if symptoms are present it is often too late to administer antitoxin, since the damage has probably already been done.

Prevention   It is easy to prevent, since botulism is killed when canned food is boiled at 100 degree C for one minute, or if the food is first sterilized by pressure cooking at 250 degrees F for 30 minutes. If you're going to eat it—heat it.

While the tightly fitted lids of home-canned food will provide the anaerobic environment necessary for the growth of botulism toxins, the spores will not grow if the food is very acidic, sweet, or salty (such as canned fruit juice, jams and jellies, sauerkraut, tomatoes, and heavily salted hams).

Even though botulism spores are invisible, it's possible to tell if food is spoiled by noticing if jars have lost their vacuum seal; when the spores grow, they give off gas that makes cans and jars lose the seal. Jars will burst or cans will swell. Any food that is spoiled or whose color or odor doesn't seem right inside a home-canned jar or can should be thrown away without tasting or even sniffing, since botulism can be fatal in extremely small amounts.

botulism, infant Unlike botulism in adults, which occurs after eating contaminated food, infant botulism occurs in babies under six months of age and is less serious. While all botulism are caused by toxins given off by *Clostridium botulinum* bacteria, in infant botulism the baby does not ingest the toxin. Instead, the spores from botulism bacteria reproduce the toxin in the baby's digestive tract, which then travels to the baby's nerve cells.

Fortunately, most babies will recover with prompt hospital treatment.

Cause This rare disease may be difficult to trace, since the spores may survive for a long time in the environment. It is clear that about 10 percent of commercial honey contains botulism spores and occasionally, light and dark corn syrup also harbors the bacteria. For this reason, parents are advised not to feed either food to infants under a year of age. The illness is found in all races in North and South America, Asia, and Europe. In 1993, there were only 65 reported cases in the United States.

Although an infected baby will excrete toxin for weeks in feces, the baby cannot pass on the infection to others.

Symptoms Infant botulism symptoms include constipation, facial muscle flaccidity, sucking problems, irritability, lethargy, and floppy arms and legs.

Complications Some experts believe that infant botulism may be responsible for up to 5 percent of all cases of Sudden Infant Death Syndrome.

Treatment The antitoxin used to treat adults with botulism is not safe for infants. Antibiotics may be used to treat secondary infections. In severe cases, the baby may need breathing assistance; while recovery may be slow, most usually completely recover.

Prevention Babies under age one should not be fed honey or corn syrup. They should be kept away from dust (both from vacuum cleaners and from the outdoors), especially around construction sites.

bouba See YAWS.

bovine spongiform encephalopathy The medical name for MAD COW DISEASE, an infectious illness of cows that may have emerged in the human population. BSE was first identified in Britain in 1986, and is one of a group of similar neurologically degenerative diseases that occur in several animal species. The disease is thought to have been transmitted to a dozen people via contaminated meat and bone meal.

Eleven human deaths from this disease in Great Britain were traced to exposure to beef that contained a piece of protein called a PRION, thought to be the cause of bovine spongiform encephalopathy. The United Kingdom appears to be the only country with a recent incidence of the disease, and the cases there seem to have been associated with the recycling of affected cow material back to cattle in their food prior to 1988. The incidence of the disease declined significantly in the United Kingdom, although the epidemic has not yet been clearly defined as such. The worldwide distribution of BSE is not precisely known, but it has been reported at a much lower incidence than in the U.K. In the United States, officials restricted imports of live cattle and meat from countries with bovine spongiform encephalopathy in 1989.

brain abscess A pocket of infection, most commonly found in the frontal and temporal lobes, usually caused by the spread of infection from another part of the body, such as the sinuses. A brain abscess also may result from spread of an infection in the bones, the nervous system outside the brain, or the heart. These abscesses cause symptoms due to increased pressure and local brain injury.

About 10 percent of cases are fatal; the remaining patients often have some brain function impairment. A seizure disorder is a common complication.

Cause Brain abscesses are almost always caused by infection spreading from somewhere else in the body. About 40 percent of abscesses are from middle ear or sinus infections. Blood-borne infections may also cause multiple brain abscesses.

Symptoms The most common symptoms are headache, sleepiness, and vomiting. There may be visual problems, with fever and seizures. There may be evidence of local brain damage as well, including partial paralysis or speech problems.

Diagnosis Brain scans (CT scans or magnetic resonance imaging) of the brain can diagnose a brain abscess.

Treatment High doses of antibiotics and usually surgery; the abscess may be accessible via a small hole in the skull.

Brazilian purpuric fever A serious systemic illness that may be caused by bacterial infection, it was first recognized in 1984 in Brazil. Since then, scientists have identified other cases, including an outbreak of 17 illnesses in a town in a neighboring Brazilian state. Cases have appeared in other states of Brazil, as well.

It is not known whether the disease occurs in areas other than southern Brazil. Cases being treated for presumed meningococcemia may in actuality be cases of BPF. In many areas a blood culture may not have been drawn to determine the diagnosis. Researchers caution that the occurrence of clusters in areas separated by 250 miles suggests the potential for spreading of the disease.

Cause Brazilian purpuric fever appears to be related to *Haemophilus aegyptius* (*H. influenzae*, biotype III). If untreated, the infection spreads and can lead to fatal purpura (bleed-

ing into the skin), release of toxins, and overwhelming shock.

Symptoms The illness typically begins with eye infection caused by *H. influenzae* III; in a small number of patients, the bacteria spread throughout the body, causing fever and bleeding into the skin. If untreated, this bleeding continues; the bacteria release a toxin that overwhelms the body's defenses and ends in death. Symptoms resemble meningococcemia.

Treatment Systemic antibiotics to treat BPF (usually ampicillin with or without chloramphenicol) before the skin bleeding begins may prevent progression of the disease.

breast cancer and virus New evidence has contributed to a controversial claim that suggests breast cancer may be linked in some form to a virus. Cancerous breast cells often contain genetic sequences similar to an infectious virus that triggers mammary tumors in mice, according to research by virologists at Mount Sinai medical school in New York City. These findings raise decades-old questions of whether some infectious virus plays a role in at least some types of breast cancer.

Over the last few decades, investigators have linked a number of viruses (specifically retroviruses) to cancer in animals and people. A retrovirus can transform a normal cell into a cancer cell by inserting its genetic material into the cell, disrupting the function of crucial genes. For example, mouse mammary tumor virus (MMTV) produces cancer in about 95 percent of the mice it infects.

The idea that viruses may cause some types of breast cancer dates to the 1930s, when scientists identified viruslike particles in mothers' milk. While mice can transmit MMTV to their babies through milk, no evidence was found that children who were breast-fed by mothers with breast cancer had a higher chance of developing the disease themselves.

Still, over the decades since then, research groups have reported some genetic evidence that an MMTV-like virus is associated with breast cancer. The problem with those reports was that in those days, scientists couldn't tell the difference between MMTV-like viruses and human endogenous retrovirus (HER), an ancient virus whose genetic code is integrated into everyone's genome.

In recent years, however, scientific procedure has become more sophisticated. Scientists have sequenced many of MMTV's genes and found regions of various genes that differ quite a bit from those of HER. The new research looked at samples of human breast tissue for MMTV-specific gene fragments. In 1995, the group reported that in almost 40 percent of breast cancer tissue tested, they found sequences similar to those in one of the MMTV's genes. Less than 2 percent of normal breast samples yielded this so-called env gene. This env gene encodes a protein that helps form the outer surface of the virus.

In 1996, the group reported that they found a different sequence of the env gene in 13 of 19 breast cancer samples, and in none of the normal breast tissue samples. Interestingly, hormones such as estrogen stimulate the activity of an MMTV-like env gene in a cell line derived from breast cancer cells.

The findings are far from conclusive proof that a virus may cause some forms of breast cancer. Other scientists are trying to replicate the Mount Sinai research.

bronchiolitis   An acute viral infection of the small airways in the lungs that primarily affects infants and young children. Winter epidemics tend to occur every two or three years, affecting thousands of children in the United States. A virus that may induce only a mild head or chest infection in an adult can cause a severe bronchiolitis in an infant. With prompt treatment, even the sickest infants usually recover completely within a few days.

Cause   The smaller airways that branch off the bronchial tubes become inflamed, usually because of the RESPIRATORY SYNCYTIAL VIRUS (RSV INFECTION), although other viruses may be responsible. Adult attacks may follow BRONCHITIS brought on by INFLUENZA. The viruses may be transmitted from person to person through airborne drops and are highly contagious. Hospitalized patients will be placed in respiratory isolation.

Symptoms   Cough, shortness of breath, and (in severe cases) blue-purple skin color. A physician can hear bubbling noises in the lungs. A baby or young child with a cold and cough that suddenly gets worse should see a physician.

Treatment   Sometimes no treatment is needed, but in severe cases the child may need to be hospitalized for oxygen and respiratory therapy to clear the mucus. Antibiotics and CORTICOSTEROID DRUGS won't work against this viral infection, although antibiotics may be prescribed anyway to prevent a secondary bacterial infection. Sometimes a child may need to be placed on artificial ventilation until normal breathing returns.

bronchitis   Inflammation of the airways that connect the windpipe (trachea) to the lungs, resulting in persistent cough with quantities of phlegm or sputum. Attacks usually occur in the winter among smokers, babies, the elderly, and those with lung disease, although anyone can get bronchitis.

Bronchitis presents in one of two forms: acute (of sudden onset and short duration) and chronic (persistent over a long period, and recurring several years).

Cause   *Acute bronchitis* is usually a complication of a viral infection (such as a cold or the flu), although it can also be caused by air pollution. A bacterial infection also may lead to acute bronchitis. Attacks occur most often in winter.

Cigarette smoking is the primary cause of *chronic bronchitis*, because it stimulates the production of mucus in the lining of the bronchi and thickens the bronchi's muscular walls and those of smaller airways in the lungs, narrowing those passages. The passages then become more susceptible to infection, which cause further damage. Air pollution can have the same effect. The disease is most prevalent in industrial cities and in smokers, and more common in manual and unskilled workers.

Symptoms The symptoms of both chronic and acute bronchitis are the same. As the bronchial tubes swell and become congested, symptoms appear: wheezing, breathlessness, and a persistent cough that produces yellow or green phlegm. There also may be pain behind the breastbone. Acute bronchitis is also characterized by fever.

In chronic bronchitis, symptoms don't quickly clear up, and there is usually no fever. The persistence of symptoms also differentiates this disease from chronic asthma, in which wheezing and breathlessness vary in severity from day to day. As the disease progresses, emphysema may develop. The lungs become more resistant to the flow of blood, leading to pulmonary hypertension. Those with chronic bronchitis usually have two or more episodes of acute viral or bacterial infection of the lungs every winter. Occasionally, blood may be coughed up.

Treatment Humidifying the lungs either with a humidifier or by inhaling steam will ease symptoms. Drinking plenty of fluids also helps bring up phlegm. Most acute bronchitis clears up on its own without further treatment. If there is a suspicion of an underlying bacterial infection, antibiotics will be prescribed.

In chronic bronchitis, an inhaler containing a bronchodilator may relieve breathlessness. In specific cases, the patient may improve by inhaling oxygen from a cylinder. Antibiotics may treat or prevent any bacterial lung infection.

Complications Pleurisy or PNEUMONIA may rarely occur in cases of acute bronchitis.

A physician should be consulted if any of the following symptoms appear:

- severe breathlessness
- audible wheezing
- no improvement after three days
- blood is coughed up
- fever over 101 degrees F
- if patient has underlying lung disease

Chronic bronchitis often leads inexorably to increased shortness of breath; eventually, the patient may become housebound.

Brucella A genus of gram-negative spherical or rodlike parasitic bacteria that cause BRUCELLOSIS (undulant fever) in humans, and contagious abortion in animals. The principal species include *B. abortus* and *B. melitensis*. The genus was named after David Bruce, a surgeon who first identified the bacteria in 1887.

brucellosis A chronic bacterial disease, carried by farm animals, that may be transmitted to humans, affecting various organs of the body. It is also known as undulant fever, Malta fever, Gibraltar fever, Bang's disease, or Mediterranean fever.

Anyone is susceptible to the bacteria, and may get the disease if exposed, but it is more likely to be found among those who work with livestock. Up to 200 cases of brucellosis are diagnosed in the United States each year. In areas where milk pasteurization is not widely practiced (such as in Latin America and in the Mediterranean) the disease is contracted from eating unpasteurized dairy products. Untreated, the disease may persist for years.

Cause The disease is caused by several different species of bacteria of the genus BRUCELLA. *B. abortus* is found in cattle. *B. suis* is most often isolated in hogs and is more deadly when contracted by humans than the version found in cattle. *B. melitensis* is found in goats and sheep and causes the most severe illness in humans. *B. rangiferi* occurs in reindeer and caribou, and *B. canis* in dogs.

The bacteria are transmitted to humans by contact with an infected animal (through a cut or breathing in bacteria) or by consuming nonpasteurized contaminated milk or fresh goat cheese. It is also found in the afterbirth from infected cattle or goats that have aborted a fetus. It is not likely that the disease spreads from person to person or that a person will be reinfected after recovery. In the United States the disease is primarily confined to workers at slaughterhouses. President Richard Nixon suffered from brucellosis as a child.

Symptoms The disease is not usually fatal, but the intermittent fevers (a source of the name, "undulant fever"), can be debilitating. Symptoms usually appear within 5 to 30 days after exposure. The acute form of the disease includes a single bout of high fever, shivering, aching, and drenching sweats that last for a few days. Other symptoms include headache, poor appetite, backache, weakness, and depression. Mental depression can be so severe that the patient may be suicidal. In rare, untreated cases, an acute attack is so serious it can cause fatal complications such as PNEUMONIA or bacterial MENINGITIS. *B. melitensis* can cause abortions in women, especially during the first three months of pregnancy.

Chronic brucellosis is characterized by symptoms that recur over a period of months or years.

Diagnosis Blood tests can diagnose the disease.

Treatment Prolonged treatment with antibiotics (including tetracyclines plus streptomycin) and sulfonamides is effective. Bed rest is imperative. After an apparent recovery, the disease sometimes recurs a few months later, requiring another course of treatment.

Prevention Immunization of livestock that have first been checked to make sure they are not already infected will prevent human disease. Infected animals are usually destroyed.

bubonic plague See PLAGUE.

bunyavirus One of a group of mosquito-borne viruses that can infect humans, causing California ENCEPHALITIS, RIFT VALLEY FEVER, and others. Symptoms include headache, weakness, low-grade fever, facial pain, and rash. Outbreaks have occurred in North America, South America, Africa, and Europe.

C

California encephalitis See ENCEPHALITIS, CALIFORNIA.

camp fever See TYPHUS.

Campylobacter A genus of bacteria responsible for between 5 and 14 percent of all diarrhea, the most common cause of diarrhea in the world. For many years, scientists had thought the bacteria were related to the VIBRIO germs that cause intestinal illnesses and CHOLERA. In fact, the bacteria are much less dangerous, but much more common.

The bacteria were first identified in 1909 by two English veterinarians who were studying aborted cattle fetuses and who named the bacterium *Vibrio fetus*. The same bacteria were then isolated in 1947 in a woman's blood, but it was not until 1972 that researchers identified it as a new genus and named it *Campylobacter* for its characteristic shape from the Greek for "curved rod."

The bacteria survive best at body temperatures of humans and cattle, poultry, horses, and pets. They are one of the four most important types of disease-causing organisms that infect the intestines; the others are *Shigella, Salmonella,* and GIARDIA LAMBLIA. All are ingested in much the same way, via tainted food and water in places where proper sanitation, hygiene, or cooking methods are not strictly observed. See also DIARRHEA AND INFECTIOUS DISEASE; ANTIDIARRHEAL DRUGS; TRAVELER'S DIARRHEA.

campylobacteriosis A form of food-borne illness, first recognized in the 1970s, that causes gastroenteritis—one of the many so-called TRAVELER'S DIARRHEA. Much more common than either *Salmonella* or *Shigella*, campylobacteriosis is responsible for between 5 to 14 per-

cent of all diarrheal infections in the world. It may affect between 2 and 4 million Americans each year. Although anyone can get an infection, children under age 5 and young adults aged 15 to 29 are more frequently afflicted.

In the 1970s, more than 3,000 residents in Bennington, Vermont, became ill with diarrhea when their town's water supply was contaminated by a dog cadaver, which exuded the rod-shaped bacterium *Campylobacter jejuni*. It has subsequently spread everywhere.

Without treatment, the stool is infectious for several weeks, but three days of antibiotics will eliminate the bacteria from the stool. While the illness can be uncomfortable and even disabling, deaths among otherwise healthy patients are rare. See also DIARRHEA AND INFECTIOUS DISEASE; ANTIDIARRHEAL DRUGS.

Cause While there are several different forms of *Campylobacter*, the most common is *Campylobacter jejuni*, which accounts for 99 percent of all *Campylobacter* infections. Campylobacteriosis is caused by eating or drinking food or water contaminated with the bacteria; only a small amount is necessary to cause illness. It can survive in undercooked food such as chicken, lamb, beef, or pork, in water, and in raw milk. The disease may also spread throughout a child care center or from the diarrhea of affected young dogs or cats.

The most common source of *Campylobacter* infection is in contaminated poultry (between 20 percent and 100 percent of all raw chicken on the market is contaminated), which is not surprising considering that many healthy chickens carry the bacteria in their intestines. Raw milk is also a source of infection. Consumers get sick when they eat undercooked chicken or when the organisms are transferred from the raw meat or raw meat drippings to the mouth. The bacteria are common among healthy chickens on chicken farms, where they may spread undetected among the flocks (perhaps through drinking water supplies). When the birds are slaughtered, the bacteria are transferred from the intestines to the meat.

Other forms of *Campylobacter* are harder to diagnose and appear to be much more rare than *C. jejuni;* it is not yet clear what the source of those infections are.

Symptoms Symptoms begin between 2 to 10 days after tainted food or water is consumed and may last up to 10 days. They include nausea and vomiting and abdominal pain followed by watery or bloody diarrhea. Other symptoms may include headaches, fatigue, and body aches.

Diagnosis The infection is diagnosed when a stool is sent to the lab and cultured using special techniques.

Treatment Unless antibiotics are taken at the very beginning of the illness they won't affect symptoms, although they will shorten the infectious period. For mild cases, rest and fluids should be sufficient. Young children are usually given antibiotics (usually erythromycin) as a way of reducing the risk of passing the infection on to other children via infected stool.

Prevention Hands should be washed after using the toilet. Anyone with diarrhea should use a separate towel and washcloth and should not prepare food (especially uncooked food). Properly cooking chicken, pasteurizing milk, and chlorinating drinking water will kill the bacteria.

Complications Infection with campylobacteriosis may provoke a paralyzing neurologic illness (Guillain-Barre syndrome) in a small percentage of patients.

Campylobacter jejuni A slender type of bacteria, of the genus CAMPYLOBACTER, now recognized as the leading cause of bacterial diarrheal illness (called CAMPYLOBACTERIOSIS) in the United States, causing more disease than *Shigella* and *Salmonella* combined.

Although this bacterium is not carried by healthy individuals, it is often isolated from healthy cattle, chickens, birds, and flies. It may be found in nonchlorinated water (such as in ponds and streams). Not all strains of *C. jejuni* cause disease, but so far it is not possible to differentiate them.

Campylobacter pylorii The former name for HELICOBACTER PYLORII.

Candida albicans The yeast that causes the infection called candidiasis (THRUSH), often found within the vagina or on other mucous membranes (such as the inside of the mouth). The infection is also known as moniliasis.

Because it is so commonly found in the body, it is a problem only when it grows too abundant due to changes in the mucous membranes. It is also the cause of diaper rash, which has nothing to do with a baby's immune system but simply a result of the perfect yeast environment. Thrush, which causes patches that look like cottage cheese in the mouth, may be a sign of AIDS in young adults, but it is also common among healthy children or among those who take inhaled steroids in the treatment of asthma.

Candida albicans, while it is a yeast, has nothing to do with the food-grade yeast used to bake bread (*Saccharomyces cerevisiae*). See also CANDIDA LUSITANIAE INFECTION.

Candida lusitaniae infection A rare but emerging human pathogen that can cause fungal infection in meninges, lung, lower urinary tract, kidney, gastrointestinal tract, bone, skin, and soft tissue. It concerns scientists because it appears to resist antifungal drugs, including amphotericin B. *C. lusitaniae* was first isolated in 1959 from the gastrointestinal tract of mammals, but it wasn't recognized as a cause of human disease until 1979. Twenty-two cases of this type of fungal infection have been reported in English medical journals, most in the past 10 years. While this infection is very rare, there is evidence that it is becoming more of a problem, especially among hospital-acquired infections.

Because of its growing drug resistance—especially to the antifungal amphotericin B—scientists expect this fungal infection to be an increasing problem, especially among those patients with impaired immune function.

The infection can affect people of all ages; as with other *Candida* species, the main risk factors seem to be the use of antibacterial drugs, having an intravascular catheter, and having an impaired immune function.

Cause The *C. lusitaniae* infection usually begins in the throat or gastrointestinal tract.

Diagnosis The presence of the fungus can be determined via blood tests.

Treatment Since the pathogen is resistant to amphotericin B, flucytosine is often used together with other antifungal drugs. Still, 30 percent of patients with this disease died. See also CANDIDA ALBICANS.

candidiasis See THRUSH.

canker sore A small painful ulcer, on the inside of the mouth, lip, or underneath the tongue, that heals without treatment. About 20 percent of Americans at any one time experience a canker sore, which occur most commonly between ages 10 and 40. The most severely affected people have almost continuous sores, while others have just one or two per year.

Cause Because hemolytic streptococcus bacteria have so often been isolated from canker sores, experts believe they may be caused by a hypersensitive reaction to the bacteria. Other factors often associated with a flareup include trauma (such as biting the inside of the cheek), acute stress and allergies, or chemical irritants in toothpaste or mouth-

wash. More women than men experience canker sores, which are more likely to occur during the premenstrual period and are more likely to occur if other members of the family suffer from them. Interestingly, the older a person gets the less likely a canker sore will occur. Some experts believe there may be an underlying immune system defect similar to an allergy.

Symptoms A canker sore is usually a small oval ulcer with a gray center surrounded by a red, inflamed halo, which usually lasts for one or two weeks. They are similar but not identical to COLD SORES (or "fever blisters"), which also appear on the mouth. Both usually cause small sores that heal within two weeks. However, canker sores aren't usually preceded by a blister. Canker sores are usually larger than fever blisters, but they don't usually merge to form one large sore as fever blisters do. Finally, canker sores usually erupt on movable parts of the mouth (such as the tongue and the cheek or lip linings) whereas cold sores usually appear on the gums, roof of the mouth, lips, or nostrils.

Treatment While the ulcers will heal themselves, topical painkillers may ease the pain; healing may be speeded up by using a corticosteroid ointment or a tetracycline mouthwash. Victims may also cover the sore with a waterproof ointment to protect it. A canker sore should heal within two weeks; if not, or if the sufferer can't eat, speak, or sleep, seek medical help.

Over-the-counter medication containing carbamide peroxide (Cankaid, Glyoxide, and Amosan) may be effective in treating the sore. Other treatment possibilities include medications in liquid or gel form of benzocaine, menthol, camphor, eucalyptol, and/or alcohol or pastes (such as Orabase) that form a protective "bandage" over the sore. For short-term pain relief, rinse with a prescription mouthwash containing viscous lidocaine, an anesthetic.

Prevention Avoid coffee, spices, citrus fruits, walnuts, strawberries, and chocolates if you are prone to canker sores. Instead, try eating at least four tablespoons daily of plain yogurt containing *Lactobacillus acidophilus;* this introduces helpful bacteria into the mouth to fight canker sore bacteria.

Also, avoid commercial toothpastes and mouthwashes; instead brush teeth with baking soda for a month or two, and rinse your mouth with warm salt water. Specifically, scientists found that toothpaste with the detergent sodium lauryl sulfate was linked to canker sores in susceptible people. In a study of 10 people prone to sores, brushing with SLS-free paste for three months led to a 70 percent decrease in the number of canker sores. Scientists suggest the detergent may dry out the mucous layer of the mouth, leaving gums and cheeks vulnerable to irritants.

carbuncle A cluster of BOILS (pus-filled inflamed hair roots) infected with bacteria, commonly found on the back of the neck and the buttocks.

Cause Carbuncles are usually caused by the bacterium *Staphylococcus aureus.*

Symptoms Carbuncles usually begin as single boils that spread, but they are less common than single boils. They primarily affect patients with lowered resistance to infection or irritation of an area of skin.

Treatment Carbuncles are treated with oral and topical antibiotics and hot compresses. These may relieve the pain by causing the pus-filled heads to burst; if this occurs, the carbuncle should be covered with a dressing until it has healed completely. The lesion must often be cut and drained. The cavity may then need packing to keep the drainage complete.

In some cases, draining is not necessary, but this is rare. Antibiotics given by mouth don't usually help, but they may prevent spread of bacteria from the pus pockets into the bloodstream or surrounding tissues.

Prevention Recurrent carbuncles usually mean that patients are constantly reinfecting themselves. Regular washing with antibacterial soap (especially around rashes, irritations, shaving, or areas of heavy sweating) can help get rid of the infection. Also, hands and bedding should be washed often.

carditis Inflammation of the heart muscles usually caused by viral infection. Most of the time, more than one layer of the heart is involved. Symptoms include chest pain, circulatory failure, heart beat irregularities, and damage to the structures of the heart. Types of carditis include endocarditis (inflammation of the internal lining of the heart chambers and valves usually caused by bacteria); myocarditis (inflammation of the heart muscle, usually caused by a viral infection); and pericarditis (inflammation of the outer lining of the heart caused by a viral or bacterial infection).

cats and infectious disease Cats may spread multi-drug-resistant bacteria that can cause serious illness, according to researchers at the Public Health Laboratory Service in London, England. Scientists there found that of 110 cases of infection by *Salmonella* bacteria in cats, 78 were the species *S. typhimurium.* Of these, 40 were of a type that resists six common antibiotics in humans, which would make infection in humans hard to treat.

Researchers suspect the cats pick up infection from their food (maybe by eating scraps of contaminated human food or from eating raw or undercooked meat). Cats should not be given free access to unprotected food and cooking areas, they warn, and people who touch cats should wash their hands before eating or preparing food. See also PETS AND INFECTIOUS DISEASE; CAT-SCRATCH DISEASE.

cat-scratch disease (CSD) A mild illness following the scratch or bite of a kitten or cat, caused by a small bacterium recently identified as *Bartonella* (formerly *Rochalimaea*) *henselae.*

Three-quarters of cases occur in children and occur more often in fall and winter.

While the disease causes few problems in healthy individuals, in those with a weakened immune system the infection can become dangerous and life-threatening. There are about 22,000 cases of CSD in the United States each year.

Cats with the bacteria have no symptoms and don't appear to be harmed. The disease was first recognized in the 1950s, but the organism that causes it has only been recently discovered.

Cause The bacteria are transmitted between cats by the common cat flea, according to a new study by University of California researchers. The animal itself does not appear to be ill, and about 90 percent of cases are caused by kittens; the rest result from grown cats, dogs, and other animals.

Researchers still don't understand how the bacteria can live in the bloodstream, since blood is normally sterile and bacteria are usually killed by the immune system. While cats with the disease aren't ill, many have large numbers of organisms in their blood.

The disease cannot be transmitted from one person to another, and it is not clear if one episode confers immunity.

Symptoms The symptoms of CSD resemble the early stages of other infectious diseases, such as TUBERCULOSIS. About two weeks after a bite or scratch, the victim reports a red round lump at the site of infection and one or more swollen lymph nodes near the scratch, which may become painful and tender, with an occasional discharge. Symptoms sometimes include fever, rash, malaise, and headache. In most cases, symptoms disappear on their own.

Diagnosis It can be diagnosed by symptoms, history, and negative tests for other diseases that cause swollen lymph glands. A blood test, developed in 1992 by the Centers for Disease Control, detects antibodies to the bacteria. The test is available free to doc-

tors and state health departments. Biopsy of a small sample of the swollen lymph node is not necessary unless there is question of cancer of the lymph node or some other disease.

Treatment There are no antibiotics effective against CSD, although they are often prescribed for children with severe pain or swelling. A severely affected lymph node or blister may have to be drained, and a heating pad may help swollen, tender lymph glands. Acetaminophen may relieve pain, aches, and fever over 101 degrees F. In most cases, the illness fades after one or two months.

Complications In HIV patients, the bacteria can cause a rare, potentially fatal (yet curable) infection called BACILLARY ANGIOMATOSIS that causes blood vessels to grow out of control, forming tumorlike masses (in bone, liver, and skin) that look like those of KAPOSI'S SARCOMA.

Another rare complication is ENCEPHALITIS, or cat-scratch disease of the brain, which appears about one or two weeks after the first symptoms of CSD.

Signs of complications include unusual spots or bruises on the skin, eye infections, unusual pain, high fever (more than 103 degrees F), stiff neck, severe headache, or severe vomiting. This mimics other more serious causes of meningitis and is often treated with antibiotics.

Prevention Other than avoiding cats, there is no way to prevent the disease. However, cats only carry the infecting organism for a few weeks during their lifetimes, so the likelihood of being reinfected, or infected by just one pet in the home, is minimal.

Patients with weakened immune systems don't need to get rid of their cats, but they should inform their physicians that they own cats and avoid getting scratched. If a scratch does occur, it should be washed thoroughly with soap and water. It is also important to control fleas. See also CATS AND INFECTIOUS DISEASE; PETS AND INFECTIOUS DISEASE.

cellulitis   A bacterial infection of the skin and the tissues underneath it. Untreated, the disease may lead to BACTEREMIA and SEPTIC SHOCK. Facial cellulitis may spread to the eye and even the brain. Before the advent of antibiotics, the disease was sometimes fatal. Today, any form of cellulitis is likely to be more serious in those with impaired immune systems.

Cause   Cellulitis is usually caused by B-hemolytic streptococci bacteria following a minor injury, although many other bacteria may be responsible. Very rarely, cellulitis develops after childbirth and may spread to the pelvic organs.

Symptoms   The affected area (usually the skin of the face, neck, or legs) is usually hot, tender, and red; other symptoms include fever and chills, with swollen lymph glands. Perianal cellulitis may occur with itchy, painful bowel movements. A rash may appear on face, arms, or legs, with raised borders. Infection may recur, causing chronic swelling of arms or legs.

Diagnosis   The organism is hard to culture from skin lesions, but it may be identified in blood. Antibodies can be found in blood.

Treatment   The infection may resolve spontaneously on its own. Cold compresses and aspirin may bring relief. Antibiotics effective against the organism causing the infection must be taken for up to two weeks to clear the infection. At the beginning of antibiotic treatment, symptoms may temporarily get worse because of the abrupt death of many organisms. Often, antibiotics must be given intravenously for a period of time, especially if the infection is spreading quickly or is located on the face.

Centers for Disease Control and Prevention
The federal organization charged with the responsibility of preventing and controlling infectious diseases for nearly 50 years. Established as the Communicable Disease Center in 1946 in Atlanta, Georgia, the CDC has led efforts to prevent MALARIA, polio, SMALLPOX, TOXIC SHOCK SYNDROME, LEGIONNAIRES' DISEASE, LYME DISEASE, hospital infections, and more recently, HIV/AIDS.

The center's responsibilities have expanded over the years and continue to evolve as the agency addresses other threats to health such as injuries and environmental and occupational hazards.

CDC supports surveillance, research, prevention efforts, and training in the area of infectious diseases through its NATIONAL CENTER FOR INFECTIOUS DISEASES.

In 1946, the mission of the agency was to protect Americans from germs, including TYPHUS, dengue, PLAGUE, malaria, and other infectious diseases. Today, its public mission is more than germs and ranges far beyond the U.S. border. Fighting disease today is a global effort using the talents of public health officials in every country, state, city, and county.

CDC epidemiologists continue to study microbes, from EBOLA in Africa to CRYPTOSPORIDIUM in Milwaukee, but the agency also combats health threats such as gun violence, poverty, and poor nutrition. In so doing, it has been criticized by those who believe the agency should stick to bugs and keep out of social policy.

Today, the CDC maintains 11 centers, institutes, and offices, including the National Center for Infectious Diseases; the National Center for Chronic Disease Prevention and Health Promotion; the National Center for Environmental Health; the National Center for Health Statistics; the National Center for HIV, STD and TB Prevention; the National Center for Injury Prevention and Control; the National Center for Occupational Safety and Health; the Epidemiology Program Office; the International Program Office; the Public Health Practice Program Office; and the National Immunization Program. It has about 6,900 employees in 170 locations in Anchorage; Atlanta; Cincinnati; Fort Collins, Colorado; Morgantown, West Virginia; Pittsburgh; Research Triangle Park,

North Carolina; San Juan; Spokane; and Washington, D.C.

The infectious disease center houses the famed maximum containment lab, one of only six in the world that can handle the most deadly organisms. High-tech filters keep the microbes inside from getting outside, and scientists at the lab wear spacesuits so microbes don't get in. The lab is locked, guarded, and under constant video surveillance. It is here that one of the last two samples of smallpox on earth survives. Smallpox was eradicated in 1977, in large part by activities supported by the CDC.

cephalosporins Antibiotics used to treat infections that occur in a variety of places in the body. They are usually used after other (less expensive) antibiotics have proven unsuccessful or when the infection is unusual. They can be used to treat most common URINARY TRACT INFECTIONS (UTIs) and upper respiratory infections such as PHARYNGITIS or TONSILLITIS. The cephalosporins include cefadroxil, cefixime, cefuroxime axetil, cefaclor, and cephalexin. As with other antibiotics, some cephalosporins can treat certain bacterial infections better than others.

They can be taken either with food or on an empty stomach; in case of nausea, they should be taken with food or milk. Liquid suspensions should be refrigerated (except for cefixime suspension). Any unused suspension should be thrown away after 14 days.

These drugs should always be taken at the same time of day and for the exact amount of time prescribed, *even if the patient feels better.* The infection may return if the drug is not taken for the full amount of time. Heart or kidney complications can result if a STREPTOCOCCUS infection is not completely treated.

If the infection is caused by a type of bacteria that responds to cephalosporins, the symptoms should improve within a few days, although sometimes it may take longer to get relief. If the symptoms remain after all the drug is taken or gets worse during the medication period, a physician should be contacted.

Cephalosporins appear to be relatively safe to use during pregnancy. They do pass into breast milk in small amounts. The drugs also may cause diabetics to get a false-positive reading for glucose in the urine if copper sulfate urine test tablets are used.

Side effects Common side effects include mild stomach cramps, nausea, vomiting, and diarrhea that go away with time. Like other antibiotics, cephalosporins may encourage the growth of fungus normally found in the body, causing a sore tongue, mouth sores, or a vaginal yeast infection.

More serious (but rarer) side effects include allergic reactions ranging from itchy, red, or swollen skin rash to severe breathing problems and shock. A patient allergic to penicillin may also be allergic to a cephalosporin.

Specific allergic reaction to cephalosporin can include skin rash, joint pain, irritability, and fever. Another rare side effect is serious colitis, with severe watery diarrhea, stomach cramps, fever, weakness, and fatigue.

cerebrospinal fluid analysis See SPINAL TAP.

cereus A type of food poisoning caused by the *Bacillus cereus* bacteria, which multiplies in raw foods at room temperature. The *B. cereus* bacteria produces toxins most often found in steamed or fried rice. It is believed that poisoning with *B. cereus* is underreported because its symptoms are so similar to other types of food poisoning (especially staphylococcal and *CLOSTRIDIUM PERFRINGENS* poisoning).

Symptoms This bacterium produces two distinct types of food poisoning: The first features a short incubation period after eating tainted food (usually less than six hours), causing cramps and vomiting, and occasionally a short bout with diarrhea. Almost 80 percent of patients with these symptoms who test positive for *B. cereus* poisoning have eaten steamed or fried rice at Chinese restaurants.

The second type of *B. cereus* poisoning is very similar to *C. perfringens* poisoning; it appears within 8 to 24 hours after ingestion of tainted food and causes abdominal cramps and diarrhea with very little vomiting.

Treatment   Treatment of both types of the disease is aimed only at making the patient comfortable. There are no medications which will shorten the course of the disease.

cestode   See TAPEWORM.

Chagas disease   A parasitic disease also known as American TRYPANOSOMIASIS transmitted by the bite of blood-sucking insects and rarely by blood transfusions. Named for 19th-century Brazilian physician Carlos Chagas, the disease is endemic in Central and South America, where it is recognized as a serious public health problem. Officials there rank their need to control this disease third, behind MALARIA and SCHISTOSOMIASIS.

More than a quarter of the total population in Central and South America are at risk, with more than a million cases each year. Of these, 45,000 people will die and up to 18 million people may be currently infected. Of these, 3 million may have already developed chronic complications, and more than 3 million are still in the incubation period. The disease is also known as Brazilian trypanosomiasis, Chagas-Cruz disease, Cruz trypanosomiasis, and South American trypanosomiasis.

Cause   The disease is caused by the single-celled parasite *Trypanosoma cruzi*, very similar to those that cause sleeping sickness in Africa. The parasite infects bugs commonly known as "assassin bugs" or "cone-nosed bugs" (reduviid); when the bugs defecate, the excrement includes the parasite, which can then enter a human through a break in the skin or through a mucous membrane. The parasites live in the bloodstream and can also affect a person's heart, intestines, or nervous system.

Symptoms   The disease may occur in an acute or chronic form. The acute form (common in children, rare in adults) is marked by a lesion at the site of infection, together with fever, weakness, enlarged spleen and lymph nodes, facial and leg swelling, and rapid heartbeat. This form disappears on its own in about four months, unless complications (such as ENCEPHALITIS) set in.

About 10 to 20 years after the initial acute phase, incurable lesions of the disease develop. In addition, 27 percent of those infected develop a chronic heart disease problem. Six percent have chronic lesions in the digestive tract, and about 3 percent may have neurological problems. Patients with chronic disease become progressively sick and ultimately die, usually as a result of heart failure.

Treatment   Nifurtimox is available from the CDC for the treatment of short-term Chagas disease. There is no accepted anti-parasitic treatment for chronic illness.

Prevention   The best prevention is to avoid potential reduviid habitats (mud, adobe, and thatch buildings, especially those with cracks or crevices). If this isn't feasible, infection may be prevented by spraying infested areas with insecticide, using fumigant canisters and insecticidal paints, and using bed nets. Housing improvements have also helped. In addition, screening blood donors at blood banks helps to control the spread of the disease via blood transfusions.

In 1991, the health ministers of Argentina, Bolivia, Brazil, Chile, Paraguay, and Uruguay began a program to eliminate Chagas disease by the end of this century. Since then, house infestation has declined 75 to 98 percent in some areas, according to the Pan American Health Organization.

Chagres fever   An arbovirus infection transmitted to humans through the bite of the sandfly. The disease, which is rarely fatal, is most common in Central America. It was named after the Chagres River in Panama and is also known as Panama Fever.

Symptoms It is characterized by fever, headache, and muscle pain of the chest or abdomen, with nausea and vomiting, giddiness, weakness, photophobia (sensitivity to light), and pain on moving the eyes. It usually passes within a week.

Treatment Bed rest, fluids, and painkillers.

chancroid A sexually transmitted disease rarely seen in the past 30 years but making a comeback since the early 1980s. In some subtropical and tropical countries, the disease is more common than SYPHILIS. There have been outbreaks in the United States in large cities in California and parts of the south over the past 15 years.

Those most at risk are men under age 24, men and women with multiple sex partners, those with other STDs (especially syphilis), prostitutes and their customers, and those in tropical areas. However, any sexually active person can be infected with chancroid. It is more commonly seen in men than women, especially in uncircumcised males.

Cause Chancroid is caused by *Hemophilus ducreyi,* a rod-shaped bacterium that grows only in the absence of oxygen (much like GONORRHEA bacteria). The bacteria are transmitted from the draining sores of an infected person during sex. It is more likely to be transmitted to another person with a small cut or scratch in the genital area. The chances of transmission are greater if a person is very active sexually and doesn't practice personal hygiene.

Symptoms Symptoms usually appear within a week of infection. In some women, there may be a small pimple with a reddish base that will gradually fill with pus, opening and hollowing. Eventually, several ulcers usually appear that are very painful and soft. About a week later, the pelvic lymph gland on one side of the groin may become enlarged and painful. Other women don't notice sores but have pain during sex or while urinating. Still others never notice any symptoms, especially if ulcers are on the vaginal walls or cervix.

Men experience painful sores under the foreskin or on the underside of the penis that fill with pus and turn into ulcers. About 50 percent of infected men will go on to develop painful, enlarged lymph glands in the groin.

Both men and women are infectious until the lesions are completely healed, which may take up to two weeks. It is not possible to become immune.

Diagnosis The disease is diagnosed by symptoms and negative test results for other more common causes of genital ulcers (such as syphilis or HERPES). About half the time, microscopic examination of the fluid from a draining ulcer will correctly diagnose the infection; a culture of the drainage will provide a correct diagnosis, but the bacteria aren't easy to grow and many labs aren't equipped to do the test.

Treatment Antibiotics for both partners, such as azithromycin or erythromycin, or a shot of ceftriaxone, will cure the disease in about a week. Lesions and ulcers will heal in about two weeks.

Complications Untreated chancroid often causes ulcers on the genitals that may persist for weeks or months. The infection does not harm the fetus of a pregnant woman. However, the lesion does increase the chances of contracting HIV if a person has sex with an HIV-infected partner.

chicken pox (varicella) A common childhood infectious disease characterized by a rash and slight fever. It affects about 4 million children each year in the United States. About 90 percent of cases occur in children under age 10, primarily in winter and spring. Chicken pox is also known as varicella, after the virus that causes the disease (varicella zoster, or VZV). The name *varicella* dates to the 1700s and derives from the Latin term for "little pox."

Most people throughout the world have had the disease by age 10, and chicken pox is rare in adults. When it does occur after childhood, it is a far more serious illness.

Cause VZV is a member of the family of herpesviruses similar to the herpes simplex virus (HSV); the same virus that causes chicken pox also causes SHINGLES. Once a person has chicken pox, the virus stays in the body in a latent stage, hiding in the nerves of the lower spinal cord for the rest of the person's life. When reactivated (in old age or during times of stress), it can lead to shingles.

Symptoms The VZV virus, which is spread by airborne droplets, is extremely contagious. The incubation period ranges from 10 to 23 days. One to three weeks after exposure, a rash appears on the torso, face, armpits, upper arms and legs, inside the mouth, and sometimes in the windpipe and bronchial tubes, causing a dry cough.

The rash is made up of small red itchy spots that grow into fluid-filled blisters within a few hours. After several days, the blisters dry out and form scabs. New spots usually continue to form over four to seven days. Children usually have only a slight fever, but an adult may experience fever with severe pneumonia and breathing problems. Adults usually have higher fevers, more intense rash, and more complications than children.

The average child will have between 250 and 500 blisters over about five days; the more blisters the child has, the harder the body has to fight to make enough antibodies to destroy the virus. The fight between the virus and the immune system causes fevers, fatigue, and poor appetite. Those who catch the disease from a sibling instead of a classmate usually have a more severe illness, from 300 to 5,000 blisters. This is because the close contact at home causes a much larger amount of virus to enter the system.

The patient is infectious from five days before the rash erupts until all the blisters are completely healed, dried, and scabbed over. This can take from 6 to 10 days after the rash appears.

Complications In children, these may include bacterial infection and, rarely, Reye's syndrome, or in even rarer cases, ENCEPHALITIS. Immunocompromised patients who are susceptible to VZV are at high risk for having severe varicella infections with widespread lesions.

Between 40 and 200 people die every year in the United States; half are previously healthy people and the other half are those with impaired immune systems.

Treatment In most cases, rest is all that is needed for children, who usually recover within 10 days. Adult patients take longer to recover. Acetaminophen may reduce the fever, and calamine lotion, baking soda baths, and oral antihistamines ease the itch. Compresses can dry weeping lesions. *Never give aspirin to a child who has flulike symptoms or has been exposed to (or has recently recovered from) chicken pox;* aspirin in these cases has been linked to Reye's syndrome.

The drug acyclovir may be prescribed for chicken pox patients who are not pregnant and who have any of the following: chronic skin or lung disorders, required regular administration of aspirin or steroids, overwhelming chicken pox, a compromised immune system (such as AIDS). Unlike the herpes-simplex viruses, VZV is relatively resistant to acyclovir, and doses required for treatment are much larger and must be administered intravenously. While the drug may shorten the length of the illness and lessen symptoms, its high cost and marginal effectiveness have prompted the American Academy of Pediatrics not to recommend it as a routine treatment.

Scratching should be avoided, as it may lead to secondary bacterial infection and increase the chance of scarring.

If possible, don't bring a child with suspected chicken pox into the doctor's office where others will be exposed to the disease; it can be very dangerous to newborns or those with suppressed immune systems. The virus can be spread both through the air and by direct contact with an infected individual. Instead, call the physician on the phone and describe the symptoms, if you suspect it could be chicken pox.

Prevention An infected child should not play with anyone at risk for serious disease from chicken pox, and should be kept away from infants younger than six weeks of age. They should also stay away from crowded public places where high-risk people might congregate.

Passive immunity that offers only temporary protection is available for high-risk susceptible patients via varicella-zoster immune globulin. This can abort or modify infection if administered within three days of exposure. Passive immunization is the administration of antibodies from donor's blood; since a person's blood is completely replaced every three months, the immunity lasts only that long.

There is some disagreement about the value of giving passive immunity to susceptible pregnant women in the first trimester; some fear that while it may prevent symptoms, the virus may still be in the mother's blood and thereby infect the fetus.

Vaccine Active immunization is provided by a vaccination that stimulates the immune system to make protective antibodies that last for life. The chicken pox vaccine is made from a live weakened virus that works by creating a mild infection similar to natural chicken pox, but without the related problems. The mild infection spurs the body to develop an immune response to the disease. These defenses are then ready when the body encounters the natural virus.

The development of a vaccine against the disease has been studied and used in clinical trials with children and adults in the United States since the early 1980s; it has been used in Japan for some time. It protects 70 to 90 percent of children, but it doesn't work well on adults.

In March 1995, the U.S. Food and Drug Administration licensed the vaccine for general use; the American Academy of Pediatrics has recommended the vaccine for all children and teenagers. Children younger than 12 require one dose; children 13 and over require two shots four to eight weeks apart.

Not all physicians agree on the benefits of the vaccine for healthy children, however. While proponents of the vaccine point out that suffering children and parents' considerable lost work time are good reasons to use the vaccine, some researchers are uncertain about how long the vaccine confers immunity. Critics warn that if the vaccine wears off in later life, the adult could then be vulnerable to infection at an age when chicken pox can be serious.

Other experts are concerned about possible side effects of the vaccine. Since the chicken pox virus belongs to the herpesvirus group, there are concerns that the vaccine might cause periodic reactivation of the varicella zoster virus, causing shingles.

Recent reports also note that the vaccine may cause birth defects when given to pregnant women or to women who conceive within three months after vaccination. Doctors already know that having chicken pox while pregnant increases the risk of bearing a child with birth defects. To determine the link (if any) between birth defects and immunization of mothers, the U.S. Centers for Disease Control and Merck (the company that makes Varivax, one of the vaccines) have set up a registry of women who receive the vaccine while pregnant or in the three months before conception. Patients and health care workers should report Varivax vaccinations to this group at 1-800-986-8999. Reports may also be mailed to Merck Research Labs, Worldwide Product Safety & Epidemiology, BLA-31, West Point, PA 19486.

For a free brochure, "What Parents Need to Know About Chickenpox," send a SASE to the National Foundation for Infectious Diseases, 4733 Bethesda Ave., Suite 750, Bethesda, MD 20814.

chiggers The larva of *Trombicula* mites, which, in summer, live in tall grass and weeds and can stick to the skin and cause irritation and severe itching. Chiggers are also called harvest mites or red mites. The swelling they cause may turn into an itchy blister that can persist for weeks.

chikungunya fever An infectious disease taken from the Swahili for "that which bends up," in reference to the stooped posture of patients afflicted with the severe joint pain associated with this disease. The disease was first recognized in epidemic form in East Africa in 1952–53.

The virus is found in eastern, southern, western, and central Africa and southeastern Asia, where it has caused illnesses in thousands of people. Epidemics have occurred in the Philippines, Thailand, Cambodia, Vietnam, India, Myanmar (Burma), and Sri Lanka.

Cause The *A. aegypti* mosquitoes carry the chikungunya virus, which they pass on to humans when they bite. Epidemics are sustained by human-mosquito-human transmission, similar to the way that epidemics of DENGUE FEVER and urban YELLOW FEVER are maintained.

Symptoms The fever is characterized by sudden onset of chills and fever, headache, nausea and vomiting, joint pain, and rash that lasts up to a week. While chikungunya is often confused with dengue fever, chikungunya has a shorter period of fever, persistent joint pain, and lack of fatalities.

Treatment There is no specific treatment; painkillers can lower fever and ease joint pain.

child care centers and infectious disease Since young children are often vulnerable targets for infectious disease due to their immature immune systems, it stands to reason that grouping many infants and preschoolers together in day care centers should contribute to the spread of infectious disease. The problem is exacerbated by the fact that young children are not particularly concerned with good hygiene and that many day care centers include care for children who are not yet toilet trained.

Still, day care centers don't have to be breeding grounds for infectious diseases. In fact, recent research indicates that after the first year, children in child care get sick at about half the rate as do youngsters who are cared for at home. This is because youngsters at day care are simply exposed to germs sooner, and their immune systems sooner learn to cope with the onslaught of exposure.

Many studies have shown that if the center staff understand, are supervised, and educated about infection control, there is much less infectious illness spread among the youngsters than before. Simply by emphasizing hand washing, some centers have managed to cut diarrhea spread in half.

Before a child care facility can be licensed, they must meet certain hygiene standards, in a variety of areas, as set by local and state licensing authorities. Among other things, centers should clean all surfaces with a safe disinfectant. Surfaces should be dried with paper towels after being sprayed. Adequate ventilation and sanitation are necessary. Chemical air fresheners should not be used because many people are allergic to them.

Many infections in child care centers are spread by fecal contamination. When diapers are changed, tiny amounts of feces on hands can be transferred to countertops, toys, and door handles, so that if one child is shedding an infection in the feces, it isn't long before the infection spreads. Some infectious viruses will appear in feces before the diarrhea starts and remain in feces until more than a week after symptoms disappear.

To head off these problems, diapers should be checked every hour. Diaper-changing areas should not be located where food is prepared, stored, or served. The changing table should

TRANSMISSION OF INFECTIONS IN CHILDREN

Children catch infectious diseases in a variety of ways.

In the air:
• chicken pox
• colds
• fifth disease
• influenza
• meningitis
• TB

By direct contact:
• cold sores
• cytomegalovirus
• head lice
• scabies
• strep infections (strep throat, scarlet fever, and impetigo)

Fecal-oral route:
• diarrheal disease
• hepatitis A

By contact with infected blood:
• hepatitis B

be cleaned after use. Soiled diapers should be disposed of in separate covered waste containers. Staffers should wash hands before and after changing diapers. If a child has diarrhea, staff should don disposable gloves before changing the diaper.

Hands should be washed after using the toilet or handling diapers; after helping a child at the toilet; before preparing, handling, or serving food; before feeding an infant; before setting the table; after wiping or blowing noses; after touching blood, vomit, saliva, or eye secretions; after handling pets; and before and after eating.

chlamydia   The most common sexually transmitted disease (STD) in the United States, infecting more than 4.5 million people each year. It is a serious but easily cured disease that is 3 times more common than GON-

ORRHEA, 6 times more common than genital HERPES, and 30 times more common than SYPHILIS. Between 1988 and 1992, the rate of reported cases of chlamydia more than doubled. Sexually active teens have high rates of chlamydia infections.

The organism that causes chlamydia (*CHLAMYDIA TRACHOMATIS*) is classified as a bacterium, even though it is similar to a virus. A parasite that—like a virus—can't reproduce outside living cells, it's enough like bacteria to be vulnerable to antibiotics.

Those at highest risk for contracting the disease are women under age 24, women who take birth control pills, men and women who have had more than one sex partner, and people with other STDs (especially gonorrhea).

In women, the bacteria centers on the cervix, where they cause an inflammation known as mucopurulent cervicitis, which can cause a yellow thick discharge, white blood cells, or bleeding from the cervix that a doctor can diagnosis during a pelvic exam.

Cause   A person catches chlamydia during sexual intercourse with a person infected with *C. trachomatis,* or a baby can contract the disease from an infected mother during birth. (The disease can be transmitted only during birth as the baby passes through the infected birth canal, not during the previous nine months of pregnancy.)

The disease does not confer immunity; some studies suggest that if you have ever had chlamydia, you are more likely to be reinfected sometime in the future.

Symptoms   Most women experience no symptoms at all; but even if a woman has no symptoms, she can infect her sex partner. About 20 percent notice a heavy, yellow vaginal discharge. If chlamydia affects the urinary tract, there may be pain, burning, or a frequent urge to urinate.

Many men have symptoms that are so mild they are ignored. The rest experience burning or pain during urination, or notice a watery, milky, or thick discharge from the penis. This is caused by an inflamed urethra.

Some studies suggest that a person can become infected between one to two weeks after exposure. The person remains infectious until the complete course of antibiotics has been taken. Untreated infected people may be infectious for years.

Diagnosis The most reliable test in women is a culture taken from the cervical cells. The current test (90 percent accurate) can identify antibodies in 24 hours. For men, doctors assume that any man with the above symptoms who does not have gonorrhea has chlamydia. Some doctors may try to identify white blood cells in the discharge. A man should be treated for chlamydia if his sex partner has a positive chlamydia test, whether or not he has symptoms.

Tests using urine samples have also recently been developed.

Complications Untreated women may go on to develop infected tubes (salpingitis) or an infected uterus lining (endometritis). PELVIC INFLAMMATORY DISEASE (PID) can lead to a buildup of scar tissue that will block the fallopian tubes, causing infertility or tubal pregnancy. Some studies have linked chlamydia with a higher risk of premature birth or a low-birth-weight baby.

About two-thirds of babies born to infected mothers go on to develop CONJUNCTIVITIS within two weeks of birth, although permanent damage to the baby's eyes is rare. A treated baby is in no risk of permanent damage. About 10 to 20 percent of exposed newborns may develop chlamydia pneumonia in the first three to four months of age. While it is usually mild, some babies may be quite ill and are at risk for developing lung problems later in childhood.

Treatment The disease can be cured by taking antibiotics for seven days (doxycycline) or a one-gram single dose of azithromycin. Pregnant women can take ery-

thromycin for several days. Penicillin is not effective against chlamydia.

Prevention All sexually active young women should be tested for chlamydia; many college health services and family planning clinics routinely test for chlamydia during physical exams. Between 5 to 10 percent of female college students have the disease.

Anyone who is treated for any STD should also be tested for chlamydia. (In some areas of the United States, half of the patients with gonorrhea also have chlamydia.)

The sex partner of anyone with chlamydia must also be treated at the same time; otherwise, reinfection will occur.

Condoms reduce the risk of transmission, but they do not provide complete protection.

All pregnant women should be tested for chlamydia; pregnant women with more than one sex partner or with a partner who has multiple partners should be retested in the third trimester. While many hospitals routinely put erythromycin ointment in the eyes of all newborns to guard against both chlamydia and gonorrhea infections, many babies born to infected mothers still develop chlamydia conjunctivitis

chlamydial pneumonia See PNEUMONIA, CHLAMYDIAL.

Chlamydia pneumoniae infection This disease is caused by infection with *Chlamydia pneumoniae,* one of the varieties of *Chlamydia* organism that has been linked to respiratory illness and coronary heart disease—specifically, heart attack or atherosclerosis (hardening of the arteries). Because it can be killed by antibiotics, this link to heart disease could be of enormous importance for public health. Up to 10 percent of community-acquired PNEUMONIA may be caused by this bacteria.

Most people are first infected during childhood or early adolescence. Up to 60 percent of all adults around the world have antibodies to

C. pneumoniae, and reinfection may be common. There is suspicion that this organism may also be related to the development of asthma.

Cause Unlike *C. psittaci,* this organism is spread from person to person by coughing or sneezing. Outbreaks of infection have been reported in families, schools, military barracks, and nursing homes. Often, there is a simultaneous infection with other bacteria or with a virus such as INFLUENZA or RESPIRATORY SYNCYTIAL VIRUS.

Symptoms Between 7 to 21 days after exposure, symptoms of upper respiratory infection appear. Infection is usually mild, but it may be severe, especially among the elderly.

Diagnosis A variety of lab tests can reveal the infection.

Treatment Clarithromycin or azithromycin are the drugs of choice.

Chlamydia psittaci infection Infection with an organism that infects birds and causes a rare type of PNEUMONIA in humans known as psittacosis (ORNITHOSIS). *C. psittaci* is carried by infected birds, especially parrots.

Cause The infection is acquired through breathing in droplets of bacteria from infected birds and is an occupational hazard for employees of pet shops and poultry processing plants. Birds can be healthy carriers of the organism; increased shedding of bacteria and susceptibility to disease occur during stress, starvation, or egg laying. Person to person transmission is rare, but there have been instances where it has occurred. In the *C. psittaci* pandemic of 1929–30, infected Argentine birds were shipped to different parts of the world, causing sporadic outbreaks with death rates of up to 40 percent. Since then, the bacterium has been isolated from more than 130 species of birds. All avian species should be considered potentially infectious.

Outbreaks of psittacosis in duck and turkey processing plants show that the infections continue to be a public health concern, despite diagnostic testing, medicated feed, and poultry screening.

Sources of human infection other than infected birds have been identified and may be more common than had previously been thought. *C. psittaci* has been identified in cats and breeding catteries, for example, which suggests that human infection from pets other than birds may occur.

Symptoms Within 6 to 19 days after exposure to infected birds, the patient experiences a flulike illness with fever, chills, headache and cough, facial pain, rash, joint pain and swelling. In severe cases, there may be an atypical pneumonia.

Diseases associated with exposure to infected animals include spontaneous abortion, symptoms of kidney and liver disease, and heart inflammation. There have also been reports of eye infections and heart problems from people exposed to infected cats and pigeons.

Diagnosis Blood tests can reveal the infection.

Treatment Recommended treatment is tetracycline for three weeks. The death rate is low but many patients experience a lengthy recovery and high incidence of relapse.

Chlamydia trachomatis An organism that lives in the conjunctiva of the eye and the cell layer of the urethra and cervix and is responsible for some types of CONJUNCTIVITIS, nonspecific urethritis, PELVIC INFLAMMATORY DISEASE, and TRACHOMA. It causes one of the most common sexually transmitted diseases in North America (CLAMYDIA) and is a frequent cause of sterility, infecting more than 4.5 million people each year. The World Health Organization estimated 89 million new cases of genital chlamydial infections worldwide in 1995. In the United States, each year an estimated 4 million new cases appear and 50,000 women become infertile as a result of infection.

Chlamydia is a serious but easily cured disease that is 3 times more common than GONORRHEA, 6 times more common than genital HERPES, and 30 times more common than SYPHILIS. Between 1988 and 1992, the rate of reported cases of chlamydia more than doubled. Sexually active teens have high rates of chlamydia infections.

The chlamydia organism is classified as a bacterium, even though it is similar to a virus and was once identified as such by scientists. A parasite that—like a virus—can't reproduce outside living cells, it's enough like bacteria to be vulnerable to antibiotics. It is known as an "energy parasite," since it possesses all the biological features needed for independence except the ability to generate its own energy.

There are three types of the chlamydia organism that are of medical interest; *C. trachomatis*, *C. PSITTACI*, and *C. PNEUMONIAE*. Of these, *C. trachomatis* is the most important, since it is the cause of the sexually transmitted disease that can cause problems with reproduction. *C. trachomatis* was first described in China and in the Ebers papyrus in Egypt thousands of years ago; it continues to be a major cause of preventable blindness, with an estimated 500 million cases of active trachoma in the world.

The organism *C. trachomatis* has two strains; one infects the eyes and/or genitals, and the other causes a swelling and ulceration of the lymph tissue near the groin. This disease, called LYMPHOGRANULOMA VENEREUM has been dropping in the United States except among gay men. It is still common in tropical regions of Africa, Central America, and Asia. The first strain attacks the eyes, causing a disease known as TRACHOMA, now rare in the United States and Europe but one that remains the leading cause of blindness in the Third World.

The second strain has been steadily increasing since the 1960s, causing a range of symptoms from conjunctivitis (inflammation of the rim of the eyes) to infertility. When transmitted sexually, it can cause a range of urinary tract infections in men and women, pelvic inflammatory disease, and ectopic pregnancy. The disease may be passed from an infected mother to a newborn, causing pneumonia. Like other genital organisms, it is often found among young nonwhite, unmarried poor people. More than half of its victims have no symptoms. Antibiotics can kill this pathogen, but condoms are the best protection.

cholera   This infection of the small intestine characterized by profuse, painless, watery diarrhea has been one of the great social and political forces in history. If untreated, severe cases can cause rapid dehydration and death within a few hours. If patients are given enough fluids, most will recover. The death rate soars in pandemics when there is not enough clean water, or if so many people become ill that there are not enough healthy people to care for the sick. After one infection, resulting antibodies will protect the patient from reinfection with the same strain.

There has been a dramatic increase in cholera in the United States and its territories, and many cases may go undetected by physicians who are not familiar with the disease, according to the National Center for Infectious Diseases. The disease thrives in places without running water or treated sewage disposal. This is why in the United States and Canada, cholera does not spread from one person to the next; any cholera organisms in infected feces are killed by sewage treatment and chlorinated water. See also TRAVELER'S DIARRHEA; DIARRHEA AND INFECTIOUS DISEASE; ANTIDIARRHEAL DRUGS.

The spread of cholera in the Western world is tied to the problems of 19th-century urbanization, with its lack of sewage control, public water supply, and burgeoning population. While tainted water supplies carry the bacillus, it is also passed in human feces. Therefore, preparing food with unwashed hands, contamination by roaches or flies, and the location of homes and buildings near raw sewage compounds the problem. During the industrialization of the 19th century, families crowded together in dirty tenements and those struggling in coal mining districts were especially at high risk, as were nurses and laundresses who handled soiled linen.

History For centuries cholera thrived only in northeast India, where outbreaks still occur regularly, because of the lack of clean water. In 1784, 20,000 pilgrims died from cholera at an Indian holy place known as Hurdwar. As the world trade routes opened in the 1800s, cholera spread throughout the world, killing millions of people in six distinct pandemics since 1817. The second pandemic reached England in the early 1800s, where London physician John Snow began his investigation of the Broad Street pump, a public source of water drawn from a well near a Soho cesspool. Snow, a general practitioner, was convinced that cholera was found in water and carried by the excretions of victims, and it was Snow who correctly identified sewage-contaminated drinking water as the source of the epidemic. In his research, he compared the incidence of cholera in a neighborhood with two different sources of water, one of which was contaminated with sewage. After he convinced authorities to remove the pump's handle (shutting off the water supply) the neighborhood's outbreak stopped.

In Paris, the pandemic of 1848–49 killed 18,000 people out of a population of 785,000. It was not until the fifth pandemic in 1881 that German and French scientific teams discovered the source of the disease. German microbiologist Robert Koch identified the "comma bacilli" (now called VIBRIO CHOLERAE) under the microscope as the actual cause of cholera.

For the first half of the 20th century, cholera was confined to Asia, and not a single case was reported anywhere in the entire Western Hemisphere between 1911 and 1973. Then between 1974 and 1988, a few cases appeared in U.S. states bordering the Gulf of Mexico (Florida, Louisiana, and Texas). In 1989, no cases were reported.

All cases today are part of a pandemic that began in Indonesia in 1961 with a new strain, called *V. cholerae*, 01 biotype El Tor. Unexpectedly, in 1991 this cholera epidemic spread to Peru when a ship arrived from the Far East dumped cholera-infected bilge water into the Lima harbor. The bacteria contaminated the fish and shellfish, which Peruvians ate raw; from there the bacteria got into the sewers and from there into the water supply. The disease then spread throughout South and Central America, where the epidemic continues to this day. The particular bacterium can survive in water for long periods. By September 1994, more than a million people in 20 countries had contracted the disease, and more than 9,000 had died.

In most years, there are only a handful of cases in the United States, usually among people who have traveled to Asia or Africa. Cases appear in areas bordering the Gulf of Mexico and around the Mediterranean are usually caused by eating tainted shellfish. From 1961 to 1991, there was an average of five cases per year in the United States; 31 percent of these infections were acquired abroad. From 1992 to 1994, 160 cholera cases were reported in the United States (about 53 per year); this is compared to a total of 136 cases reported in the previous 26 years. Experts suggest the reported cases are probably only a fraction of the actual incidents of cholera, since as many as 90 percent of people with the disease have only mild diarrhea.

Another new strain (*V. cholerae 0139*) moved across India and Bangladesh into Thailand in 1993, killing thousands of patients on its way. It was carried to California that year by someone who had traveled to India.

Cause Cholera is caused by the comma-shaped bacterium *Vibrio cholerae*, which is acquired by swallowing food or water contaminated with human feces. A person may also contract cholera from eating fruits or vegetables that are washed in tainted water and eaten raw, by eating raw or undercooked shellfish harvested from contaminated water, or by eating food prepared by someone with contaminated hands. Sometimes, flies can carry the bacteria to food.

The rapid fluid loss that is the primary symptom of cholera occurs because of the action of a toxin produced by the bacterium. This boosts the passage of fluid from the blood into the large and small intestines.

Still, unless there is a huge source of germs (such as contaminated water or the clothes of victims), the disease is fairly hard to acquire. Chlorination can kill the bacteria, and acids in saliva and the stomach are a natural defense.

Symptoms   Up to three fourths of all victims show no symptoms. But severe forms of the disease known for hundreds of years as "cholera morbus"—usually among people who have been drinking contaminated water—can be quickly fatal. Between a few hours and five days after infection, symptoms appear suddenly, beginning with incessant diarrhea and vomiting, with severe muscular cramps and prostration. Worse yet, facial features and soft body tissues shrink because of the radical loss of fluid, and discoloration of the skin from ruptured capillaries turns the shriveled victim black and blue. Over a pint of fluid may be lost hourly, and if this is not replaced, death will occur within a few hours. Because the bacteria are inhibited by stomach acid, those with high levels of gastric acid will have only a mild infection. Those who are poorly nourished and have less gastric acid, may have more severe diarrhea.

Many people (especially those living in areas where cholera is common) may have no symptoms, but they can still spread the disease to others. If the diarrhea is very bloody, the cause is probably not cholera but may be *Shigella, E. coli*, or CAMPYLOBACTER.

Treatment   Cholera is treated by quickly replacing the lost fluids with water containing salts and sugar, together with intravenous fluids (if needed). Antibiotics (such as tetracycline) may shorten both the period of diarrhea and the infectiousness. While it is usually taken by mouth, IV tetracycline may be needed for very sick patients. Antidiarrheal medicine should not be taken.

As soon as vomiting stops, the patient should eat a bland diet rich in carbohydrates and low in protein and fats. Airlines are required to carry onboard packets of oral rehydration solution if they carry passengers to and from cholera-infected areas so that anyone developing severe diarrhea on a long flight won't get dehydrated. With proper treatment, most patients will recover with no permanent damage.

Diagnosis   A positive stool culture will confirm the diagnosis. Stool specimens must be cultured on special culture media designed to find cholera. A blood test taken a few weeks after the illness begins will show antibodies to cholera.

Complications   Patients experience profuse watery diarrhea and without prompt treatment, half the people with severe cholera will die from profound dehydration within a few hours. Symptoms include extreme thirst, lack of urination, cramps, wrinkled skin, sunken eyes, and weakness. Because there will not be enough fluid in the body to maintain circulation, shock, coma, and death can follow.

Prevention   A vaccine is available for those traveling to cholera-infested areas but is no longer recommended because it is only 50 percent effective and protects for only three to six months. The vaccine is no help against controlling epidemics. A new, more effective oral vaccine is being tested. The new vaccine is produced in Vietnam, where cholera afflicts more than 3,000 people each year; about 30 of whom will die. Because of its low cost, the new vaccine may be within the limited health care budgets of poor countries.

The bacteria are killed by chlorine or boiling. Contaminated shellfish must be boiled or steamed for 10 minutes to kill all bacteria. The core temperatures of cooked food should be 158 degrees F. Unless all the bacteria are killed by cooking, they will multiply rapidly at room temperature in cooked shellfish.

Cholera can be controlled by improved sanitation, especially by maintaining untainted water supplies. Travelers to high-risk areas (affected areas in Latin America, Africa, and Asia) must follow these guidelines:

- don't bring perishable seafood back to the United States
- don't consume unboiled or untreated water or ice
- don't eat food or beverages from street vendors
- don't eat raw or partially cooked fish or shellfish
- don't eat raw vegetables or salads
- treat unbottled water with chlorine or iodine tablets
- drink carbonated bottled water or bottled soft drinks (the carbonation destroys the bacteria)
- drink tea and coffee made only with boiled water
- eat only fruits that you peel yourself
- eat only foods that are cooked and hot

chromomycosis   An invasive, chronic fungal infection of the top two layers of the skin on the feet and legs. The infection almost always begins in the skin at the site of trauma, and is most common in the tropics. Called chromomycosis or verrucous dermatitis, the infection may remain localized, or become a generalized infection throughout the body.

Cause   This uncommon tropical infection is caused by a group of closely related molds that are found in the soil, affecting people involved in manual labor with soil or its products. While it is not clear why the infection occurs only in the tropics, it is believed that in colder climates, workers wear shoes, which protect feet from contracting chromomycosis. Still, even in the tropics this disorder is not common.

Symptoms   The disease begins with an itchy, watery, warty nodule on the leg or foot that develop in a cut or break in the skin. Appearing first as a small dull red lesion, it gradually develops into a large ulcer; over a period of weeks or months, more warty, foul-smelling growths appear in other parts of the skin along the path of lymphatic drainage of the foot, ankle, knee, elbow, or hand. As the ulcer spreads, the central area becomes scarred. Many patients develop secondary bacterial infections.

Treatment   Bed rest, elevation of the affected part, and antibiotic therapy to control secondary infections are recommended. Surgical excision of the affected area, destruction of the affected tissue, or drug treatment (potassium iodide, flucytosine, thiabendazole, ketoconazole, and topical heat) may be successful.

Complications   This condition is chronic and may last for years or decades, leading to the necessity of amputation, the development of ELEPHANTIASIS, or to squamous cell cancer.

chronic fatigue syndrome   A group of symptoms including fatigue, weakness, poor concentration and memory, once derisively dismissed as a new "yuppie flu." Contrary to popular notions, however, the disease is not new; clinical reports of the condition have appeared for more than 100 years. The modern stereotype of "yuppie flu" began because those who sought help in the early 1980s were primarily affluent, well-educated women in their 30s and 40s. Since then, however, physicians have realized the disease strikes those of all ages, races, and social classes in countries around the world, although it is still diagnosed two to four times more often in women than in men.

In the 1860s, it was called "neurasthenia," and considered to be a neurosis characterized by weakness and fatigue. In the 1960s it was called "Icelander's disease." Since then, physicians have blamed the symptoms variously on "iron-poor blood" (anemia), low blood sugar (hypoglycemia), allergies, or a body-wide yeast infection (CANDIDIASIS). In the mid-1980s, the disease was believed to be caused by the Epstein-Barr virus, after scientists found signs of the EBV antibodies in affected patients. Since then, scientists realized that the EBV is so common, it is actually found in the blood of many healthy Americans, while some people with no EBV antibodies have the symptoms of chronic fatigue syndrome.

The degree to which patients are disabled varies widely. Some can still function at home and work, but others become severely disabled and can't perform many of the routine activities of daily living. The total number of affected people in the United States is unknown.

In other countries, CFS is known as myalgic encephalomyelitis, post-viral fatigue syndrome, chronic fatigue and immune dysfunction syndrome.

Cause No one knows the cause of CFS, and no virus or antibody has been identified. This has made it more difficult to determine how many people actually have the illness. Based on the first three years of an ongoing surveillance study in four U.S. cities, the Centers for Disease Control estimates the minimum rate of CFS in the United States to be 4 to 10 cases per 100,000 adults.

Recent research at Johns Hopkins suggests that at least some CFS sufferers may in fact have a condition in which inadequate upper-body blood pressure causes fainting spells. For these patients, treatment with drugs and high-sodium diets to raise blood pressure resolved the CFS symptoms. In one of the most recent studies, 16 of 23 people with CFS were found to also have this low-blood-pressure problem. After treatment with salt supplementation and drugs, nine patients were completely recovered and seven others had marked improvement in symptoms. This plus many other remedies have been tried.

Scientists have also studied a range of other possible causes, including EPSTEIN-BARR and other HERPES infections, the yeast organism CANDIDA ALBICANS, and immune system or hormone regulation problems. Many of these problems are found among CFS patients, but scientists have not yet been able to establish any of them as the source of CFS.

Symptoms To be diagnosed with chronic fatigue syndrome, a patient must have an unexplained persistent fatigue that is not caused by exertion or alleviated by rest; it must severely curtail activities. In addition, the patient must have any four of the following symptoms for at least six months that were not present before the fatigue:

- impaired memory or concentration
- sore throat
- tender lymph nodes in neck or under arms
- muscle pain
- multi-joint pain
- new headache
- sleep that isn't refreshing
- malaise following exercise

Many of these symptoms mimic the flu, but the flu goes away while CFS symptoms persist or recur frequently for more than six months. Many people first notice symptoms after an acute infection (cold, BRONCHITIS, HEPATITIS, MONONUCLEOSIS, or intestinal flu).

The course of the disease varies from one patient to the next. For most, the disease hits a plateau early on and ebbs and flows thereafter. Some get better, but are not completely well. Others spontaneously recover.

Treatment Although no specific treatment has been identified for CFS, there have been anecdotal reports of success with small numbers of patients using a range of treatment, including antiviral drugs, antidepressants, or drugs that boost the immune system. Many physicians prescribe tricyclic antidepressants, since these drugs help people with fibromyalgia (a disease much like CFS). Some patients improve with benzodiazepines (a class of drug used to treat anxiety and sleep problems).

Nonsteroidal antiinflammatory drugs may help ease body aches and fever; nonsedating antihistamines may help relieve allergic symptoms.

For a packet of information on chronic fatigue syndrome, contact: NIAID, Office of Communications, Building 31, Rm. 7A50, 9000 Rockville Pike, Bethesda, MD 20892.

ciguatera A common clinical syndrome caused by eating certain tropical marine reef fish (mostly barracuda, red snapper, amberjack, surgeonfish, sea bass, and grouper). The fish are toxic at certain times of the year when they ingest a certain type of dinoflagellate called *Gambierdiscus toxicus,* which contains "ciguatoxin," an odorless, tasteless poison that can't be destroyed by either heating or freezing.

Ciguatera occurs most often in the Caribbean Islands, Florida and Hawaii, and the Pacific Islands. Recent reports cited 129 cases over a two-year period in Dade County, Florida, alone. It appears to be occurring more often, because we now recognize it.

Cause Ciguatera occurs after eating any of more than 300 species of fish that may contain ciguatoxin, which is found in greatest concentration in internal organs, but it can't be detected by inspection, taste, or smell. The likelihood that ciguatoxin is present is greater with larger, more predatory coral reef fish.

Symptoms Eating a fish contaminated with ciguatoxin produces both stomach and neurologic symptoms. Patients often report a curious type of sensory reversal, so that picking up a cold glass would cause a burning hot sensation. Other symptoms include a tingling sensation in the lips and mouth followed by numbness, nausea, vomiting, abdominal

cramps, weakness, headache, vertigo, paralysis, convulsions, skin rash; coma and death from respiratory paralysis occur in about 12 percent of cases. Subsequent episodes of ciguatera may be more severe.

Treatment Effective antidotes are available.

clonorchiasis A parasitic infection caused by flatworms in raw or improperly cooked or pickled freshwater fish. Saltwater fish don't carry these parasites. Clonorchiasis occurs in China, Hong Kong, Vietnam, Korea, Japan, and Taiwan. The infection is rarely fatal, and most victims recover completely.

Cause The infestation begins when the worm eggs are eliminated into water in human or animal feces and are eaten by certain snails. The eggs hatch inside the snail, where they develop into many free-swimming larval organisms that escape into the water and penetrate under the scales or in the flesh of freshwater fish. Humans become infected when they eat the fish raw or undercooked. Once inside a human host, the organism migrates to the human bile ducts, where they mature and remain for their life span, shedding eggs into the bile.

Symptoms Most people aren't infected with many parasites, and have no symptoms. If acute symptoms do occur, they include fatigue, fever, and abdominal pain. Chronic symptoms include weakness, lack of appetite, abdominal pain, diarrhea, prolonged low-grade fever, and jaundice.

Treatment Medication is available to get rid of the parasites.

Prevention Pickling, smoking, or drying fish may not destroy these infective organisms in freshwater fish. Thorough cooking is the best way to prevent the infection.

clostridial myonecrosis See GANGRENE.

Clostridium A genus of spore-producing bacteria, named for the Greek word meaning "spindle," found in earth throughout the world. Some forms of the bacteria are found in the intestines and stools of different mammals (including humans). Others produce toxins as they multiply. These germs, which can't thrive in the presence of oxygen, can cause food poisoning and wound infection.

The genus includes the deadly CLOSTRIDIUM BOTULINUM, cause of BOTULISM. CLOSTRIDIUM PERFRINGENS is a more common and much less dangerous cause of food poisoning in the United States and is found most often in cooked beef and poultry. It is found widely in nature, and its spores can survive high cooking temperatures; if the food cools slowly, the spores germinate and the bacteria become activated. If the tainted food is served without reheating properly, live toxin-producing bacteria can be consumed, causing cramps and diarrhea in about 16 hours. Two separate outbreaks were traced to tainted corned beef served on a 1993 St. Patrick's Day.

CLOSTRIDIUM TETANI is a third deadly member of this bacterial family. The toxin produced by this bacteria causes TETANUS, not as often when eaten as when entering the body via a wound.

C. difficile is a recently identified cause of colitis linked to the administration of antibiotics. About 3 percent of healthy adults carry this bacterium in the intestines. When a patient takes antibiotics, the drugs can alter the balance of bacteria in the intestines and stomach, allowing *C. difficile* to reproduce to the point where its toxins cause diarrhea.

However, not all the types of bacteria in the genus are deadly. *C. pasteurianum* is a type of bacteria found in the soil that helps plants acquire nitrogen, a fundamental requirement in producing food. See also DIARRHEA AND INFECTIOUS DISEASE; ANTIDIARRHEAL DRUGS.

Clostridium botulinum A species of spore-producing bacteria that cause BOTULISM in humans. Botulinus food poisoning is caused by the ingestion of food containing toxins produced by this species. The spore's resistance to heat makes the spores an important cause of poisoning in improperly cooked or canned foods. In addition, the bacteria are commonly found in soil, where the spores can survive for years.

Clostridium difficile A species of bacteria that has emerged as an increasing threat to hospitals in Europe and North America, since it produces two toxins that lead to pseudomembraneous colitis among those taking antibiotics aimed at another infection.

The bacteria are not easily eradicated and represent a significant challenge to hospital staff. The spores are highly resistant and can last for months on surfaces within the hospital. In one study, the most common sites of contamination were hospital floors and utensils associated with the disposal of feces, such as bedpans, steam flushers, and toilet seats.

Patients who are infected with this bacteria should stop taking antibiotics, and take either vancomycin or metronidazole instead.

Clostridium perfringens A species of anaerobic gram-positive bacteria (bacteria which grow in the absence of oxygen) capable of causing gas GANGRENE in humans, and a variety of digestive and urinary tract disease in livestock. The oval spores of this bacteria, also known as *Clostridium welchii*, are found mainly in soil and in human intestines.

Clostridium perfringens infection A mild food-borne illness caused by multiplying toxins produced by *Clostridium perfringens* type A bacteria in human and animal feces and in soil and water. These bacteria are also normally found in meat that hasn't been cooked.

This type of food poisoning is among the most common in the United States, with an estimated 10,000 cases each year, according to the U.S. Centers for Disease Control. Most cases go unreported.

Cause The toxin-producing organism is found in undercooked meat (such as rare beef; meat pies; burritos; tacos; enchiladas; reheated meats; or gravies made from beef, turkey, or chicken). The bacteria multiply quickly in reheated foods; once ingested, the bacteria produce illness in the digestive tract 8 to 24 hours later. A large amount of the bacteria must be ingested in order to cause illness. Outbreaks have often been traced to restaurants, caterers, and cafeterias.

The bacteria have a spore form, a dormant state that is not killed by cooking; the spores can't reproduce into bacteria at temperatures below 40 degrees F or above 140 degrees F.

Symptoms The illness appears suddenly (within 8 to 24 hours after eating), causing severe colic or cramps and abdominal gas pains followed by a 24-hour bout of watery diarrhea. There may be nausea but usually not vomiting or fever. While usually a mild illness, it can be dangerous to infants and the elderly, who may become dehydrated. Having the disease does not confer immunity, but patients are not infectious.

In injuries, this type of bacteria causes the potentially fatal gas GANGRENE by proliferating in the injured tissues.

Diagnosis Recently, scientists at the University of Illinois at Urbana-Champaign produced a test that can detect the presence of the bacterium. The bacteria will also grow on a culture plate in a lab from either a food or a stool sample.

Treatment Because this is technically not an infection but an intoxication, no antibiotic will cure it. Patients should try to replace fluid losses by drinking clear liquids. If dehydration is suspected, seek medical help. If food poisoning is suspected, local health departments should be notified.

Clostridium tetani One bacterial member of the genus CLOSTRIDIUM that cause TETANUS, dangerous not in itself but because of the toxin it releases. Spores of this bacteria are found in soil that can enter the body via any type of wounds, from the classic deep puncture cuts to injuries as innocuous as a splinter injury.

As the bacteria are activated by decomposing tissue, the toxin travels though the nervous system into the spinal cord, triggering spasms, giving rise to the common name for this syndrome, "lockjaw." A terrible grin, called RISUS SARDONICUS, can transform the face of any untreated victim.

CMV See CYTOMEGALOVIRUS.

Coccidioides immitis The infectious fungal spores that cause the acute or chronic illness COCCIDIOIDOMYCOSIS.

coccidioidomycosis The medical name for valley fever, an infectious fungal disease caused by inhaling bacterial spores, which may be either acute or chronic. It is endemic in hot, dry areas of the U.S. Southwest—Central and San Joaquin valleys and desert areas of California, as well as the arid areas of Nevada, Utah, Arizona, West Texas, and New Mexico. A person who lives in one of these areas is quite likely to be affected by valley fever. For example, almost 60 percent of the residents of Bakersfield, Kern County, California, have positive skin tests for valley fever. (A positive skin test means the person has had an infection and has developed immunity to the fungus, and will never contract valley fever again.) The disease is also found in Mexico, Central America, and South America. It is a disease associated with AIDS.

Animals can develop the disease—especially horses, cattle, dogs, and llamas. Cats are not usually affected. Coccidioidomycosis is also known as desert fever, desert rheumatism, or San Joaquin fever.

Cause The bacterial spore *Coccidioides immitis,* which is carried on windborne dust particles, is the cause of the disease. The cocci fungus lives in a sort of hibernation in alkaline soil, blooming when weather conditions are good. When it blooms, the tiny spores are stirred by wind or other movement and become airborne, floating in the air for many miles. When a person or animal who is not immune breathes them in, the spores enter the lungs and cause an infection. In general, the more spores inhaled, the more serious the infection.

Symptoms About two weeks after inhaling the spores, the lungs become infected. At first, the disease resembles a flulike illness that primarily involves the lungs, with fatigue, aching, chills, sweats, fever, headache, and cough. Symptoms can be mild, never amounting to more than a slight cold (about 60 percent of cases are the mild variety). The remaining 40 percent have more severe symptoms, eventually spreading throughout the body. Along with the flulike symptoms, these patients experience skin rash and joint aches (especially the knees). Dark-skinned patients appear to have more severe symptoms and to have the disease spread to other parts of the body. However, the most serious form that valley fever takes— when it infects the lining of the brain, called cocci meningitis—is most likely to occur in Caucasian males. Cocci meningitis is the form most likely to end in death.

Diagnosis The diagnosis can be confirmed if the patient has recently visited an endemic area, and if the fungus has been identified in sputum, body fluid, or tissue.

Treatment Most patients with valley fever don't need to be treated. However, those whose disease has spread to other parts of the body need medication. Ketoconazole, fluconazole, and itraconazole are all antifungal agents approved for the treatment of valley fever. The most effective medication for treating valley fever infections is amphotericin B.

Abscesses in soft tissue, bone, and joints may need to be drained, and bone infections may need to be removed.

cold, common An upper respiratory infection caused by one of at least 200 different types of viruses. Colds are most likely to occur during "cold season," which begins in the fall and continues throughout the spring; tropical areas tend to encourage cold viruses during the rainy months. While cold viruses are found throughout the world, they infect only humans with what are considered to be upper respiratory infections, which means they are limited to the nose and throat. After one bout with a particular virus, the victim will develop an immunity to that precise virus. This is why adults have fewer colds than young children, and why the oldest Americans have the fewest colds of all.

A person who smokes or lives in a polluted atmosphere has a higher chance of coming down with a cold. This is because air pollution and the nicotine and tars in tobacco smoke can irritate the lining of the nose and throat, making it easier for a cold virus to enter the cells and cause an infection. This irritation can also prolong the length of the infection. This is why people who live in heavily polluted areas or who smoke (or live with smokers) have more colds and have them longer than those who don't.

The common cold costs Americans millions of days of missed work and school every year and more than $2 *billion* for over-the-counter and prescription remedies, none of which will cure the infection.

Cause Different types of viruses proliferate at different times; in the fall and late spring, a cold may be caused by one of the more than 100 types of rhinovirus. These are the most common villains, and appear to be related to crowding indoors, school openings, and seasonal variations. Between December and May, several types of coronaviruses are responsible for most cases. Besides these two types of viruses, colds may also be caused by PARAINFLUENZA, RSV, ADENOVIRUS, ENTEROVIRUS, and INFLUENZA. All of these viruses seem to be able to change their characteristics from one season to the next.

A cold is NOT transmitted by sitting in a draft, getting wet feet, or going outside without a jacket. Because the cold viruses are so specific, a person can only get a cold if the virus travels high up inside the nose, into the nasopharynx. A cold virus can only reach this area by touch, or (less often) through the air. One study found that while saliva didn't pass on germs, even a very brief contact with a nasal mucous-contaminated hand (as quick as a 10-second touch) led to transmission of virus in 20 of 28 cases.

While cooling the body doesn't seem to bring on a cold, fatigue, stress, and anything else that weakens the body's immune system *can* influence susceptibility. It's possible to catch a cold from other people who have colds or from the things they use or touch: faucets, phones, doorknobs, light switches, straps on buses or subways, office equipment. A virus can survive for many hours on these objects, unless someone washes it off with alcohol, a household disinfectant, or hot, sudsy water. Everyone who touches one of these contaminated objects and then touches their nose, eyes, or mouth can get the virus. Once the virus is on the hands, others can be exposed by shaking hands or by touching other things that they touch.

Cold viruses are NOT carried very far through the air, however. If someone with a cold sneezes across the room, neighbors won't come down with the cold, too—but if someone should cough or sneeze right into a person's face, the person could get sick.

Healthy people have a film of mucus lining the nose and throat; tiny hairs called cilia move this mucus from sinuses and throat to the stomach. As the mucus is moved along, it traps harmful bacteria and viruses and carries them along to the stomach, where they are broken down by acids. A healthy mucous membrane can snag germs trapped in the nose and throat, then breathe, cough, or sneeze them back out. The mucus around the tonsils and adenoids can trap these germs, where they can be destroyed by the immune system.

If a person is not so healthy, the mucous membranes in the nose will be either too thick (causing a stuffy nose and congested throat) or too thin (runny nose). The germs won't be cleared away. Once the viruses enter the nose, they set up housekeeping in the mucous layer of the nose and throat, attaching themselves to cells found there. The viruses drill holes in the cell membranes, inserting their own genetic material to enter the cells. Soon, the virus takes over and forces the cells to pump out thousands of new little virus particles.

In response to this invasion, the body's immune system swings into action. Injured cells in the nose and throat release chemicals called prostaglandins, which trigger inflammation and attract infection-fighting white blood cells. (The throat will begin to feel scratchy and swollen.) Tiny blood vessels stretch, which allows spaces to open up and specialized white cells to enter. Body temperature rises and histamine is released (causing a fever), which steps up the production of mucus in the nose, trapping and removing viral particles. The nose starts to run. As the nose and throat stimulate the extra mucus production, it irritates the throat and triggers a cough. Cold viruses are also responsible for congestion in the sinuses.

All of this activity comes at a price, of course—the unpleasant symptoms experienced as "a cold." Actually, by the time a person starts feeling sick, the body has already been fighting the invader for a day or two. When people are in the process of catching a cold, they probably feel fine. It's not until they're actually getting better that they feel ill.

In order to break through the body's defenses (hair, mucus, and other barriers in the human nose) viruses must attack in huge numbers in order to successfully cause a cold.

Most of the time, a brief encounter with a sick stranger won't cause disease, even if a person sits in a doctor's office filled with sick patients for 10 or 20 minutes.

On the other hand, working all day in an office building filled with people who have colds could be a risk. Traveling on a plane carrying sick passengers is an even bigger risk for catching a cold, since the recirculated air in a pressurized cabin evenly distributes viruses to everybody, while drying out mucous membranes that would normally trap viruses and get rid of them.

Symptoms A stuffy congested nose, sneezing, sore scratchy throat, cough, headache, runny eyes, and (possibly) a low fever. Viruses that attack the lower respiratory tract—the windpipe, bronchial tubes, and lungs—are more serious but less common and are responsible for PNEUMONIA and BRONCHITIS, among others.

The symptoms of a cold (scratchy throat, runny nose, and congestion) aren't caused by the virus itself but are the result of the immune system's fight to get rid of the invader.

Because the symptoms of a cold are actually caused by the body's attempt at healing itself, there are times when the patient should not interfere. It's best to let a fever below 103.5 degrees burn itself out, for example, since this type of fever will also help the body burn up viruses and toxins. And mucus from a runny nose is a good way of getting rid of germs (and spreading the disease).

Treatment There is no treatment that will cure a cold, which is caused by a virus. Symptoms may be treated by a wide variety of over-the-counter medications and many different home remedies. While the use of vitamin C to treat colds is still controversial, several well-controlled studies demonstrate that it can lessen a cold's symptoms and duration. Other studies have shown that zinc lozenges can shorten the duration of symptoms.

Complications A cold usually lasts for about 10 days, although it can range from three days to several weeks. A doctor should be consulted if the patient still feels sick after 10 days. A person should call even sooner if the face starts to swell or teeth become extremely sensitive, because these symptoms can signal a bacterial infection in the sinuses or middle ear.

When the sinuses become clogged with nasal secretions, they may become infected with bacteria. While antibiotics won't touch a cold, they *will* be effective in treating this secondary bacterial infection.

Colds may also trigger asthma attacks in those who suffer with this condition. In children, colds may also lead to middle-ear infections (the most common complication of colds).

PNEUMONIA may also set in at the end of a cold; if you suddenly develop a fever after the symptoms seem to be going away, see a doctor.

Prevention A person remains infectious from 24 hours before symptoms appear until five days *after* the cold starts. A person is most infectious for the first three days, from the time when the first symptoms show up. Young children are infectious for a longer period of time (up to three weeks), since it takes their immune systems longer to fight off the virus.

It may not seem practical, but a person with a cold should stay home. While most adults feel that they should force themselves to go to work if they have a cold, in fact it would be much better for everyone if they would isolate themselves to decrease the spread of the virus.

The most important factor in reducing the transmission of colds is to keep hands away from nose and eyes. By scratching the nose or rubbing the eyes with a contaminated hand, the virus can easily be inhaled higher up in the nose or enter the nasopharynx through the tear ducts of the eye. According to research, most people touch their nose or eyes about once every three hours.

Since most people find it difficult *not* to touch their face occasionally, washing hands often may help prevent colds. It's especially important for people who already have colds to wash their hands, since they are even more likely to be wiping, blowing, scratching, or touching the nose area. Washing the hands vigorously with soap and water for 20 seconds will remove the virus. Disposable towelettes are a good alternative.

Hands should be washed:

• after sneezing or coughing
• before eating
• after wiping, blowing, or touching your nose
• after using the toilet
• before touching another person

Disposable tissues should be used instead of cloth handkerchiefs when coughing, sneezing, or blowing the nose and thrown away immediately afterward. A used tissue is filled with virus just waiting to be passed on to someone else.

In addition to not touching the face and washing the hands, it's also a good idea to disinfect areas likely to be contaminated with germs, such as door handles, telephones, light switches, etc.

By being careful, it is really possible to stop the spread of colds, even if you're living in a household where others are sick.

Since plane travel brings a higher risk of catching someone else's cold, it's a good idea to drink at least 8 ounces of water for each hour spent on a plane to rehydrate the nose.

Diet   There is some evidence that certain strains of rhinoviruses can be destroyed by high levels of vitamin C. Several German studies have suggested that the herb echinacea (*E. purpurea*, *E. angustifolia*, or *E. pallida*) appears to be mild stimulant of the immune system that may help fend off colds. Because its effect appears to fade when used on a daily

basis for longer than eight weeks, it's best to use it intermittently.

Stress   There is a definite link between emotions and infections, according to studies reported in the *New England Journal of Medicine*. In one study by Sheldon Cohen, Ph.D., professor of psychology at Carnegie-Mellon University in Pittsburgh, it is reported that a high level of psychological stress lowers resistance to viral infections and nearly doubles the chance of getting a cold. Other studies have found that mental and emotional stress impairs the ability to fight off viruses and doubles the risk of catching a cold.

Studies found that about 25 percent of those who were infected with the rhinovirus *didn't* develop cold symptoms; the reason, studies suggest, may be that some people have healthier immune systems than others.

Humor may also help. Levels of protective chemicals (such as IgA) jumped significantly when volunteers watched comics, according to a study by psychologist Kathleen Dillon, Ph.D., at Western New England College in Springfield, Massachusetts. Those who watched a documentary had no rise in IgA levels.

Humidity   Studies suggest that the relative humidity of the air may affect the risk of colds. During the winter and the start of winter heating (with its lowered humidity), there is a sharp increase in the number of colds. This low humidity causes dry throats and nose, which increases the chance of infection.

The nose, throat, and lungs work best when the air has a relative humidity of about 45 percent. If the air during the winter falls below that level, moisture will be absorbed into the heated air from the mucous membranes. Since dried mucous membranes can't clean themselves they become more vulnerable to invasion from cold viruses.

Air circulation   Good ventilation can also help disperse germs and hinder the spread of colds.

The closed circulation systems of airplanes are another potential danger for the transmis-

---

IS IT A COLD, THE FLU, OR AN ALLERGY?

A cold is *not* the same thing as the flu. Head colds are just what they say they are—limited to the head, whereas the flu will affect your entire system. A cold will come on gradually, beginning with a vague feeling of unease; the sore throat may be slight; chills or aches will not be severe, and fever won't usually rise above 100 degrees F. The common cold causes

- scratchy throat
- runny nose
- itchy eyes

On the other hand, INFLUENZA strikes fast and hard, with symptoms that are much more severe than those characterized by a simple cold. The flu often causes

- nausea
- vomiting
- diarrhea
- high fever (from 101 to 104)
- body aches (especially in the back)
- chills
- cough
- eye pain
- light sensitivity
- headache

Allergies share a few symptoms with colds, but they have significant differences. If your cold seems to be hanging on for months, it could be an allergy. Winter allergies (known as perennial allergic rhinitis) cause

- itchy eyes
- itchy, runny, stuffy nose
- itchy throat
- postnasal drip
- coughing
- sneezing
- season-long symptoms

others (especially babies). The sick person should use a separate set of towels and washcloths and change the bedding more often. (Actually, bedding should be changed more often for *everyone*, healthy or sick, during the winter months to help cut down on virus transmission.)

It's not likely that rhinovirus (the most common cold virus) can cause illness by hitching a ride on a toothbrush—they must get into the nose to cause a cold. However, viruses such as the enteroviruses (found in the stomach/intestines) can occasionally cause a cold. To be safe, experts suggest replacing a toothbrush every three months. A

WHEN TO CALL THE DOCTOR

Call your doctor with these warning signs:

- fever of 101 degrees F or above that stays up after fever medication has been given
- fever of 102 degrees F in children
- any fever that lasts more than three days
- difficulty breathing, very rapid breathing, shortness of breath, wheezing or stridor (rattling or crackling noises in the chest or high-pitched sounds when inhaling)
- blue or dusky color around mouth, nail beds, or skin
- extreme pain (ears, headache, throat, sinuses, teeth)
- skin rash
- white or yellow spots on tonsils or throat
- coughing episode lasting longer than interval between coughs
- cough that produces thick yellow-green, gray, or bloody sputum or that lasts longer than 10 days
- shaking chills
- delirium
- enlarged, tender glands in neck
- symptoms that get worse instead of better
- extreme difficulty swallowing
- headache and stiff neck with no other symptoms (could be meningitis)
- headache and sore throat with no other symptoms (could be strep throat)

sion of colds. Airplane air usually has very low humidity. To combat this, passengers should drink lots of fluids on planes and avoid alcohol, which can dehydrate the body.

Personal hygiene If there are cold germs circulating in a household, members should not share eating or drinking utensils with toothbrush should not be shared with anyone else.

Rest/exercise   Plenty of exercise and sufficient rest will improve circulation, lymphatic system, organs, and emotions. In one study, volunteers who exercised regularly showed improved immune function, and only half as many days of cold symptoms. But too much of a good thing can be harmful—those who exercised too strenuously depressed their immune systems and actually increased their risk of getting colds. Any moderate noncompetitive exercise can work. Experts recommend exercise several times a week—*not every day.*

cold sore   A small skin blister, also known as a "fever blister," that appears on the mouth during a cold. Cold sores are extremely common and are usually first transmitted during childhood. The term *fever blister* comes from the fact that such blisters often appeared during fevers.

Cold sores are harmless in healthy children and adults, although they are painful to the touch and can be unattractive. They are similar, but not identical to, CANKER SORES, which also appear on the mouth. Both usually cause small sores to develop in the mouth but that heal within two weeks. However, canker sores aren't usually preceded by a blister, and they are usually larger than fever blisters, without merging to form one large sore as fever blisters do. Finally, canker sores usually erupt on movable parts of the mouth (such as the tongue and the cheek or lip linings) whereas cold sores usually appear on the gums, roof of the mouth, lips, or nostrils. Cold sores may occur on any part of the body.

People are most infectious when the sores first appear, but the virus is shed in the saliva for a long time (up to two months after the sores have healed). Cold sores can be spread to others during this entire time. Patients with an active cold sore should limit contact with newborns or anyone else with a weakened immune system.

Once a person has been infected, the virus remains in a latent stage in the body and may be reactivated when the immune system is stressed.

Cause   Cold sores are caused by the HERPES SIMPLEX virus. The viral strain usually responsible for cold sores is herpes simplex Type 1 (HSV1); up to 90 percent of all people around the world carry this virus. This strain usually appears on the mouth, lips, and face.

The virus is highly contagious when the blisters are present; it is often transmitted by kissing. The virus can also be spread by children who touch their blister and then touch other children. About 10 percent of oral herpes cases in adults are acquired by oral-genital sex with a person with active genital herpes.

Cold sores tend to appear when the victim is stressed, exposed to sunlight, a cold wind, another infection, or feels run down. Women tend to experience more cold sores around their menstrual periods, but some people are afflicted at regular intervals throughout the year. People with compromised immune systems may experience prolonged attacks.

One study suggests that the tendency for relapses might be inherited.

Symptoms   Most people have their first infection before age 10, although most won't have symptoms. About 10 percent will go on to develop many fluid-filled blisters inside and outside the mouth about five days after exposure, together with fever, swollen neck, and aches. This is followed by a yellow crust that forms over the blister, healing without scars in about two weeks. Once the infection occurs, the virus remains in a nerve located near the cheekbone. There it may remain, forever inactive, or it may travel down the nerve to the surface of the skin to cause a new blister. Recurrent attacks tend to be less severe.

The first attack may not even be noticed; the first infection in childhood usually causes no symptoms. However, about 10 percent of newly infected children experience a mild to fairly severe illness with fever, tiredness, and several painful cold sores in the mouth and throat.

Subsequent outbreaks are often signaled by a tingling in the lips, followed by a small water-filled blister on a red base that soon grows, causing itching and soreness. Within a few days the blisters burst, encrust, and then disappear. The virus then retreats back along the nerve where it lies dormant in the nerve cell; in some patients, however, the virus is constantly reactivated.

Treatment   There is no cure for recurrent fever blisters. For mild symptoms, the sore should be kept clean and dry and it will heal itself. For particularly virulent outbreaks, the antiviral drug acyclovir may relieve symptoms. Otherwise, there are a range of nonprescription drugs available containing some numbing agent (such as camphor or phenol) that also contain an emollient to reduce skin cracking.

Some studies have suggested that zinc may help prevent outbreaks because the zinc interferes with herpes viral replication. Studies found that both zinc gluconate and zinc sulfate helped speed up healing time, but zinc gluconate was less irritating to the skin. Both zinc products are available at health food stores.

Sores can be protected with a dab of petroleum jelly (applied with a clean cotton swab); don't dip the swab that touched the affected area back into the jar. Patients should avoid drinks with a high acid content (such as orange juice).

Complications   Anyone with an impaired immune system is at risk of complications; the virus may spread throughout the body, causing a severe illness.

Prevention   While there is no effective preventive treatment, some patients find applying a lip salve before going out in the sun prevents outbreaks. Research has shown that the virus can live up to seven days on a toothbrush, causing a reinfection after the sore heals. Once a sore develops, an infected toothbrush can also lead to multiple sores, so a new toothbrush should be used after the sore heals. It's also better to use small tubes of toothpaste, since the paste can transmit germs, too.

An infected individual should not touch sores, which could spread the virus to new sites (such as the eyes or the genitals). Kissing should be avoided during an outbreak if the blisters will come in contact with the lips.

coliform count   A method of determining the level of fecal coliform bacteria (such as *E. coli*) in water. While these bacteria are abundant in the lower intestines of warm-blooded animals (including humans), they are rare or absent in unpolluted waters. As a result, their presence serves as a reliable indication of sewage or fecal contamination in water.

Total coliform measurements include all types of coliform bacteria strains. Various methods are available for determining the presence and amount of coliform bacteria in water. Results are usually given as the number of bacteria per 100 mL of water, or by the "presence" or "absence" method. Because the bacteria are too small to count directly, a basic method is used to "magnify" their presence using a special broth that can detect acidity formed during lactose fermentation by the bacteria.

Commonly, ocean water along public beaches is regularly tested in the summer for coliform bacteria; contaminated water can result in beach closings, since the bacteria can cause disease.

communicable/contagious disease   Any disease that is transmitted from one person or animal to another, either directly—by contact with feces or urine or other bodily discharges—or indirectly, via objects or substances such as contaminated glasses, toys, or water. It may also be transmitted via fleas, flies, mosquitoes, ticks, or other insects.

Control of a communicable disease rests on properly identifying the organism that transmits it, preventing its spread to the environment, protecting others, and treating the infected patients.

By law, many communicable diseases must be reported to the local health department. Communicable diseases include those caused by BACTERIA, such as CHLAMYDIA, FUNGI, PARASITES, rickettsiae and VIRUSES.

Not all communicable diseases must be reported, since they are not all considered to be a danger to society. Some diseases which must be reported include bacterial MENINGITIS, AIDS, FOOD POISONING, MEASLES, HEPATITIS, RABIES, LYME DISEASE, SYPHILIS, MALARIA, and TUBERCULOSIS.

condylomata acuminata   A type of wart that commonly occurs in the genital area. Found throughout the world, the condition is readily spread by sexual contact. The warts are also known as acuminate warts or veneral warts.

Cause   This type of wart is caused by infection with human PAPILLOMAVIRUS (HPV).

Symptoms   The warts primarily appear in the moist genital folds and creases, and while just one wart may appear, they are commonly found in heaped-up bunches that form cauliflower-like masses. The warts are subject to injury and can bleed, although they are generally painless. Women who are pregnant or who take birth control pills tend to have more vigorous growth of these warts.

Giant condylomata acuminata can invade local tissue, which may rarely develop into a form of skin cancer.

Treatment   There is no known treatment that will eradicate human papillomavirus from the skin, and the virus has survived even laser treatment; recurrence, therefore, is common. Treatment is aimed at removing

warts; sexual partners should be examined for warts. Condoms should be worn to reduce the chance of transmission.

Most lesions in moist areas can be treated with a chemical (podophyllin) that is painted on the lesion and then washed off several hours later. Extensive areas should not be treated at one time, since absorption of the resin can be toxic. For the same reason, pregnant women should not be treated. Dry lesions do not respond as well to the resin treatment.

Burning off the wart with liquid nitrogen is often effective, nontoxic, and does not require anesthesia. If done properly, it does not scar. Cutting out the wart may also be successful. While alpha interferon is available for treatment of resistant cases, it is not recommended because of its high likelihood of toxicity, low effectiveness, and expense.

A carbon dioxide laser and more conventional surgery may also be helpful in cases of extensive growths, especially for those who have not responded to other treatments.

In pregnant patients, freezing is most effective. Women taking birth control pills must stop taking the pills before the warts can be successfully treated.

Prevention   Because these warts are easily spread, sexual contact should be avoided when warts are present. Because there is a strong association between cancer of the cervix and HPV, a woman with HPV should be screened often. Not all HPV strains cause cancer, but several of the more than 100 types are believed to be linked to malignancy.

congenital infectious disease   Any infectious disease present at birth that was acquired by the infant either before birth or during its passage through the birth canal.

A wide variety of bacteria, viruses, and microorganisms can cross the placenta from the mother's blood into the infant's body. Organisms that cause particularly serious diseases include RUBELLA, SYPHILIS, TOXOPLASMO-

SIS, and CYTOMEGALOVIRUS. Often, the effect these microorganisms have on the fetus depends on the stage of pregnancy at which the infection was acquired. For example, a rubella infection at the 9th or 10th week of pregnancy may cause deafness, heart disease, and other damage. If the same infection occurs much later in pregnancy, no harm usually results.

The infant is also vulnerable to maternal infection while passing through the birth canal. At this time, any active infection in the mother's genital area can have serious repercussions to her child. Conditions acquired in this way include CONJUNCTIVITIS, genital HERPES, or chlamydial infection. Staph or strep infections, MENINGITIS, HEPATITIS B, or LISTERIOSIS may also be passed on.

Some of these diseases may be prevented by proper medical care. All girls should be immunized against rubella and pregnant women should have any sexually transmitted diseases treated immediately.

A baby who is born with an infectious disease is treated immediately, although some diseases that occurred in the uterus cannot be reversed at birth.

Congo fever (Congo-Crimean hemorrhagic fever) An infectious disease (associated with a tick bite) that causes a fever and bleeding from mucous membranes and the skin. The disease, which was first observed in the Crimea by Russian scientists in 1944 and 1945, is fatal in about 30 percent of cases. The virus that causes this disease was isolated in Africa in the mid-1960s and named Crimean, but African researchers found the same organism and named it Congo; therefore, it is called either Congo fever or a combination of both names.

Cause The viral infection is usually transmitted to humans by a tick in the genus *Hyalomma.* The virus has been classified as a Nairovirus in the genus *Bunyavirus.* (The Nairovirus group includes the Hazara virus isolated from ticks in Pakistan, and to Nairobi sheep disease virus.) In Africa, the virus has been isolated from a variety of animals, including cattle, sheep, goats, hares, and hedgehogs and from a number of ticks found on these animals. More and more cases have been reported among medical and nursing staffs caring for patients in hospitals and in lab personnel studying these patients. In these cases, the infection was apparently acquired by contact with the patient's blood or blood-contaminated specimens. Exposure to the blood of infected animals (especially cattle and sheep) has led to severe, often fatal, infections.

Antibodies to the disease have been widely found in farm workers, cattle, sheep, and small mammals in southern Africa without evidence of disease.

Symptoms Within two to seven days after exposure, the onset of illness begins suddenly with fever, chills, severe muscular pains, headache, and vomiting. Between the third and fifth day of the infection, a red rash or hemorrhages in the skin appear, and blood pours from all body orifices. At this stage, the face is flushed and the tongue is dry and often coated with dried blood. As blood loss continues, the pulse starts to race and blood pressure drops. This is followed by signs of shock and collapse, with massive hemorrhage and cardiac arrest. In fatal cases, death usually occurs between seven and nine days after onset.

Among patients who recover, the fever falls between 10 and 20 days after infection begins and bleeding stops. However, recovery may take more than a month in these cases.

Diagnosis The diagnosis may be confirmed in the lab by a variety of methods for testing the blood for presence of the virus and its antibodies.

Treatment There is no cure. Treatment is aimed only at easing symptoms.

conjunctivitis The medical name for "pink eye," an inflammation of the transparent membrane covering the white of the eye and the lining of the eyelid. This common infection of childhood, also referred to as a "cold in the eye," causes redness, discomfort, and a discharge from the eye.

Cause Most conjunctivitis is caused by bacteria (staphylococci) spread by hand-to-eye contact or by viruses associated with a cold, sore throat, or illness such as measles. Viral conjunctivitis can spread like wildfire through schools and other group settings.

Newborns sometimes contract a type of conjunctivitis called neonatal ophthalmia, caused by infection in the mother's cervix during birth from either GONORRHEA, genital HERPES, or CHLAMYDIA. The infection may spread to the entire eye and cause blindness.

Symptoms All types of conjunctivitis lead to redness, itchy, scratchy, or painful feelings; discharge; and photophobia (discomfort from bright lights). There may be so much discharge that the eyelids stick together in the morning.

Treatment Antibiotic eye drops or ointments are given if a bacterial infection is suspected; however, this will not cure a viral infection. Warm water may wash away the discharge and remove crusts; in babies, the eye may be washed with sterile saline. In addition to eye drops, the discharge must be cleaned from the eyes (on an hourly basis for the first day).

Complications A doctor should be called immediately if any of these symptoms appear: swollen red eyelids, blurry vision, severe headache, fever higher than 101 degrees F, or a very painful eye. A doctor should be seen within 24 hours for any of the following symptoms: no improvement after drops or ointment, eye pain, decreased vision, or eyes that get more red or itchy *after* drops or ointment (which may be an allergic reaction).

Prevention Careful hand washing may prevent conjunctivitis, since the disease is spread from hand to eye very easily. Anyone with the disease should have separate washcloths and towels. It is also important that swimming pools and hot tubs be properly chlorinated. Children with conjunctivitis should be kept at home until 24 hours after antibiotics have been taken or until the eye is better.

contagious disease Any communicable disease. (Previously, the term referred to any disease transmitted by direct physical contact.) Some of the contagious diseases are ACTINOMYCOSIS, AMEBIASIS, CANDIDIASIS, CHICKEN POX, CHOLERA, COLDS, CONJUNCTIVITIS, DIPHTHERIA, GASTROENTERITIS, GIARDIASIS, HEPATITIS, HERPES, INFLUENZA, MENINGITIS, MONONUCLEOSIS, MUMPS, PARATYPHOID FEVER, PEDICULOSIS, PNEUMONIA, RINGWORM, ROUNDWORM infection, RUBELLA, SHIGELLOSIS, STREP THROAT, SYPHILIS, TUBERCULOSIS, TYPHOID FEVER, and WHOOPING COUGH.

coronavirus Any one of a family of viruses that includes several types capable of causing respiratory illness and the common COLD, especially during the winter and spring. Coronaviruses rarely cause fatal illness in humans. Named for their appearance, which includes a sort of thorny crown when visualized under an electron microscope, they are among the most common of the cold viruses.

It takes only about three days after exposure to these viruses for symptoms to appear, and they last up to about a week (a few days shorter than is typical for a cold caused by a RHINOVIRUS). However, the coronavirus tends to cause more nasal congestion and is capable of reinfecting the same person.

corticosteroid drugs An extremely important group of drugs, commonly called steroids, that are similar to the natural corticosteroid hormones produced by the adrenal glands. These drugs, which are used to fight a variety of inflammatory conditions, include beclomethasone, betamethasone, cortisone, dexamethasone, hydrocortisone, predniso-lone, and prednisone.

Side effects The severity of effects depends on the dose, the form of the drug, and the length of treatment. The effect of the steroids is to prepare the body for stress; they do this by increasing blood pressure, blocking histamine release, increasing sugar in the bloodstream, reducing the body's response to infection or inflammation, boosting appetite, and storing more fat. Short-term use of steroids, therefore, can produce beneficial "side effects," especially by decreasing inflammation (such as in the case of the asthmatic who stops wheezing).

Long-term treatment, which is often necessary in certain diseases, can cause high blood pressure, obesity, diabetes, and soft bones. High-dose steroid use can cause acute psychosis, which stops when the medication is discontinued.

Corynebacterium diphtheriae A bacterium that causes DIPHTHERIA, found in the mouth, throat, and nose of an infected individual. The bacteria are easily transmitted to others during coughing or sneezing or through close contact with discharge from nose, throat, skin, eyes, and lesions.

Diphtheria is usually a disease of the throat that mimics STREP THROAT (although diphtheria may be more severe), characterized by a dense white membrane over the tonsils and the back of the throat.

In the United States, diphtheria is uncommon because of childhood immunizations. The immunity of adults is kept current by the practice of giving diphtheria vaccine whenever a tetanus booster is given.

cowpox An infection that usually affects cows caused by the VACCINIA virus. An attack of cowpox in humans used to confer immunity against SMALLPOX, since the two viruses were so similar. In fact, this was the basis for the smallpox vaccination. Vaccinia virus (for which the term *vaccine* was named) continued to be used as a smallpox vaccine until smallpox was eradicated in the 1970s. See also MONKEYPOX.

Coxiella burnetti Another name for *Rickettsia burnetti,* the organism that causes Q FEVER.

coxsackievirus Any of 30 different entero-viruses associated with a variety of symptoms that primarily affect children during warm weather. The germ resembles the POLIO virus (especially in size).

Among the diseases associated with these viruses are herpangina; HAND, FOOT AND MOUTH DISEASE; MYOCARDITIS; and aseptic MENINGITIS. There is no known way to prevent infection with these viruses other than avoiding infected patients. Treatment is usually aimed at easing symptoms.

crabs The popular term for pediculosis pubis, or lice in the pubic hair. The pubic louse may also be found in eyebrows, beards, eyelashes, chest hairs, and armpits, but it is not found in hair on the head.

While the scientific name for the pubic louse is *Phthirius pubis,* it gets its common name from its crablike appearance; it even has tiny pincer claws that it uses to hang onto the hairs. The pubic louse is a cousin of the body louse and the head louse and infects only humans.

Pubic lice don't live more than a few days away from humans, which makes reinfestation less likely.

Cause Crabs are caught through close body contact with an infected person (usually a sex partner) although it is possible to catch lice by sharing a bed, clothing, or towels with someone who has lice. Pubic lice are more common among those who live in crowded places with poor laundry facilities.

The pubic louse lays tiny round eggs (called "nits") that hatch in about a week; 8 to

10 days after that, the louse matures. Once it is attached to the hair, the louse hangs upside down and bores into the skin to feed on the blood vessels close to the skin's surface.

Symptoms Severe itching begins in the pubic area about a week after exposure to lice, with reddened skin as a result of scratching. Nits are visible attached to the base of the pubic hairs, and the lice leave a bluish stain on the skin on the upper thigh. In particularly bad infestations, there may be swelling of the lymph glands in the groin. The longer the infestation has been going on, the more lice there will be and the worse the itching.

Diagnosis Inspection of the pubic area will reveal nits. Tests are not necessary.

Treatment Pubic lice are eliminated the same way as other types of lice, using permethrin 1% that is available without prescription or pyrethrins; over-the-counter shampoos are available with RID. Lindane 1% is no longer considered to be the treatment of choice because of concerns about side effects.

After treatment, all visible nits should be removed with a nit comb. The patient should be checked daily for the first week after treatment to make sure all nits are gone. If itch remains after seven days, another treatment is needed. Close physical contact (including sex) should be avoided until the treatment is complete. Nits in eyebrows or eyelashes should not be treated (they are too close to the eyes); instead, nits in these areas should be removed with tweezers. All bedding, towels, and clothing should be washed in hot sudsy water, then dried in the dryer for 20 minutes on high. Anything that can't be washed should be left isolated for three to four days, since lice can't survive long without a human host.

Prevention All sex partners and roommates should be treated, since lice can be passed on to others as long as there are live, unhatched nits attached to the pubic hairs. Vigilant checks for nits should continue for one week.

croup Inflammation and narrowing of the air passages (in young children), causing a hoarse, barking cough and a wheezing on breathing in. Once very common in children up to age four, croup is a frightening but not terribly serious illness. In older children and adults, the air passages are too wide and the cartilage in the air passages too stiff for swelling or inflammation to cause the walls to collapse.

One bout of croup does not confer immunity, and some children get several attacks. However, most cases are mild and children recover uneventfully.

Cause Croup is caused by one of several different types of viral infections (often a cold) that affect the larynx, windpipe, and airways into the lungs. The most common is PARAINFLUENZA VIRUS (which usually occurs in late fall). RESPIRATORY SYNCYTIAL VIRUS (RSV) and INFLUENZA may appear in winter and early spring. ADENOVIRUSES, RHINOVIRUS, and sometimes MEASLES may lead to croup. While croup can't be passed on to anyone else, it is possible to catch a virus that can cause croup.

Some babies appear to be more likely to get croup than others, possibly because of a sensitive larynx; premature infants may also be prone to croup. Twice as many boys get croup as girls; some infants never get it, and others get it every time they have a cold.

Children outgrow the tendency toward croup, but there is no immunity.

Symptoms Croup begins like a cold. About one to seven days later, fever, cough, and breathing problems often appear at night. The child may awake with the characteristic barking cough, with shallow, fast, and noisy breathing. The high-pitched sounds occur during inhaling, not exhaling.

The child may feel better during the day but suffer the barking cough during the night for three or four nights.

Diagnosis A doctor can diagnose croup from the symptoms; tests are not needed, although a neck X-ray may be used to rule out foreign bodies or obstructions.

Treatment Cool mist vaporizers or cool night air help a child to breathe; the child should be kept upright while breathing in the cool air. Steam from a shower will work if no vaporizer is available.

A doctor should be called if the coughing doesn't get better or if the illness is severe (fever over 101 degrees F and severe breathing problems). For serious cases, doctors may check oxygen levels in the blood and provide oxygen together with epinephrine. A tube may be inserted down the throat or they may insert a tube through the throat (tracheostomy). The infant may be placed in a croup or mist tent, but such a tent should not be constructed at home.

Complications Croup that enters the windpipe and small airways leading into the lungs is called acute tracheobronchitis, a more serious condition that can interfere with breathing and may require hospitalization.

Epiglottitis is a rare (but dangerous) condition that may be confused with croup. Epiglottitis is caused by a sudden bacterial infection of the epiglottis that causes so much swelling in the upper throat that the child's airway is blocked. A doctor should be called if there are any of these warning signs of epiglottitis:

- fever higher than 103 degrees F
- drooling with open mouth
- agitation, restlessness, flaring nostrils
- bluish lips, skin, or nail beds
- muffled speech
- rapid, difficult breathing
- respiratory noise
- failure to breathe
- movement in and out in the areas between the ribs during breath
- severe sore throat
- refusal to swallow

Prevention If the child has a tendency toward developing croup, there are some ways to prevent the disease from occurring:

- keep a cool-mist vaporizer in the room during sleep
- don't smoke in the house
- give clear fluids to baby with a cold

cryptococcosis A rare fungal infection caused by inhaling *Cryptococcus neoformans*, a type of fungus found throughout the world, especially in soil contaminated with pigeon droppings. Untreated, this infection may be progressive and ultimately fatal. The disease is also known as Buschke's disease or European blastomycosis.

Cause Although the infection usually affects adults, it can occur at any age. In North America, it is most likely to be found among those already ill with cancer (such as leukemia or lymphoma) or those with impaired immune systems, such as patients with AIDS. Infection with this fungus is unusual in patients who are otherwise healthy.

Symptoms Cryptococcosis is characterized by the development of fever and other symptoms depending on the specific organ involved. Because the lungs are the first site of infection, initial symptoms may include coughing. The fungus spreads from the lungs to the central nervous system, skin, skeletal system, and urinary tract. After the fungus spreads to the meninges, neurologic symptoms may develop, including headache, blurred vision, and difficulty in speaking.

While MENINGITIS is the more usual and serious form of the disease, it can also cause a range of granular lesions, including ULCERS, ABSCESSES, tumors, papules, nodules, and draining sinuses into the skin, lungs, and so on.

Diagnosis The diagnosis is made by isolating and identifying the fungus in specimens of sputum, pus, spinal fluid, or tissue biopsy.

Treatment Fluconazole freely passes into the central nervous system and is the drug of choice; intravenous amphotericin B and oral flucytosine also may be helpful.

Cryptococcus A genus of yeasty fungus that reproduce by budding instead of by producing spores. Many harmless types of this fungus are found in soil, on the skin, and in the mucous membranes of healthy humans. However, there are a few disease-causing species, including *C. neoformans,* the cause of CRYPTOCOCCOSIS.

cryptosporidiosis One of the more recently discovered types of food poisoning caused by a protozoan *Cryptosporidium,* which means "hidden spore" in Greek. The tiny invisible microbe infects cells lining the intestinal tract, and it was not identified as a cause of human disease until 1976. It is a major threat to the water supply of the United States.

In the United States, the number of outbreaks that occur each year aren't well documented. However, in 1993, more than 400,000 Milwaukee residents got sick after drinking water contaminated with *Cryptosporidium.*

Some immunity follows infection, but the degree to which this immunity occurs is not clear. See also TRAVELER'S DIARRHEA, DIARRHEA AND INFECTIOUS DISEASE, ANTIDIARRHEAL DRUGS.

Cause This parasite lives its entire life within the intestinal cells; it produces worms (oocysts) that are excreted in feces. These infectious oocysts can survive outside the human body for long periods of time, passing into food and drinking water, onto objects, and spread from hand to mouth. Unfortunately, chlorine does not kill the protozoan; instead, drinking water must be filtered to eliminate it. Many municipal water supplies do not have the technology to provide this filter.

Because the parasite is transmitted by the fecal-oral route, the greatest risk occurs in those infected people who have diarrhea, those with poor personal hygiene, and diapered children.

Symptoms Between 1 to 12 days after infection, the most common symptom is a watery diarrhea together with stomach cramps, nausea and vomiting, fever, headache, and loss of appetite. Some people with the infection don't experience any symptoms at all.

Healthy patients usually exhibit symptoms for about two weeks, but those with impaired immune systems may have a severe and lasting illness. In the Milwaukee outbreak, those affected noticed symptoms between 2 and 10 days after exposure. Some deaths were reported.

Diagnosis The infection is diagnosed by identifying the parasite during examination of the stool. If cryptosporidiosis is suspected, a specific lab test should be requested, since most labs don't yet routinely perform the necessary tests.

Treatment There is no standard treatment, but some patients may respond to some antibiotics (paromomycin). Intravenous fluids may be necessary, and antidiarrhea drugs may help.

Prevention Eradication of the organism from drinking water depends on adequate filtration, not chlorination. Scientists are studying new ways to protect water supplies, including reverse osmosis, membrane filtration, or radiation.

Cryptosporidium A type of parasite that causes the waterborne infection CRYPTOSPORIDIOSIS. This organism is about 1/60th the size of an average dust particle and has been found in up to 87 percent of surface water samples across the United States.

The egglike form of the organism, called oocysts, are passed into the feces of infectious animals, finding their way into water supplies, where they can then enter human intestines. Once in the intestine, they release an infective spore that begins another reproductive cycle.

A healthy infected human will experience watery diarrhea and cramps that pass in about a week, but those with impaired immune systems may have a much more serious (or fatal) case.

Boiling water for one minute is the only way to kill this bacteria, since they can live in chlorinated water. (Consumers who live above 6,562 feet should boil water for three minutes.)

cutaneous larva migrans Also known as creeping eruption, this disease is caused by HOOKWORM larvae that normally parasitize dogs, cats, or other animals.

Cause Hookworm infestation occurs whenever human skin touches soil contaminated with cat or dog feces; shaded, moist, and sandy areas—such as beaches, children's sandboxes, and areas underneath houses—are the most likely spots to find larvae. Eggs passed in the feces hatch into infective larvae that can penetrate human skin (even through beach towels). The larvae penetrate the skin of the feet and move randomly, leaving intensely itchy red lines (sometimes accompanied by blisters).

Because several different parasites produce similar symptoms, there may be confusion about the diseases included under the umbrella of "cutaneous larva migrans." It usually refers to disorders caused by cat or dog hookworm larvae.

Symptoms Skin lesions usually appear in areas that often contact soil, such as feet, hands, and buttocks, appearing like a red papule a few hours after the larvae penetrates the skin. After a latency period of a few days to a few months, the larvae migrate, causing a red, raised, intensely itchy red line that may loop and meander all over the skin. Bacterial infection from scratching may occur. About half of the larvae die within three months even without treatment.

Treatment Thiabendazole can be administered on the skin over the tracks, and to normal-appearing skin around the lesions (because there may be larvae outside the visible lines).

Older methods of treatment such as freezing the track with carbon dioxide or liquid nitrogen is unreliable and painful.

Side effects Thiabendazole taken internally is effective but associated with a high probability of side effects such as dizziness, nausea, and vomiting.

Cyclospora cayetanensis A parasitic microbe that infects the intestine and causes intense diarrhea, weight loss, and fatigue. It was identified as a cause of human disease only in recent years. The United States is currently battling its fourth epidemic of cyclospora, which began in the spring of 1996.

In a recent outbreak, contaminated raspberries sickened more than 1,000 people in 11 states east of the Rocky Mountains. Scientists found it hard to track the source of the problem because it takes a week between ingestion and symptoms.

The first outbreak in the United States probably occurred in 1979, although it was never properly identified; it came to the attention of officials in Chicago in 1989. This was followed by reports of outbreaks in Morocco, Peru, and New Guinea. The first full description of the disease was reported in the *American Journal of Tropical Medicine and Hygiene* in 1991.

Cause Little is known about the parasite's life cycle, the way it spreads, and whether birds or animals that feed on berries are involved. The organism is a distant cousin of CRYTOSPORIDIUM, the protozoan that infiltrated a Milwaukee water supply in 1993 and caused an epidemic of stomach problems and 40 deaths, but this new organism is twice as large. Because the organism is a parasite of the small bowel, patients continue to lose weight even after the diarrhea stops because they can't absorb nutrients.

The organism does not appear to be halted by iodine or chlorine and can even elude filtration systems. The only thing that kills it is boiling the water in which it lives.

Symptoms About a week after ingestion, the disease begins with severe diarrhea, stomach cramps, nausea, and vomiting. It then progresses to weeks of mild fever, debilitating fatigue, and loss of appetite; patients can lose 15 to 20 pounds. While the disease is not normally fatal, some patients have been hospitalized because of dehydration.

Treatment The antibiotic combination of sulfa and trimethoprim can shorten the term of the illness, although most other diarrhea-causing organisms are now resistant to the drug. Those with impaired immune systems require higher doses and longer therapy.

Prevention Scientists advise those in epidemic areas not to eat strawberries or raspberries, especially for those with impaired immune systems. All fruit and vegetables should be thoroughly washed before eating.

cysticerosis See TAPEWORMS.

cytomegalovirus (CMV) infection A disease caused by cytomegalovirus, one of the HERPES family of viruses. The CMV is the largest, most complex virus that infects humans. First discovered in 1956, this extremely common infection has affected almost all children, yet rarely produces symptoms. By adulthood, up to 85 percent of Americans have been infected.

While not usually a serious disease, those with impaired immunity may have more severe symptoms. Cytomegalovirus also may cause significant problems during pregnancy if a woman has an acute infection, which would be transmitted to her unborn child. This can lead to minor impairments affecting hearing, vision, or mental capacity; a few of these babies are born with severe brain damage, including mental retardation or severe hearing loss.

Once a person has been infected, the virus remains latent in the body like other herpes viruses and can be reactivated later on during periods of stress or weakened immunity.

Cause CMV is present in almost all body fluids, including urine, saliva, semen, breast milk, and blood. It can be sexually transmitted, although most people don't get it this way. It is commonly found in day care centers, where it is passed around in children's saliva or urine-soaked diapers and transmitted from unwashed hands or shared toys.

Women with toddlers in day care are often infected, since CMV transmission happens often in these institutions. While young children rarely have symptoms, they excrete the virus in their urine and saliva for months to years. Anyone who works with young children is exposed to CMV. It is also possible to acquire CMV from transfused blood or transplanted organs, since so many individuals have an infection without having symptoms.

A person having an organ transplant or chemotherapy for cancer takes drugs that suppress the immune system; if such a patient had been infected with CMV earlier in life, the dormant virus can reactivate, resulting in life-threatening illness. If a patient taking these drugs has a first exposure to the virus, the new infection can cause a serious illness. In AIDS patients, reactivation of a CMV infection can lead to serious eye infections called RETINITIS, PNEUMONIA, HEPATITIS, ENCEPHALITIS, and colitis.

Symptoms Very few adults (including pregnant women) have symptoms when infected; if they do, symptoms will be mild, including achiness, low fever, and sore throat. Young children may experience a mild cold or flulike illness with fever.

However, if a woman is first exposed to this virus early in pregnancy, the resulting infection can cause serious fetal abnormalities. About 40,000 infants in the United States are infected each year, but almost all babies infected before birth are normal. About 10 percent of babies infected before birth are sick with the symptoms listed above. Of these 10 percent, 20 to 30 percent have a "congenital CMV syndrome" with serious symptoms that may be fatal. These symptoms include problems of major organs, including the liver, brain, eyes, and lungs together with convulsions, lethargy, and breathing problems. If such a profoundly affected infant survives, there may be permanent damage (mental retardation, water on the brain, small brain, hearing loss, eye inflammation, poor coordination, and liver disease).

Some studies suggest that a few apparently normal babies who were infected at birth may encounter health problems later in life. Babies infected before birth excrete the virus intermittently for years and are infectious when shedding the virus.

While CMV doesn't usually cause a problem for healthy people, it can sometimes lead to an acute illness resembling infectious MONONUCLEOSIS that is almost identical to the infection associated with EPSTEIN-BARR VIRUS, including a fever of two to three weeks, inflamed liver, and sometimes a rash. Healthy people with CMV mono have an excellent prognosis.

Diagnosis   Test results for CMV can be misleading. Blood can be tested for the CMV antibody, but all the presence of antibody indicates is that there was an earlier infection. The test won't reveal whether the virus is presently in blood, urine, or saliva. If a patient has symptoms that imply a recently acquired infection, sequential tests may reveal changes in antibody levels that indicate an active infection. However, since these changes can be hard to distinguish from normal fluctuations, researchers are trying to develop tests that are more specific.

The test for virus in these fluids is available in most large hospital and commercial labs, but results may take between two and six weeks.

Newborns with possible congenital CMV infection must have the virus cultured from their urine, nose, eyes, or spinal fluid to confirm CMV. This can be helpful in diagnosing potential future problems such as hearing loss. Researchers are now refining tests that would measure CMV in saliva.

In patients with impaired immunity, tests can be helpful to measure the effectiveness of therapy.

Treatment   There is no cure for congenital CMV; babies with the disease need to be hospitalized. In AIDS patients, treatment includes two intravenous antiviral drugs, ganciclovir or foscarnet. These drugs are not recommended for those with healthy immune systems because the side effects from the drugs are more severe than the risks of the illness.

Prevention   Good hygiene can reduce the risk of transmission at day care centers, but intensive infection control is not practical when dealing with a virus as common as CMV. Scientists are presently researching a preventive vaccine.

People who need organ transplants are tested for antibodies to CMV; those who do not have the antibodies will be matched to donors without antibodies as well. Because a match isn't always possible, the recipient faces a risk of serious CMV infection from the transplanted organ later.

CMV-negative organ recipients who need blood transfusions will be given special CMV-negative blood, which is rare and saved for special cases.

There is no vaccine currently available for CMV. Antibodies from those with high levels of immunity are available in the form of hyperimmune globulins for certain high-risk patients, but use of these products is expensive and of limited value. Researchers studying the feasibility of a CMV vaccine believe that widespread vaccination of children with a safe, effective vaccine is justified to protect unborn children from birth defects by reducing the risk that mothers are exposed to infected children. Researchers are studying a possible recombinant CMV vaccine.

D

dacryocystitis Inflammation of the lacrimal sac or tear gland at the corner of the eye, caused by obstruction of the duct. This causes tearing and discharge from the eye.

Symptoms In the acute phase, the sac becomes inflamed and painful. The disorder almost always occurs only on one side and is usually seen in infants.

Treatment Systemic treatment with antibiotics will cure the problem. Occasionally surgery to insert a small plastic tube to hold the duct open is necessary.

deer tick See TICKS AND DISEASE.

DEET (diethyltoluamide) A type of insect repellent that can be sprayed on the skin to repel mosquitoes, gnats, and other insects that carry disease. In low concentrations, DEET is generally considered to be nontoxic, but it is not recommended for use on children. While poisoning with DEET is rare, there have been a few cases of toxicity.

dengue fever An infectious viral disease with four distinct types, causing severe pain in the joints, fever, and rash. It is transmitted by mosquitoes. The disease is usually not serious, although there may be a prolonged convalescence. However, dengue may also cause a severe and fatal hemorrhagic disease called dengue hemorrhagic fever, in which patients' blood vessels leak, sending them into shock if they aren't promptly treated with fluids. (See DENGUE HEMORRHAGIC FEVER SHOCK SYNDROME.) Its name may be a Spanish adaptation of the Swahili *Ki denga pepo* that describes cramps that seize victims like a spirit. Others believe the term is derived from the Spanish word meaning "affectation," referring to the mincing walk adopted by untreated victims suffering from severe joint pain. For the same reason, the English called it "Dandy fever."

Dengue fever is a rapidly spreading disease now found in most tropical areas of the world. After decades of being only a minor nuisance in Latin America, as mosquito control programs shut down over the past 20 years it has become the most widespread ARBOVIRUS disease of humans. There are now 2 billion people at risk and millions of new cases each year as epidemics caused by all four types of virus have become larger and progressively more frequent. Since 1982, major epidemics have occurred for the first time in more than 30 years in Venezuela, Brazil, Bolivia, Paraguay, Peru, Ecuador, Costa Rica, and Panama; Saudi Arabia, Somalia, Kenya, Djibouti, Mozambique, Angola, and Burkina Faso in Africa; China; and Taiwan. A current outbreak in New Delhi has swept through overcrowded urban areas, bringing the death toll to 225.

Although the United States hasn't had any major epidemics of dengue since the 1940s, health authorities fear the disease may appear here at any time. A small number of people have developed dengue from local mosquitoes in Texas, and both species of mosquitoes that carry the dengue virus are firmly established in several southeastern states. In 1995, an outbreak infecting more than 200,000 people in Latin America and the Caribbean threatened thousands of Americans along the entire southern United States border. That year, Texas recorded almost 50 cases, the highest number in 10 years. Six of the patients got dengue without leaving the country. While scientists can't predict the future incidence, it is anticipated that there will be increased dengue transmission in all tropical areas of the world during the next several years.

Dengue was called "break-bone fever" by 18th-century doctor Benjamin Rush during a Philadelphia epidemic in 1780, because of the severe bone pain; others called it "break-heart" fever because of the depression that often follows the illness. Through September 1996, 140,000 cases of classic dengue have been reported in Latin America; dozens have died from hemorrhagic dengue.

During the mid-20th century, mosquito-eradication efforts almost wiped out dengue in much of the Americas. Population growth and urban sprawl, together with lax official policies, led to the return of the mosquito.

Cause Dengue fever is transmitted by urban *Aedes* mosquitoes (usually *A. aegypti*), which can be found across the United States and which prefers to feed on humans during the daytime. The mosquito may bite at any time during the day (especially indoors), in shady areas or when it is overcast. Frost wipes it out in northern areas, but the mosquito survives in many parts of the south, especially along the Gulf of Mexico.

Symptoms Typically, the virus feels like a bad case of the flu, with sudden fever and severe frontal headaches and deep-muscle aches. There may be nausea and vomiting; the rash appears three to five days after onset of fever and may spread from torso to arms, legs, and face. The rash may be accompanied by itching and scaling. Most cases are mild, treated only with bed rest and fluids.

Health officials are concerned about dengue because people who have suffered a bout with one of the viruses face a potentially life-threatening complication if they later catch any other dengue virus. The danger is dengue hemorrhagic fever, accompanied by a red rash, bruises, and bleeding from gums, nose, and gastrointestinal tract. This bleeding can trigger a loss of blood pressure that can lead to shock; as many as 1 out of 10 patients who develop the hemorrhagic fever will die.

Treatment There is no specific treatment, although vaccines are currently being devel-oped. Painkillers are given to relieve headache and other pain.

Prevention People traveling to dengue- and malaria-infested areas should use insect repellents containing DEET and stay in places with screened windows and mosquito nets for sleeping. Preventive drug therapy for malaria is also a good idea.

dengue hemorrhagic fever shock syndrome (DHFS) A grave form of DENGUE FEVER char-acterized by shock, with collapse, and hemor-rhages. The incidence of dengue hemorrhagic fever has increased dramatically in southeast Asia in the past 20 years, with major epi-demics occurring in most countries every three to four years. DHF first occurred in the Americas in 1981, with a major epidemic in Cuba. A second major DHF epidemic occurred in Venezuela in 1989–90; smaller outbreaks have occurred in Brazil, Colombia, French Guiana, and Nicaragua.

Cause Although not completely under-stood, data suggest that the type of virus, together with the patient's age, immune status, and genetic background are the most impor-tant factors for developing DHF. In Asia, chil-dren under the age of 15 who are experiencing a second dengue infection appear to have the highest risk. Although adults can also develop DHF, most international travelers from the United States appear to be at low risk.

Symptoms Cold, clammy extremities; weak, thready pulse; respiratory distress; plus all the symptoms of dengue fever. Hemor-rhage, bruises, and small red spots all indicate bleeding from skin capillaries; bloody vomitus, urine, and feces may occur and herald impend-ing circulatory collapse.

Treatment Fluid and electrolyte replace-ment and fresh blood, plasma, or platelet transfusions. Oxygen and sedatives also may be given.

dermatophytes Superficial fungi (also called tineal infections, including RINGWORM) that infect the skin, hair, and nails, usually caused by the fungi *Microsporum, Epidermophyton,* and *Trichophyton.* This type of fungi can be spread from person to person or from an animal to a person. The infections they cause usually have a Latin name using the term *tinea* with the part of the body affected (such as tinea pedis for ATHLETE'S FOOT). Although there are many different kinds of dermatophytes, seven species cause more than 90 percent of all infections.

dermatophytosis　A type of fungus infection (also called tinea) caused by *Trichophyton, Epidermophyton,* or *Microsporum* spp.

desert fever　A popular name for COCCIDIOIDOMYCOSIS.

desert rheumatism　A popular name for COCCIDIOIDOMYCOSIS.

diarrhea and infectious disease　Many infectious diseases cause diarrhea, with frequent passage of loose, watery stools that may also contain pus, mucus, blood, or fat. In addition to frequent trips to the bathroom, a patient with diarrhea may complain of abdominal cramps and weakness, nausea, and vomiting.

Acute diarrhea affects almost everyone at some time, usually from eating contaminated food or drinking contaminated water. Diarrhea is not a disease in itself, but a symptom. While it may not seem to be a serious problem, if it remains untreated severe diarrhea can lead to dehydration and electrolyte imbalance. This is a particular concern among the very young and the very old.

Diarrhea usually starts suddenly and lasts between a few hours to two or three days. Diarrhea beginning within six hours of eating usually indicates that the food has been contaminated by toxins from *Staphylococcus,* CLOSTRIDIUM, or *E. coli* bacteria. If it takes longer (between 12 to 48 hours after eating), the diarrhea is probably from contamination

of food or water by bacteria such as *CAMPYLOBACTER* or *SALMONELLA* or by a virus such as ROTAVIRUS or NORWALK VIRUS. Infective GASTROENTERITIS may be caused by inhaling droplets filled with ADENOVIRUS or ECHOVIRUS. Less often, diarrhea may be related to SHIGELLOSIS, TYPHOID, or amebic DYSENTERY.

Treatment　During a severe attack, water and electrolytes must be replaced to prevent dehydration. Drinking water with sugar and salt added is one way to do this (one teaspoon salt and four teaspoons sugar dissolved in one quart of water). ANTIDIARRHEAL DRUGS should not be taken to treat diarrhea caused by infection, since they may in fact prolong the illness. See also CHOLERA, CRYPTOSPORIDIOSIS, ENTEROVIRUS, *ESCHERICHIA COLI, ESCHERICHIA COLI* 0157:H7, GIARDIASIS, MARBURG VIRUS.

diarrhea, viral　See GASTROENTERITIS, VIRAL.

diphtheria　A preventable bacterial disease that affects the tonsils, throat, nose, or skin that was once feared throughout the world. Through the 1920s, diphtheria killed 13,000 babies and children in the United States each year and made another 150,000 sick. Today it is most common in low socioeconomic groups, where people live in crowded conditions; unimmunized children under age 15 are likely to contract the disease.

The conquest of diphtheria in modern times is one of the greatest vaccination success stories. In 1992, only four people in the United States were reported to have diphtheria, and no U.S. cases were reported in 1993 and 1994. This does not mean that the disease has been eliminated, however. Because so many Russian children did not get vaccines, a serious outbreak began in Moscow in 1990; by 1992, there were 4,000 cases in the Russian federation and 24 deaths in Moscow. The problem has gotten worse since then, spreading throughout Russia with 50,000 recorded cases and 1,100 deaths in 1994. Most of the victims are adults, but the outbreak has spread because many children had not been receiving their vaccines and adults who had been vaccinated were no longer immune. Today, the epidemic is most severe in cities on the Sea of Japan north of North Korea, where an immunization campaign has been going on at airports, hotels, and train stations.

Travelers to these areas must have completed a series of the vaccine and must have had a booster within the last five years. There is no risk if the traveler is fully immunized.

In the United States, confirmed cases of diphtheria must be reported to, and investigated by, the local and state health departments.

History Since the time of Hippocrates, periodic outbreaks of diphtheria occurred around the world, becoming more common during the 16th century. Italian physicians began to perform tracheotomies during the Naples epidemic of 1610 in an attempt to help patients breathe through the terrible swollen throat that is characteristic of the disease.

Some 50 years later, New England minister Cotton Mather described a disease he called "Malady of Bladders in the Windpipe," which was particularly deadly among Massachusetts children. A second epidemic began in New Hampshire in 1735, killing more than 1,000 citizens, most of them children. The Spanish called it *garrotillo,* after the executioner's garrotte, a string around the neck that could be tightened by twisting a stick.

The disease got its modern name during the French epidemic of 1826, when French physician Pierre-Fidele Bretonneau called it after the Greek word for leather, *dipthera,* a reference to the tough gray membrane that often formed across the back of the throat.

As the disease spread during the 19th century, it appeared to grow stronger and more deadly; fatalities in New York skyrocketed to more than 2,300 in 1872. The bacterium that caused the disease was identified in 1883, and seven years later scientists determined that a poison produced by the bacterium (an exotoxin) could be used in weakened form to trigger an immune response in humans called an antitoxin. This ability was similar to tetanus, which scientists were beginning to understand at about the same time.

Routine immunizations began in the 1920s.

Cause Diphtheria is caused by a bacterium (*Corynebacterium diphtheriae*) named for the Greek word *koryne,* meaning "club-shaped." The bacteria thrive in dark, wet places such as the mouth, throat, and nose of an infected individual and are easily transmitted to others during coughing or sneezing or through close contact with discharge from nose, throat, skin, eyes, and lesions. Bacteria don't travel very far through the air, and they infect only humans. Crowded unhealthy places help the germs spread from one person to another.

The infection can also be spread by carriers (those with the bacteria but who have no symptoms). Untreated patients who are infected can be contagious for up to two weeks, but not usually more than a month. Recovery from the disease does not always confer immunity.

Symptoms Once established in the tonsils, *C. diphtheriae* produce symptoms faster than almost any other organisms by forming a powerful exotoxin. Symptoms usually appear within two to five days of being exposed. There are two types of diphtheria; one type involves the nose and throat, and the other involves the skin.

Diphtheria usually develops in the throat, causing fever, red sore throat, weakness, and headache. There may be swelling and a gray membrane that completely covers the throat. This membrane can interfere with swallowing and talking and causes an unpleasant, distinct odor; if the membrane covers the windpipe, it can block breathing and suffocate the patient. Other symptoms include slight fever and chills. The exotoxin produced by the bacteria can spread throughout the body and can damage tissue in the kidneys, heart, or nervous system. Death often comes from an inflamed heart.

In the skin variety, skin lesions may be painful, swollen, and red.

Diagnosis A sample of the nose or throat discharge is cultured. Results may be available within eight hours.

Treatment Diphtheria is a preventable and treatable disease, but if treatment is inadequate or not begun in time, the powerful toxin produced by the bacteria may spread throughout the body. This poison may cause serious complications.

Intensive hospital care and prompt treatment with diphtheria antitoxin offers the best hope for cure. The antitoxin neutralizes the toxin if it has not yet invaded cells but is still circulating in the blood. Antibiotics (penicillin or erythromycin) can help destroy the bacteria and decrease infectiousness in the respiratory secretions. Patients are kept isolated and in bed for 10 days to two weeks, and fed a liquid or soft diet. Secretions in nose and throat must be suctioned; tube feeding may be necessary if swallowing is impossible. A tracheotomy may be necessary if the breathing muscles are paralyzed.

A person is infectious from two to four weeks, or until two to four days of antibiotic treatment. Anyone with a confirmed case must be isolated until negative results are obtained from two cultures from the nose and throat taken 24 hours apart, after completion of antibiotic treatment.

Complications If the bacteria has time to produce the toxin, its complications can include broncho-pneumonia, heart failure, or paralysis in the throat, eye, and breathing muscles. Severe paralysis of the breathing muscles or diaphragm can be fatal. The toxin will inflame the heart muscle (myocarditis), which can lead to heart failure and death. About 1 out of every 10 patients with diphtheria will die.

Prevention Diphtheria vaccine is almost always given to infants in a combination with pertussis and TETANUS (DPT), given as a shot at ages two, four, and six months. The DTaP (diphtheria, tetanus, and acellular pertussis) is given again at 15 months and once more as a booster before entering school at ages four to six.

All infants should be immunized; boosters throughout life will prevent resurgence. The vaccine is made of a toxoid (weakened form of the toxin) that stimulates the immune system to make antibodies (called antitoxin) against the toxin. However, this immunity wanes; a booster is required every 10 years.

The toxoid comes in two strengths; children under age seven need a higher concentration to develop immunity. Older patients should get the lower concentration, since it has fewer side effects yet will still boost immunity. (See also DIPHTHERIA TOXOID.)

Anyone exposed to diphtheria must receive a vaccine booster (DPT, DT, or Td) if one has not been given within five years. Exposed people must have a throat culture and be under observation for one week; anyone with a positive culture (even without symptoms) needs seven days of antibiotics.

Anyone with a high fever or serious illness should not get a vaccination until recovered, but children with mild colds and low fevers may be vaccinated.

Side effects Common side effects of the vaccine and booster include slight fever and irritability in the first 24 hours, with redness, swelling, or pain at the injection spot. Giving acetaminophen at the time of the shot may prevent a fever. A fever more than one day after the shot requires a call to the physician.

diphtheria, skin A bacterial infection common in the tropics, but also found in Canada and the southern United States, that causes a rash similar to IMPETIGO. It is found in any area of crowded conditions and poor hygiene.

Cause Skin diphtheria is caused by the same organism that causes DIPHTHERIA

(*Corynebacterium diphtheriae*), found in the mucous membranes of the nose and throat and probably on human skin. Rarely, it is caused by food contaminated with the bacteria. A person can catch skin diphtheria by touching the open sores of a patient.

Symptoms Superficial ulcers on the skin with a gray-yellow or brown-gray membrane in the early stages that can be peeled off; later, a black or brown-black eschar appears, surrounded by a tender inflammatory area. Nasal discharge may also be present.

Treatment Antibiotics and specific antitoxin; oral penicillin V potassium is effective in mild cases. Whereas the antibiotics will inhibit the bacteria, diphtheria antitoxin is required to inactivate the toxin.

diphtheria toxoid A vaccine against DIPHTHERIA that is often combined with pertussis and tetanus toxoid vaccine (DPT) and given as a series of injections during infancy and childhood. The toxoid is prepared by mixing formaldehyde with the poisonous toxin produced by *Corynebacterium diphtheriae,* rendering the toxin harmless.

Alternatively, diphtheria toxoid may be combined with tetanus toxoid alone (DT) and given to children or combined with tetanus toxoid (Td) in an adult vaccine. The Td version only contains about 15 to 20 percent of the diphtheria toxoid found in the DPT vaccine and is used for older children and adults.

The vaccine, which was introduced more than 50 years ago, led to a dramatic reduction of the incidence of diphtheria throughout the world. Primary preventive programs aimed at immunizing all infants and children in the community have almost eliminated the disease.

Yet while the reported incidence of diphtheria has been almost the same since the 1960s, it still occurs in isolated epidemics, primarily because some countries have taken a complacent attitude toward vaccination. The disease continues to represent a serious public health problem because it is possible for even fully immunized people to carry the C. *diphtheriae* bacteria in nose and throat, transmitting it to nonimmunized individuals.

diphyllobothriasis A disease caused by broad fish tapeworm infection that occurs after eating infested fish. Rare in the United States, it was formerly common in the Great Lakes area, where it was known as "Jewish or Scandinavian housewife's disease" because the preparers of gefilte fish or fish balls tended to taste their food as they prepared it, before fish was fully cooked. The parasite is now supposedly absent from Great Lakes fish; recently, however, cases have been reported on the West Coast.

Foods are not routinely analyzed for this parasite. In 1980, an outbreak involving four Los Angeles physicians occurred when the four ate sushi made of tuna, red snapper, and salmon. At the time of this outbreak, there was also a general increase in requests for niclosamide (the drug used to treat the infestation). Interviews of 39 patients showed that 32 remembered eating salmon before becoming sick.

Cause The disease is caused by parasitic flatworms *Diphyllobothrium latum* and other members of this tapeworm genus. The larva is often found in the viscera of fresh and marine fishes. *D. latum,* a broad, long tapeworm often grows to lengths between 3 and 7 feet and is potentially capable of reaching 32 feet. It is sometimes found in the flesh of freshwater fish, or fish that migrate from salt water to freshwater for breeding. Bears and humans are the final hosts for this parasite. The closely related *D. pacificum* usually matures in seals or other marine mammals and grows to only half that length.

Symptoms Distended abdomen, flatulence, cramping, and diarrhea about 10 days after eating raw or poorly cooked fish. Those who are susceptible (usually those of Scandinavian heritage) may experience a severe anemia as a result of this tapeworm infection, caused by the tapeworm's absorption of vitamin B$_{12}$.

Diagnosis The disease is identified by finding eggs in the patient's feces.

Treatment The drug niclosamide is available to physicians through the Centers for Disease Control's Parasitic Disease Drug Service.

***Diphyllobothrium* spp.** The genus of flat tapeworms that causes DIPHYLLOBOTHRIASIS.

disinfectant Chemical germicide used to disinfect surfaces; most should not be used on human skin. Any household product that is called a disinfectant contains either ethyl alcohol (ethanol), isopropyl alcohol (isopropanol), hydrogen peroxide, chlorine, ammonia, phosphoric acid, or pine oil.

- *Alcohol* sold at drug stores or supermarkets; can be used to wipe off thermometers.
- *Ammonium* Found in many household disinfectants; quaternary ammonium compounds are used in hospitals to wipe down floors, walls, and furniture.
- *Chlorine* The ingredient in household bleach that kills germs, usually found as sodium hypochlorite. It will kill bacteria and viruses and can be used to wipe down bathrooms, diaper changing tables, diaper pails, toys, and cutting boards. Chlorine can be used in solution: $\frac{1}{4}$ cup (4 tablespoons) bleach in 1 gallon water, or 1 tablespoon bleach to 1 quart water. **NEVER USE CHLORINE WITH ANY ACID PRODUCT OR AMMONIA;** the resultant chlorine gas will react with water to form hydrochloric acid, which can cause serious symptoms from eye irritation to lung damage and pneumonia.
- *Hydrogen peroxide* Three percent hydrogen peroxide can be found in drug stores. It can be useful in cleaning small surface areas and as an antiseptic.

disinfection The elimination of most germs on surfaces. Low-level disinfection is used in most hospitals for items that will only come in contact with intact skin; this is usually all that is required in the home. Alcohol, chlorine bleach, and other chemical DISINFECTANT products are used for low-level disinfection.

Household detergents or cleaners are not disinfectants or germicides; they usually contain phosphates and are good for general cleaning.

Division of Bacterial and Mycotic Diseases A division of the National Center for Infectious Diseases, part of the U.S. Centers for Disease Control and Prevention in Atlanta, Georgia.

The division is dedicated to preventing and controlling diseases caused by bacteria or fungi. These organisms are important causes of illness and death in the United States and abroad and are major causes of new and emerging diseases as well as drug-resistant diseases.

dracunculiasis (dracontiasis) A parasitic disease caused by infection with a guinea worm just beneath the skin surface in humans. Dracunculiasis, also known as guinea worm disease, is the only parasitic illness that may be totally eradicated in the very near future. At the beginning of the 20th century the disease was widely distributed; active pockets of the disease are now found only in certain parts of Africa south of the Sahara, on the Arabian peninsula, and in India.

In 1991 the World Health Assembly vowed to eradicate the disease by the end of the 1990s; by the end of 1996, the disease was eliminated from some but not all affected countries. It is expected there should be a 95 percent reduction in the number of cases, compared with the one million cases that had been reported in 1989.

Cause Humans are infected by swallowing contaminated drinking water from shallow wells and ponds found commonly in the tropics. Worm larvae penetrate the intestinal wall, develop and mature in the abdominal cavity, and finally migrate to areas just underneath the skin. The adult worm discharges embryos through an opening in the skin. The entire process (from drinking water to embryo) takes about 13 months.

Symptoms   Several hours before the worm's head appears at the skin's surface, there is local itching and burning, followed by an ulcer or blister (usually on the leg or foot) through which the embryos are produced. Other symptoms include nausea and vomiting, fever, and generalized itching. As the blister forms and ruptures, the symptoms disappear.

Uninfected ulcers heal in about six weeks, but secondary infection is common.

Treatment   Antibiotics can treat the secondary infection. Patients should stay in bed with affected limbs elevated during recovery.

Prevention   It is important for travelers to purify drinking water, boiling any water that appears impure. Uncooked food washed with contaminated water should be avoided.

dysentery   An infection of the intestinal tract that causes severe bloody diarrhea. Amebic dysentery (AMEBIASIS) is caused by the protozan *Entamoeba histolytica* and causes ulcers in the intestines and sometimes abscesses in liver, heart, brain, or testes. Bacillary dysentery (SHIGELLOSIS) is caused by bacteria of the genus *Shigella* that is spread by contact with a patient or carrier or through contaminated food or water.

The term *dysentery* was invented by Hippocrates to describe a disease known since earliest history. It was written that Horus, the son of the Egyptian gods Osiris and Isis, had dysentery. Known widely as "campaign fever," dysentery has hobbled warriors from the Peloponnesian War through Napoleon's time on to the great struggles of this century, claiming more victims than have died on all the battlefields of all the wars. Dysentery has plagued a variety of great historical figures, including William the Conqueror, Edward I, and Henry V of England (the latter two both died of the disease). George Washington also suffered from dysentery that was exacerbated by hemorrhoids so painful that he sometimes had to ride on pillows over his saddle.

It still appears today in the United States, in places that are overdeveloped or where wells have been dug too close to septic systems. It also may crop up in day care centers and preschools, on cruise ships with poor hygiene, and in poor countries with poor sanitation facilities.

Drug-resistant strains of *Shigella dysenteriae* have appeared since the 1960s in underdeveloped countries, where the fatality rate is very high. Four fifths of all children living in the tropics will get bacillary dysentery before age five.

In the United States, new strains of *Shigella* have been isolated in undercooked hamburgers served at fast-food restaurants. (See also DIARRHEA AND INFECTIOUS DISEASES, ANTIDIARRHEAL DRUGS, TRAVELER'S DIARRHEA.)

dysentery, amebic   See AMEBIASIS.

E

ear infection The common name for *otitis media,* this is an infection involving the middle ear (that cavity between the eardrum and the inner ear). A middle-ear infection can produce pus or fluid and cause severe earache and hearing loss. While an ear infection is annoying, it is not terribly serious; it is easily treated and there are not usually any long-term complications.

Ear infections are most common in children because of their short eustachian tubes (the passage that connects the back of the nose to the middle ear). This makes it easier for bacteria to enter from the back of the throat. Almost all children have had at least one infection by the time they are six years old; youngsters are most susceptible to ear infections during the first two years of life.

Some children (especially babies with ear infections within two months of birth) have recurrent ear infections. They seem to run in families and are characterized by persistent fluid in the middle ear and short-term hearing loss. These conditions may require long-term antibiotics or surgery.

Cause During a cold, the eustachian tube can swell and become blocked, allowing fluid to accumulate in the middle ear. The fluid produced by the inflammation can't drain off through the tube and instead collects in the middle ear, where it can allow bacteria and viruses drawn in from the back of the throat to breed.

The usual cause of a middle-ear infection is bacteria that are normally present in a child's throat, including *Streptococcus pneumoniae, Haemophilus influenzae,* and *Moraxella catarrhalis.*

Risk factors for the developing of an ear infection include being male, bottle-fed, native American or Hispanic, younger than two, and/or allergic. Other risk factors include living in crowded conditions, going to day care, having allergies, and inhaling household cigarette smoke.

Symptoms Acute middle-ear infection causes sudden, severe earache, deafness, ringing of the ear (tinnitus), sense of fullness in the ear, and fever. Occasionally, the eardrum can burst, which causes a discharge of pus and relief of pain. In a baby or young child, parents may notice a cold with thick discharge, irritability, pulling or tugging at the ear, crying in the middle of the night, head shaking, and poor appetite. There may be fluid draining from the ear, although this isn't always the case. The fever is not usually high; the worst symptom is ear pain.

Chronic middle-ear infection is usually caused by repeated attacks of acute otitis media, with pus seeping from a perforation in the eardrum together with some degree of deafness. Complications include otitis externa (inflammation of the outer ear), damage to the bones in the middle ear, or a matted ball of skin debris that can erode the bone and cause further damage (called a "cholesteatoma"). Rarely, infection can spread *inward* from an infected ear and cause a brain abscess.

Diagnosis Middle-ear infection can be detected by examining the ear with an instrument called an otoscope. A sample of discharge may be taken to identify the organism responsible for the infection, but it is not often done.

Treatment Acute middle-ear infection usually clears up completely with antibiotic drugs (usually amoxicillin), although sometimes there may be continual production of a sticky fluid in the middle ear known as "persistent middle-ear infection." A doctor may also remove pus and skin debris and prescribe antibiotic ear drops. Ephedrine nose drops can help establish draining of the ear in children.

One recent study found that one shot of ceftriaxone cured ear infections just as well as 10 days of amoxicillin. Since the mid-1980s, some strains of bacteria have developed resistance to amoxicillin and some other antibiotics. In areas with resistant strains, the child may need cefixime or another broad-spectrum antibiotic. Some children may not improve after 10 days of antibiotics and may need three or four more weeks of drug treatment.

Acetaminophen may be given to relieve pain or to reduce fevers above 101 degrees F. A warm towel or hot water bottle over the sore ear, or an ice pack wrapped in a towel, may ease pain. The child should lie with infected ear down to help drain the fluid.

Complication   Rarely, a middle-ear infection can lead to bacterial MENINGITIS and MASTOIDITIS (a serious infection of the air cells behind the middle ear). Warning signs of mastoiditis include high fever, severe ear pain, puslike drainage and redness, swelling and tenderness behind the ear.

Prevention   Breast-feeding prevents ear infections during the first six months. Bottle-fed babies should not drink with the bottle propped or while lying on the back. Adults should not smoke around an infant, since the smoke irritates the lining of the nose and throat. Early treatment prevents most problems.

The vaccine *H. influenzae* type b (Hib) given to prevent meningitis may also prevent ear infections that are caused by this bacterium.

Eastern equine encephalitis   See ENCEPHALITIS, EASTERN EQUINE.

Ebola (hemorrhagic fever)   Illness caused by one of the deadliest viruses known to science, the Ebola virus kills up to 90 percent of everyone who contracts the disease. The virus was discovered in 1976 in Zaire and in a nearby western equatorial province of the Sudan, where it killed almost all of the 600 people who were infected. An isolated case appeared in Tandala, Zaire, in 1977, and another outbreak in the Sudan appeared in 1979, again killing 90 percent of its victims. An epidemic in the Bandundu Region of Zaire in 1995 killed 245. Two isolated cases of Ebola hemorrhagic fever were also identified in Cote d'Ivoire in 1994–95. The most recent outbreak to date occurred in rural Gabon in February 1996.

Still, despite fears of a modern-day plague, there has been little spread of the deadly Ebola infection in developed countries. A primary reason for the spread of the disease in poorer countries appears to be the lack of clean water and adequate hospital supplies, requiring reuse of needles and syringes.

Cause   The four currently identified Ebola viruses are known as filoviruses for their long, filamentlike appearance under a microscope. The chief means of spreading Ebola virus is through direct contact with contaminated blood, vomit, feces, and urine. The virus may also be passed by touching the body of someone who has died of Ebola or from breathing in Ebola droplets in the air. Health care workers have often been infected while caring for patients. In the 1976 Zaire epidemic, every person with Ebola caused by contaminated syringes died.

The virus is also sometimes present in sweat glands and air sacs in the lungs. Its incubation period is between 2 and 21 days (and averages less than 10). Transmission of the virus may also occur via semen up to seven weeks after clinical recovery.

Scientists strongly suspect that the virus is carried by an insect, such as mosquitoes, but they have so far failed to find such a carrier in more than 1,600 tests they have done on insects. Monkey virus closely resembling Ebola filovirus was isolated from monkeys imported into the United States from the Philippines in 1989; a number of the monkeys died, and at least four people were infected, although none of them suffered symptoms.

Past studies have shown that the greatest risk of spreading Ebola virus is to those who have closest contact with an infected person, such as health care workers and spouses.

Symptoms Ebola hemorrhagic fever is characterized by the sudden onset of fever, weakness, muscle pain, headache, and sore throat. This is followed by vomiting, abdominal pain, diarrhea, rash, kidney and liver failure, and massive internal and external bleeding.

Diagnosis Specialized lab tests (not commercially available) on blood specimens can detect specific antigens or antibodies and isolate the virus. Because these tests present an *extreme* risk to lab workers, they are only conducted under maximum containment procedures. A new skin test developed by scientists at the Centers for Disease Control and Prevention has helped identify cases that otherwise would have gone undiagnosed. The test offers a safe way to send skin samples from remote African areas to labs in Europe and the United States. In the field, a health worker can put a piece of skin in a preservative that kills any virus present. After arrival in a lab, the skin is processed with chemicals and other substances. If Ebola virus is present, it turns bright red.

Treatment There is no specific treatment or vaccine that exists for Ebola hemorrhagic fever, although general good hygiene and medical precautions have helped stop the spread of the disease. Severe cases require intensive supportive care, yet there are still few survivors.

Prevention Transmission can be stopped by washing hands, wearing gloves and masks around infected patients, and avoiding reuse of needles. Suspected cases should be isolated. Since the primary method of transmitting the virus is through person-to-person contact with blood, secretion, or body fluids, anyone who has had close personal contact with patients should be kept under strict surveillance.

EBV   See EPSTEIN-BARR VIRUS.

echinococcosis   A tapeworm infection found throughout the world. The infection is most frequently found in the sheep- and cattle-raising areas of South America, South Africa, the Soviet Union, and the Middle East.

Cause The infection is caused by the larval stage of a tapeworm (*echinococcus granulosus*) whose eggs are transmitted to humans in contact with infected dogs or other canines, or by ingesting soil, vegetables, or water contaminated by feces of infected animals.

In humans, the larval phase of the adult worm forms fluid-filled sacs mostly in the liver and lungs but also in other organs. The incubation period varies from months to years.

Symptoms Many people in the early stages of infection don't exhibit any symptoms. After many years, however, victims who develop cysts in the liver may experience abdominal discomfort, nausea, and vomiting; a ruptured cyst can cause sudden pain, fever, and possibly death. Liver cysts are most often seen in middle-aged or elderly patients. Patients with cysts in the lung may spit up blood, cough, and have shortness of breath. A rupture of the cyst in a lung can cause an acute PNEUMONIA and lung abscess. These lung cysts are more often found in children and younger patients.

Diagnosis Because many of the early infections cause no symptoms, the disease may not be detected until a routine X ray, medical exam, or autopsy reveals the infestation.

Complication A very serious form of the disease is called alveolar hydatid disease and occurs throughout the world—but most often in Europe, Russia, Japan, Alaska, Canada, and the United States. The disease is transmitted to man through infected feces of fox and domestic cat and dogs. When infected, a person develops multiple cysts that spread rapidly; usually occurring in the liver, the disease is often fatal.

Treatment   Surgical removal of the cysts, when possible. Mebendazole and albendazole are two antiinfectives that can destroy the living organisms inside the cysts.

ECHOvirus   An acronym for Enteric Cytopathogenic Human Orphan, the ECHOvirus is a picornavirus associated with many syndromes but not identified as a cause of any specific disease. There are many ECHOviruses, and more than 30 types have been identified.

ECHOvirus may cause a variety of nonbacterial MENINGITIS.

E. coli infection   See ESCHERICHIA COLI.

ecthyma   A shallow ulcerative bacterial skin infection that often results in scarring. Similar to IMPETIGO, it is usually found on the legs and protected areas of the body.

Cause   The infection is caused by group A streptococci or *Staphylococcus aureus*.

Symptoms   The condition begins with one lesion, which enlarges and encrusts; beneath this crust is a pus-filled "punched ulcer." Children are more commonly affected with ecthyma, which is usually associated with poor hygiene and malnutrition and minor skin injuries from trauma, insect bites, or SCABIES.

Treatment   Antibiotics plus meticulous skin care are the treatments of choice.

ectoparasite   A parasite that lives on the skin, getting nourishment from the skin by sucking the host's blood; various types of ticks, lice, mites, and some types of fungi may occasionally be ectoparasites on humans. (Parasites living *inside* the body are called "endoparasites.")

ectothrix   A fungus that grows outside the hair shaft.

eczema, herpeticum   A rare skin condition caused by the HERPES simplex virus characterized by an extensive rash of blisters in a patient with a preexisting skin condition. Hospitalization is required, since fatalities have occurred. The disease is also called Kaposi's varicelliform eruption.

Ehrlichia   A genus of bacteria that includes several well-known species infecting domestic animals. The genus is in the same family (*Rickettsia*) as the bacterium that causes another tick-borne human disease, ROCKY MOUNTAIN SPOTTED FEVER. The species were first reported in dogs in 1935 but were only documented to cause human disease in 1986.

The genus includes *Ehrlichia chaffeensisi*, which causes human monocytic ehrlichiosis (HME); *E. canis* causes canine ehrlichiosis; *E. phagocytophila* causes tick-borne fever; *E. equi* and *E. risticii* cause equine ehrlichiosis and Potamac horse fever.

Ehrlichia chaffeensis   A type of bacterium in the genus EHRLICHIA that so far has caused an illness similar to human granulocytic ehrlichiosis in about 360 people and has been responsible for several deaths. See also EHRLICHIOSIS, HUMAN GRANULOCYTIC.

ehrlichiosis, canine   A disease caused by the bacteria *Ehrlichia canis* carried by the brown dog tick *Rhipicephalus sanguineus*. This disease of dogs and other canids was identified during the 1930s and is found throughout the world. See also EHRLICHIA.

ehrlichiosis, equine   A disease of horses caused by the bacteria *Ehrlichia equi* found in the eastern United States. No vectors have been identified. See also EHRLICHIA; ERLICHIOSIS, CANINE.

ehrlichiosis, human granulocytic   A disease identified in 1990 that is spread by the type of ticks that also carry LYME DISEASE. The newly identified illness has stricken at least 80 people nationwide, killing 4. Although the disease can be treated with antibiotics, treatment is often delayed because victims confuse it with a summer flu. If it is treated early and properly, the disease is not associated with neurological damage or arthritis.

The Centers for Disease Control and Prevention reported at least two deaths between 1990–93 from the disease in Wisconsin and Minnesota. Some researchers believe HGE is not a new disease; New York and New England patients may have had the illness but who were instead diagnosed with Lyme.

It is also possible that some patients are infected with both Lyme and HGE disease at the same time, making a proper diagnosis more difficult. For every 12 Lyme-infected ticks a person might find during an hour's walk in tick-infested areas of Nantucket, there are four HGE-infected ticks—and two ticks infected with both diseases, which raises the possibility of getting two infections from one bite.

Some Harvard University researchers believe that the HGE bacterium was first discovered by Dr. Ernest Tyzzer of Harvard in 1938 in voles and mice from Martha's Vineyard but at that time it was believed to be exclusively an infection of rodents.

Cause The bacterium causing HGE belongs to the genus *Ehrlichia;* it has not yet been assigned a species name. Scientists have isolated the HGE bacterium in a few patients and found it was almost identical to *Ehrlichia equi,* a form of the organism that causes fevers in horses. Another closely related bacterium, EHRLICHIA CHAFFEENSIS, was identified in 1990.

Diagnosis Only four labs in the nation can perform the week-long test for HGE. Diagnosis is difficult, and testing has not been standardized. If it's summer and a patient develops sudden, flulike symptoms without coughing or nasal congestion, HGE is a likely suspect—especially if the patient remembers a recent tick bite. (Lyme disease symptoms usually appear more gradually.)

Symptoms While Lyme disease often produces a telltale circular rash around the tick-bite site, HGE does not usually cause visible symptoms. Instead, about 10 days after a person has been bitten, the bacteria multiply inside white blood cells and then suddenly cause fever, chills, headache, and muscle ache. Their flulike symptoms are far more severe than those associated with Lyme disease.

While many of the symptoms overlap with Lyme, the HGE symptoms tend to peak very quickly, moving from health to severe debilitation in a few hours.

Treatment Prompt treatment is essential; the longer a case is untreated, the worse the outcome. HGE responds to doxycycline and other tetracycline antibiotics; it does not respond to amoxicillin and other antibiotics used to treat Lyme disease.

The antibiotic suppresses the growth of microbes but doesn't kill them, so the immune system must fight off the infection. Coinfection with another type of bacteria at the same time can suppress the immune system, increasing a patient's vulnerability to other infections. In these cases, treatment may need to be longer.

Signs of the disease fade away within two months, and the disease does not appear to cause the chronic, arthritislike symptoms that haunt Lyme disease patients for years.

Prevention The same precautions that prevent Lyme disease should also be taken to prevent HGE. Avoiding tick habitats is the best way to prevent tick bites. But ticks may also be found in lawns, gardens, and on bushes adjacent to homes.

When walking in the woods, people should stay on trails and avoid brushing up against low bushes or tall grass. Ticks do not hop or jump but are carried by the wind, where a person must come in direct contact with them. To prevent bites, wear protective clothing (light-colored long-sleeve shirts and light-colored pants tucked into boots or socks). The light-colored clothing allows ticks to be more easily spotted.

Use an insect repellent, preferably containing no more than 30 percent DEET (N-diethyl-metatoluamide), on bare skin and clothing. Duranon can be applied to clothing only, but not to the skin. All insect repellent should be used with caution (especially with children) and should not be applied to the hands or face.

Ticks and hosts (mice, chipmunks, voles, and other small mammals) need moisture, a place hidden from direct sun, and a place to hide. The clearer the area around a house, the less chance there will be of getting a tick bite.

All leaf litter and brush should be removed as far as possible away from the house. Low-lying bushes should be pruned to let in more sun. Rake up leaves every fall, since ticks prefer to overwinter in fallen leaves. Woodpiles are favorite hiding places for mammals carrying ticks. Keep woodpiles neat, off the ground, in a sunny place, and under cover.

Gardens should be cleaned up every fall; foliage left on the ground over the winter provide shelter for mammals that may harbor ticks. Stone walls on the property increase the potential for ticks.

Shady lawns may support ticks in epidemic areas; keep lawns mowed and edges trimmed. Entire fields should be mowed in fall, preferably with a rotary mower.

Birdfeeders attract birds that carry infected ticks; don't place feeders too close to house. Clean up the ground under the feeder regularly. Suspend bird feeding during late spring and summer, when infected ticks are most active. Building eight-foot fences to keep out deer may significantly reduce the abundance of ticks on large land parcels. Examine pets allowed outside on a daily basis; tick collars and/or dips may be needed.

Four pesticides may help; Damminix; chlorpyrifos (Dursban); carbaryl (Sevin); and cyfluthrin (Tempo). One or two applications a year in late May and September can significantly reduce the tick population. See also EHRLICHIOSIS, HUMAN MONOCYTIC.

ehrlichiosis, human monocytic The first type of ehrlichiosis that was discovered in 1985, and which is transmitted by the Lone Star tick (*Amblyomma americanum*). Since 1986, about 400 cases have been confirmed in 30 states, mostly in the southeastern and south-central United States; nine people died.

Cause The disease is caused by EHRLICHIA CHAFFEENSIS, a type of bacterium in the genus EHRLICHIA that was only identified in 1991. It is carried by the Lone Star tick.

Symptoms Symptoms are similar to human granulocytic ehrlichiosis (EHRLICHIOSIS, HUMAN GRANULOCYTIC), including fever, headache, chills, malaise, sweating, muscle aches, nausea, and vomiting. The infection may range from a mild illness to a severe, life-threatening disease. It may cause leukopenia (reduction of white blood cells), thrombocytopenia (reduction in blood platelets), anemia, or abnormal liver function.

Treatment Antibiotics are effective if begun early enough in the disease.

elephantiasis Massive swelling of the legs caused by obstructed lymph vessels, which prevents drainage of lymph from the surrounding tissues. This causes inflammation and thickening of the vessel walls, eventually blocking them.

Cause Worldwide, the most common cause of this chronic swelling is the tropical disease FILARIASIS, caused by infestation with worms (*Wuchereria bancrofti* and *Brugia malayi*).

Symptoms The syndrome gets its name from the appearance of the skin of the legs, which resembles elephant hide. While the legs are most commonly affected, the arms, breasts, scrotum, or vulva may also be affected.

Treatment There is no treatment that can reverse elephantiasis, although the massive enlargement of the scrotum may be relieved with surgery. Elastic bandages applied to the affected parts and the elevation of limbs may help. Larval forms of the worms in the blood that cause FILARIASIS are killed with diethylcarbamazine. See also EHRLICHIOSIS, HUMAN GRANULOCYTIC.

encephalitis   Inflammation of the brain usually caused by a viral infection. Often, the meninges (membranes covering the brain) are affected. An attack may be very mild, but in most cases it is a serious condition.

The most common strains of mosquito-borne encephalitis in North America include St. Louis encephalitis (SLE), Eastern equine encephalitis (EEE), California encephalitis (CE), western equine encephalitis, La Crosse encephalitis, Venezuelan equine encephalitis, and Powassan encephalitis (the only one spread by ticks, not mosquitoes). Japanese encephalitis is not found in the United States, but it is very common throughout Asia and poses a risk to international travelers.

Cause   Most of the time, the virus responsible is the HERPES simplex virus type I, which also causes COLD SORES. There is no insect cause in this. In the United States, encephalitis may be commonly caused by a virus transmitted to humans via mosquito bite, causing St. Louis encephalitis (see ENCEPHALITIS, ST. LOUIS) or other viral encephalitis. More and more cases are related to infection with HIV, the organism responsible for AIDS. Occasionally, encephalitis is a complication of other viral infections such as MEASLES or MUMPS.

Symptoms   Usually, symptoms begin with headache, fever, and prostration, often with hallucinations, confusion, paralysis of one side of the body, and disturbed behavior, speech, memory, and eye movement. There is a gradual loss of consciousness and sometimes a coma; epileptic seizures may develop. If the meninges are affected, the neck is usually stiff and the eyes are unusually sensitive to light.

Central nervous system symptoms include some (not all) of the following:

- abnormal reflexes
- changes in consciousness
- confusion
- disorientation
- dizziness
- inability to speak
- irritability
- listlessness
- loss of balance
- odor hallucinations
- seizure
- sleepiness
- spasticity
- tremor
- weakness

Diagnosis   Symptoms, signs, and a spinal tap to study the cerebrospinal fluid will help diagnose the disease. CT scans and MRIs are used to rule out other causes of headache, fever, and changes in the senses.

Treatment   The antiviral drug acyclovir administered intravenously is an effective treatment for encephalitis caused by the herpes virus. If the disease is related to other viral infections, there is no known effective treatment. Depending on the virus causing the problem, some patients will die, and some who recover will have brain damage, with mental impairment, behavioral disturbances, epilepsy, and deafness.

encephalitis, California   The most common form of a group of viruses that cause encephalitis. First discovered in Central Valley, California, in 1943, this variety is the most common type of insect-borne viral encephalitis and infects more boys than girls under age 15 in both rural and suburban areas. La Crosse encephalitis (a widespread encephalitis common in young children) belongs to this group.

The California virus belongs to a group of viruses called BUNYAVIRUS. It is a zoonosis (disease passed from animals to humans) and carried by many different types of mosquitoes, which catch the virus from and give it to both squirrels and chipmunks in wooded areas. La Crosse encephalitis is carried by the *Aedes triseriatus* mosquito.

The infected mosquitoes remain infected for life; because the virus is not present in human blood, it is not possible to transmit the virus between humans.

Most adults who live in areas where the mosquitoes live are immune because they have antibodies produced when they were bitten as children. Elderly people may be susceptible, because the immunity appears to wear off with age.

Cause   When an infected mosquito bites a human, the virus passes into the person's bloodstream and then travels to the brain and spinal cord. It multiplies in the central nervous system, inflaming and damaging nerve cells, interfering with signals sent from the brain to other parts of the body.

Symptoms   Only a small percentage of patients with the disease exhibit any symptoms, which usually begins with fever, irritability, drowsiness, headache, nausea/vomiting, and sensitivity to light. This can lead to convulsions or seizures. Most people recover completely.

Diagnosis   A spinal tap (lumbar puncture) will reveal antibodies to the specific encephalitis virus in cerebrospinal fluid. The actual virus may be found in brain tissue from those who have died from the disease. Only the antibodies will appear in blood or CSF fluid, not the virus itself.

Complications   Less than 1 percent of the children who contract the disease will die. Some may experience occasional seizures or behavioral changes (such as reduced attention span).

Treatment   There is no cure for viral encephalitis. When a person's immune system produces enough antibodies to destroy the virus, the person recovers. Generally, a person with the symptoms of encephalitis is admitted to the hospital for treatment in a darkened room and given medication to reduce fever and treat the severe headache.

Prevention   There are no drugs that prevent the California encephalitis.

encephalitis, Eastern equine (EEE)   The least common of all the arboviral infections, but the most deadly, since one third of its victims will die. This type of encephalitis primarily affects horses, donkeys, and mules along the eastern seaboard; it only affects about 5 to 10 humans each year in the United States. The viral disease is characterized by inflammation of the brain and spinal cord, often causing serious or fatal damage.

Outbreaks of the disease in horses have occurred along the east coast since 1831. The first human to die of the disease was a Massachusetts baby in 1938. EEE is related to a similar virus that infects horses and humans in the western states called western equine encephalitis (WEE).

Most recently, a 1996 outbreak in Rhode Island sent oceanside residents into panic as experts discovered that one out of every hundred mosquitoes in the area was carrying the disease. High school football and other outdoor games were moved out of town, and children were urged to stay away from woods and swamps. A state of emergency was declared as tests showed a tenfold increase in infected mosquitoes, and the state sprayed an entire town with an insecticide called resmithrin. Only four people in Rhode Island have since been recorded as having the virus, however; one of them, a teenager, died in 1993.

In 1991, five older people in northern Florida contracted EEE; two died and three partially recovered. Other cases cropped up in Georgia, Michigan, Louisiana, and South Carolina; at the same time, an epidemic in horses swept along the southeastern states, killing many animals. Two years later, only 88 cases of EEE were reported in horses and only five humans contracted the disease.

In addition to eastern equine encephalitis and western equine encephalomyelitis, there is a third type: Venezuelan equine encephalitis. Eastern equine encephalitis is a severe form of equine encephalitis; it lasts longer and causes more deaths and problems than either the western or Venezuelan versions. Venezuelan equine encephalitis occurs in Central and South America, Florida, and Texas.

Cause   Four different types of mosquitoes carry the virus responsible for EEE. The virus enters the bloodstream through the mosquito bite, traveling directly to the spinal cord and brain. As the virus multiplies in the central nervous system, it damages the nerve cells, interfering with the signals the brain sends to the body.

Despite its name, the primary natural hosts of the viruses of eastern and western equine encephalitis are birds, not horses.

Because the virus is not present in the blood of humans, it is not transmitted between people. People who live in areas where the mosquito carries the virus are immune, since they were bitten as children and developed antibodies without ever becoming sick. Since the disease is transmitted primarily by mosquitoes, it occurs most often during the insect season, especially in low marshy areas.

Symptoms   Unlike St. Louis encephalitis (see ENCEPHALITIS, ST. LOUIS) in which only a few patients have symptoms, most people with EEE get symptoms, which begin 5 to 15 days after a mosquito bite. Symptoms begin with headache, fever, chills, muscle aches, and nausea, followed by paralysis, convulsions, and coma.

In humans, the elderly are most at risk for serious cases; almost 80 percent of older patients die. Infants and young children are also at risk. Those who are sick for a few days before the paralysis and convulsions appear will probably recover completely. Chances for

a complete recovery without any permanent damage are best in adults over 40 and under 80.

Signs of the disease in horses include fever, loss of appetite, discomfort, mental deterioration, head pressing, circling, and blindness. Death occurs two to three days after infection, caused by the sudden inability to breathe.

Diagnosis   Rapid tests to identify antibodies to the EEE virus in blood and cerebrospinal fluid are now available.

Treatment   There is no cure for encephalitis. Pain medication for fever and headache may be given.

Complications   Long-term damage may include facial palsy, weakness, seizures, or mental problems such as confusion and hallucinations. Children younger than five have a poor outlook for recovery.

Prevention   A vaccine can prevent the disease in horses and should be given in areas where EEE is prevalent. All foals must be vaccinated, and older horses must be revaccinated during the EEE season. An experimental vaccine is available for those who work in labs with the virus.

encephalitis,   Japanese   A mosquito-borne version of ENCEPHALITIS that is primarily a rural disease of the Orient and does not occur in the United States. It is found primarily in China and Korea, India, Bangladesh, Nepal and Sri Lanka, and southeast Asian countries. It occurs less often in Japan, Taiwan, Singapore, Hong Kong, and eastern Russia. It is the leading cause of viral encephalitis in Asia.

Japanese encephalitis is a zoonosis a disease that primarily infects animals but sometimes moves into the human population. It belongs to a group of viruses called flavivirus (which includes St. Louis encephalitis). See ENCEPHALITIS, ST. LOUIS.

The chance that a U.S. traveler to Asia will contract the disease is small; only 11 cases among Americans traveling or working in

Asia are known to have occurred between 1981 and 1992, eight of whom were military personnel or their families.

Cause The disease is transmitted by the *Culex* mosquitoes, usually during the summer and fall as the mosquito season occurs. The mosquitoes breed in ground pools and flooded rice fields and become infected after biting infected domestic pigs and wading birds who are raised near the rice paddies. However, in areas infested with mosquitoes, only a small portion of the insects are actually infected with the virus.

After the mosquito bites, the virus enters the bloodstream and travels directly to the brain and spinal cord, where it multiplies, causing inflammation and damage to nerve cells. This damage interferes with the signals the brain sends to the body, thus causing the symptoms of encephalitis.

Because the virus is not present in human blood, it can not be transmitted between humans. Most adults who live in an area where the mosquitoes carry the disease are immune because they were infected as children.

Symptoms Most people who are infected with the virus have only mild symptoms or no symptoms at all. However, those who develop encephalitis as a result of the virus are usually gravely ill. Within six to eight days after the bite, the disease begins with a flulike illness, with headache, fever, and stomach problems. Confusion and behavior problems appear early; in one third of cases, the encephalitis is fatal. Another third survive with serious types of brain damage, including paralysis. The last third recover without any further problems.

Infection during the first and second trimesters of pregnancy have been associated with miscarriages. Most deaths occur in children aged 5 to 9, and in people over age 65.

Diagnosis The disease can be diagnosed by a rapid test that looks for antibodies to the virus in the blood and cerebrospinal fluid. Sometimes the actual virus is found in brain tissue from patients who have died.

Treatment There is no treatment for this viral disease. Anyone with the symptoms of this disease is admitted to the hospital and given pain relievers and medicine to lower the fever. Intensive care is often necessary.

Complications Up to one quarter of survivors have long-term nervous system damage; the rest recover quickly. Children have a better chance of long-term recovery.

Prevention There is a vaccine for Japanese encephalitis currently available in the United States through most traveler's health clinics. It is about 85 percent effective in anyone over age one. The U.S. Centers for Disease Control recommends the vaccine only to those Americans who work in or visit at risk rural areas for more than four weeks. The risk is low to most travelers who stay in cities or who travel through the country only for short periods. People over age 55 may be at higher risk and should consider vaccination if they travel to areas of risk.

The vaccine is given in three doses, and protection begins about 10 days after the last dose. A booster shot may be required in two years. Serious allergic reactions (hives and dangerous swelling of mouth and throat) have been reported in a few people, which may not appear until several days after vaccination. Patients with multiple allergies (especially to bee stings and drugs) appear to be at higher risk for side effects. Fever and local redness and swelling are reported in about 10 percent of those vaccinated.

The vaccine is also available in many Asian countries; travelers should contact the local U.S. embassy or consulate for a list of reputable clinics that may have the vaccine. With or without the vaccine, it is important to try to avoid mosquito bites while traveling.

encephalitis lethargica An epidemic form of encephalitis that has not occurred in the United States in epidemic form since 1920, although an occasional sporadic case occurs now and then. The symptoms in this case are the same as for other ENCEPHALITIS, with the addition of extreme lethargy and drowsiness.

During the major epidemics, about 40 percent of the victims died. Many of those who survived later developed a movement disorder known as post-encephalitic parkinsonism, characterized by tremors, rigidity, immobility, and disturbed eye movements.

A few survivors of the last epidemic were still alive in the 1970s when a new antiparkinsonism drug (levodopa) remarkably improved their condition. Unfortunately, after almost 50 years of immobility, most sufferers did not appear to be able to cope with their awakening and lapsed back into their former stupor.

encephalitis, St. Louis   An ARBOVIRUL INFECTION of the brain transmitted from birds to humans by the bite of an infected mosquito. It is found most often in the central and southern United States and can sometimes be fatal. Areas with open drainage ditches, old tires, or stagnant water are most likely to experience an outbreak. (See also ENCEPHALITIS, CALIFORNIA; ENCEPHALITIS, JAPANESE; ENCEPHALITIS, EASTERN EQUINE.)

More than 3,000 people were infected in a 1933 outbreak in St. Louis, from which this version of the disease was named. Since then, it has caused similar outbreaks through the 1930s, and every 10 years after that. The last large outbreak in 1975 sickened 2,800 people in 31 states. Los Angeles has experienced outbreaks every year since 1984. Outbreaks usually occur in August and September.

St. Louis encephalitis is a disease that primarily affects animals, but as the above numbers indicate, it occasionally crosses the species barrier.

Most adults who live in mosquito-prone areas are immune because they were bitten as children, and their immune systems produced antibodies that protect them later. By old age, however, these antibodies have usually disap-

peared, and the elderly are once again susceptible to infection.

Cause   The virus enters the human bloodstream from an infected mosquito bite, where it travels to the brain and spinal cord, multiples in the nervous system and inflames and damages nerve cells.

Symptoms   Only a few people (1 percent) who have this type of encephalitis ever develop symptoms. Most of those who do report a flulike illness characterized by headache, malaise, fever, stiff neck, delirium, and convulsions. There may be visual and speech problems, walking difficulty, and personality changes. Symptoms typically appear between 5 and 15 days after a mosquito bite.

Elderly patients are most at risk for serious symptoms; 20 percent of them die. Those at risk include patients with high blood pressure or heart disease, but most people—even those who are seriously ill—recover completely.

Complications   After an infection, a few patients will experience long-term damage such as weakness, seizures, facial palsies, or mental deterioration. These symptoms may improve gradually.

Diagnosis   A doctor may perform either an EEG or CT brain scan, which will reveal abnormalities but will not pinpoint the cause of the encephalitis (brain inflammation). Antibodies can be found in the blood and cerebrospinal fluid, and sometimes the virus itself is found in brain tissue of those who have died from the disease.

Treatment   There is no cure or vaccination for this viral disease. Public health officials monitor the mosquito activity and infection rates in birds; when rates are high, a mosquito alert is issued.

encephalitis, tick-borne   A viral infection of the central nervous system caused by a tick bite, usually in people who visit or work in forested areas. Tick-borne ENCEPHALITIS occurs in eastern Europe, Russia, and the former Soviet republics from April through August, when the ticks are alive. (See also ENCEPHALITIS, EASTERN EQUINE; ENCEPHALITIS LETHARGICA; ENCEPHALITIS, CALIFORNIA.)

Cause In addition to the bite of ticks, this type of encephalitis can be transmitted by consuming unpasteurized dairy products from infected animals.

Symptoms Symptoms appear between one to two weeks after the bite of an infected tick or after ingesting infected dairy products and resemble symptoms of mosquito-borne encephalitis.

Treatment Treatment is symptomatic.

Prevention Vaccines have been developed and are available in most endemic areas; no such vaccine is available for use in the United States.

encephalomyelitis Also called equine encephalitis (ENCEPHALITIS, EASTERN EQUINE), this disease is an inflammation of the brain and spinal cord (as opposed to ENCEPHALITIS, which refers to inflammation of the brain alone). There are various applications of the terms *encephalitis* and *encephalomyelitis*. *Encephalomyelitis* is now the usual term in animal diseases.

While encephalomyelitis is now also called "sleeping sickness," it should not be confused with the African sleeping sickness (TRYPANOSOMIASIS) caused by a protozoan.

The agents most often involved in human infections are the viruses of St. Louis encephalitis (ENCEPHALITIS, ST. LOUIS), western equine encephalomyelitis, California encephalitis (ENCEPHALITIS, CALIFORNIA) and MUMPS virus, ECHOviruses and COXSACKIEVIRUS.

Encephalomyelitis also sometimes occurs in domestic animals. Avian encephalomyelitis (also called "crazy chick disease" or "epidemic tremor") is a viral disease of young chickens, characterized by profound weakness, paralysis, and head and neck trembles.

Sporadic bovine encephalomyelitis ("Buss disease") is an uncommon infection of cattle by the bacterium CHLAMYDIA. Porcine encephalomyelitis is a viral infection of pigs that doesn't usually cause symptoms.

Symptoms The most common symptoms of encephalomyelitis in humans and horses is mental impairment. In humans, symptoms include weakness, discomfort, headache, nausea before drowsiness, confusion, stiff neck, and seizures. Permanent complications are common in infants and children who survive. Signs of the disease in horses include fever, loss of appetite, discomfort, mental deterioration, head pressing, circling, and blindness. Death occurs two to three days after infection, caused by the sudden inability to breathe.

Treatment There is no specific treatment for viral encephalomyelitis in animals or humans. Disease caused by bacteria, fungi, or protozoa—which is much more rare—involves cause-specific therapy.

Prevention Horses and poultry can be vaccinated against viral Venezuelan equine encephalomyelitis.

endothrix A dermatophyte (superficial fungus) whose growth and spore production are confined primarily within the hair shaft, without forming conspicuous spores on the outside of the hair.

endotoxin shock See SEPTIC SHOCK.

Entamoeba histolytica A species of amoeba that cause amoebic dysentery and hepatic AMEBIASIS in humans.

enteric fever See TYPHOID FEVER.

enteritis Inflammation of the lining of the intestine from a variety of causes, including bacterial or viral infections. If both the large and small intestines are involved, the problem is known as enterocolitis. Gastroenteritis, on the other hand, refers to an inflammation of the stomach and intestines and accompanies a variety of disorders.

enterobiasis A parasitic infestation of the intestines by the common pinworm (*Enterobius vermicularis*).

Cause As the worms infect the large intestine, the females deposit eggs in the perianal area. Often, the eggs are transferred to the mouth and the patient is reinfected. Airborne transmission is also possible, since the eggs remain alive for up to three days in contaminated bedcovers.

Symptoms Itching and sleeplessness caused by the presence of the worm crawling in the perianal area to lay its eggs.

Diagnosis Tape is applied to the skin around the perianal area and then examined under a microscope for the presence of worm eggs.

Treatment An entire household may need to be treated to make sure all pinworms are destroyed. Therapy may include treatment with one of a variety of medications: piperazine, pyrantel pamoate, pyrvinium pamoate, or thiabendazole.

Prevention Disinfection procedures in the home do little good in preventing infection. There is no good way to prevent pinworms.

Enterobius vermicularis A common parasitic nematode (known also as pinworm, seatworm, or threadworm) that resembles a small, thin white thread. See also ENTEROBIASIS.

Enterococcus The former term for several *Streptococcus*-like bacteria that inhabit the human gastrointestinal tract. The bacteria are now grouped in their own genus, since they differ from more traditional strep germs.

Enterococcus faecium and *E. faecalis* are two that are particularly dangerous, since they are now becoming highly resistant to antibiotics. These antibiotic-resistant organisms first appeared in the 1980s in New York City hospitals, where they led to the death of 19 out of 100 patients infected with the bacteria.

By 1994, 8 percent of all reported *Enterococcus*-related illness were caused by drug-resistant strains. Scientists are concerned as the resistant strains of enterococcus transfer their resistance to other germs that inhabit the gastrointestinal system, such as *Streptococci* and *Staphylococci*.

enterotoxin A type of bacteria-released poison that inflames the lining of the intestine, causing vomiting and diarrhea. Staphylococcal food poisoning is caused by eating food contaminated with an enterotoxin produced by staphylococci bacteria. The toxin is resistant to heat and is not destroyed by cooking. The severe diarrhea and vomiting associated with CHOLERA is also caused by an enterotoxin produced in the intestine by the cholera bacteria.

enterovirus A group of viruses that multiply primarily in the intestinal tract. This group includes the COXSACKIEVIRUS, ECHOVIRUS, and polio virus. Others can trigger MENINGITIS, ENCEPHALITIS, respiratory illness, diarrhea, CONJUNCTIVITIS, and a host of other diseases, including the common COLD.

Any one of the enteroviruses can produce a wide variety of symptoms that may mimic symptoms produced by other enteroviruses. They are very difficult to kill and are not affected by antibiotics or most disinfectants. They can survive temperatures of up to 122 degrees F and are found throughout the tropics and subtropics; however, they appear to prefer late summer or early fall in cooler climates. While they can be inactivated in the presence of chlorine, the smallest amount of organic matter will protect them so that they can survive most attempts at public water purification. Most children are infected with some types of enteroviruses at a young age;

in general, these viruses cause older people to suffer more serious symptoms, with infection.

Enteroviruses have been found along beaches miles from the nearest offshore dump site; swimmers are at high risk for infection, since the easiest way into the human body is through the mouth. See also DIARRHEA AND INFECTIOUS DISEASE; ANTIDIARRHEAL DRUGS; TRAVELER'S DIARRHEA.

epidemic The occurrence in a population of more cases of disease than one would expect under normal circumstances. The term also describes the pattern of certain diseases that markedly ebb and flow over a short period of time. (For example, prior to the development of the measles vaccine, large numbers of measles cases would occur in waves.)

When a disease sweeps over broad geographic areas at one time, creating widespread epidemics, the disease is referred to as being *pandemic*. The INFLUENZA virus of 1918 was a pandemic as HIV is today.

In Europe during the Middle Ages at least one fourth of all deaths were caused by epidemic diseases. Major epidemics have included AIDS, EBOLA, PLAGUE, CHOLERA, polio, TYPHUS, SMALLPOX, and YELLOW FEVER. Some epidemics, such as the yearly sweep of flu viruses, are relatively harmless if the patient's immune system is healthy and/or patients have been properly vaccinated. Other epidemics have become more of a concern, including the AIDS outbreak, the 1993 outbreak of HANTAVIRUS, and regular outbreaks of a new and deadly strain of ESCHERICHIA COLI that has sickened and killed people throughout the world who ingested contaminated meat. Since 1985, TUBERCULOSIS has been more prevalent in the United States due in part to emergence of drug-resistant forms of the disease. Mutated forms of pneumococcal PNEUMONIA have become resistant to antibiotics and are a rising epidemic concern.

epidemiology The scientific discipline that seeks to detect disease causes and to determine preventive measures. The focus of epidemiology is on diseases as they occur in defined groups, rather than as they affect individuals.

epiglottitis Inflammation of the epiglottis, a thin flap of cartilage, lying behind the root of the tongue, that covers the entrance to the larynx during swallowing. Acute epiglottitis is a severe form of the condition that usually affects children. The condition is also called epiglottiditis.

Cause Epiglottitis is caused by *Haemophilus influenzae* type B.

Symptoms The severe form is characterized by sore throat, fever, noisy breathing, croupy cough, and a swollen epiglottis. The patient may turn blue and require an emergency tracheostomy to maintain breathing.

Treatment Antibiotics, rest, oxygen, and supportive care.

Epstein-Barr virus (EBV) One of the most common universal human viruses, the EBV causes infectious MONONUCLEOSIS. A member of the HERPES family, EBV was named for the two scientists who discovered it in 1964. It infects most people sometime during their lives, usually after childhood; as many as 95 percent of American adults between ages 35 and 40 have been infected. In the United States and other developed countries, many children are not infected by the virus; if they are, they will not usually have any symptoms. If a child becomes infected during adolescence, the virus causes infectious mononucleosis. About 10 percent of high school and college students become infected each year in the United States, of which more than half develop infectious mononucleosis. In poor countries with lower standards of hygiene, however, most children are infected by the time they are six years old, when the disease is mild and almost unnoticeable.

Transmission of the EBV is not understood but is believed to require contact with saliva of an infected person, since the virus is not normally transmitted through air or blood. EBV does not leave the body. It establishes a lifelong dormant infection in some of the body's immune system cells. A very few carriers will go on to develop Burkitt's lymphoma and cancer of the nose and throat, two rare cancers that are not normally found in the United States. EBV appears to play a major role in the development of these cancers, but it is not considered to be the only cause.

Complications During the 1980s, the virus was linked to a syndrome featuring severe fatigue diagnosed as CHRONIC FATIGUE SYNDROME (CFS), because some sufferers had above-average levels of Epstein-Barr virus antibodies in their blood. Scientists suspected that the virus's ability to reactivate after long periods of time could mean it had something to do with the debilitating condition of CFS. This theory has since been abandoned.

Prevention At least one drug company is currently testing a vaccine against the EBV.

equine morbillivirus (EM) A rare, emerging infectious disease caused by a previously unknown morbillivirus—a viral group that includes MEASLES, canine distemper virus, seal plague virus, rinderpest virus, and peste des petits ruminats.

In the first known outbreak, EM surfaced in Australia in the fall of 1994, killing 13 of 17 infected horses and one of two humans before it was identified.

Cause As mysterious as the African EBOLA virus, scientists do not know where the virus came from or where it will reappear next. Until its natural host is identified, scientists cannot predict its future path. They suspect that the benign virus may be found in some type of Australian animal that rarely comes in contact with horses or humans and that it only causes disease when it moves into the horse or human groups.

Symptoms They do know that the virus is extremely virulent, killing 70 percent of infected horses. The virus induces cells lining the blood vessels to clump, creating holes in the vessel walls, thus allowing fluid to leak into the lungs and tissues. As the fluid pours into the lungs, the patient—horse or human—drowns in its own fluid.

Diagnosis There is a test for antibodies to the virus.

Treatment There is no known treatment.

erysipelas Contagious infection of the facial skin and subcutaneous tissue caused by *Streptococcus pyogenes* and marked by rapid-spreading redness and swelling. The bacteria are believed to enter the skin through a small lesion. Although this disease is contagious, it does not produce huge epidemics like those of SCARLET FEVER.

Before the advent of antibiotics, this disease could be fatal (especially for infants and the elderly). Today, it is quickly controlled with prompt treatment.

Symptoms After a five to seven day incubation period, the patient experiences a sudden high fever with headache, malaise, and vomiting. The skin feels tight, uncomfortable, itchy, and red, with patches appearing most often on the face, spreading across the cheeks and bridge of the nose. It also occurs on the scalp, genitals, hands, and legs. Within the inflammation, pimples appear, blister, burst, and crust over.

Treatment Penicillin will cure the infection within seven days. Bed rest, hot packs, and aspirin for pain and fever may also help.

erythema annulare centrifugam This is one of a group of "reactive erythemas" characterized by expanding ring-shaped plaques. The lesions, which are usually found on the trunk, enlarge slowly. Although the disorder can occur at any age, most patients are young adults when stricken. Symptoms may last for only a short time, or they may persist for decades, depending on the cause.

Causes This type of erythema may be caused by a DERMATOPHYTE infection, fungus infection (CANDIDA ALBICANS), blue cheese ingestion, cancer, parasitic bowel disease, or autoimmune disorder.

Treatment Treating the underlying cause (such as fungus or parasite) will effectively cure the erythema (redness).

erythema chronicum migrans This is a skin lesion that is the initial sign of LYME DISEASE. It begins as a small papule and spreads, extending by a raised red margin and clearing in the center. It marks the site of a deer tick bite.

erythema infectiosum See FIFTH DISEASE.

erythema nodosum An inflammatory skin disease associated with an infectious agent or drug sensitivity to sulfonamides, penicillin, salicylates, or others. The eruption of reddish-purple swellings on the skin may also be a result of another illness, such as inflammatory bowel disease, collagen disease, lymphoma, leukemia, or some other condition. It occurs most often in women between ages 20 and 50, although the disease can appear in both sexes at any age.

Pain may be severe and disabling, but permanent problems from this disease are rare. Lesions usually disappear within one or two months, although the disorder can recur.

Cause Streptococcal throat infection is the most common underlying cause, although this disorder is also associated with TUBERCULOSIS. About 30 percent of the time no cause can be found. The exact mechanism behind the disease is not known, although it is believed to be some type of immune reaction around large blood vessels in the subcutaneous fat.

Symptoms Shiny, tender swellings of up to four inches across appear suddenly on shins, thighs, and sometimes arms. There is usually also fever and pain in muscles and joints, and there may be other symptoms including chills, malaise, headache, or sore throat.

Treatment The underlying illness should be treated. Bed rest with the legs raised is important; for ambulatory patients, support stockings may help. Warm water compresses may be soothing, and tenting the bedcovers may relieve discomfort from lesions rubbing against material. Otherwise, treatment may include painkillers or sometimes nonsteroidal antiinflammatory drugs to reduce inflammation. While corticosteroids may also be used, they reduce the patient's resistance if the erythema is caused by infection; the drugs may also interfere with diagnostic tests. Even when the cause is not known, the prognosis for recovery is good.

erythrasma A bacterial infection (of the toe web, groin, and underarms) that causes mild burning and itching. It is more common in warmer climates and among diabetics.

Cause The infection is caused by *Corynebacterium minutissimum*. Recurrences are common.

Treatment *C. minutissimum* is very sensitive to a wide variety of antimicrobial drugs; extensive cases may also require oral administration of erythromycin. Tolnaftate and Whitfield's ointment are also beneficial.

Escherichia A genus of gram-negative rod-like bacteria that are found in the intestines of humans and other animals.

Escherichia coli (E. coli) A species of coliform bacteria of the family Enterobacteriaceae that is normally found in the intestines, milk, water, and soil. Part of the reason it can be dangerous is that it comes in many different strains capable of reproducing at extraordinary rates, doubling their population every two hours (if enough food were available, one *E. coli* cell could reproduce into a mass bigger than the earth in three days). Fortunately, most of the strains are harmless to the majority of people most of the time.

Named for the 19th-century German physician Theodor Escherich who identified it, the bacterium is the most frequent cause of urinary tract infections and is commonly found in wounds. *E. coli* blood poisoning can be rapidly fatal as a result of shock because of the action of an endotoxin released by the bacteria.

There are five groups of *E. coli* whose toxins can cause TRAVELER'S DIARRHEA. The worst is *ESCHERICHIA COLI* 0157:H7 that can cause a DYSENTERY-type of fatal bloody diarrhea. See also DIARRHEA AND INFECTIOUS DISEASE; ANTIDIARRHEAL DRUGS; COLIFORM COUNT.

***Escherichia coli (E. coli)* 0157:H7** One of the most deadly of the hundreds of strains of the bacterium *Escherichia coli.* Although most strains of *E. coli* are harmless and live in the intestines of both humans and animals, the 0157:H7 strain produces a powerful toxin that can cause severe illness. It has emerged during the past 10 years as a cause of food-borne illness that can cause kidney failure and death.

This mutation, which was discovered in 1982, has at least 62 subtypes. The combination of letters and numbers in the name of this bacterium refers to specific markers found on its surface and distinguishes it from other types of *E. coli.* The number of this type of *E. coli* food poisoning cases appears to be increasing, as has the frequency of complications from infection.

An estimated 10,000 to 20,000 cases of infection occur in the United States each year, most associated with eating undercooked, contaminated ground beef. The disease was first recognized as a cause of illness in 1982 during an outbreak of bloody diarrhea, which was traced to contaminated hamburgers. During this outbreak, scientists discovered that the *E. coli* 0157:H7 strain had somehow acquired the gene for Shiga toxin, caused by the organism *Shigella dysenteriae.* This strain of *E. coli* caused three outbreaks in 1982 among scores of patients who came down with an alarming type of bloody diarrhea.

The strain continued to appear sporadically until, in 1993, four children died and hundreds more fell ill after eating *E. coli*–tainted hamburger in a fast-food restaurant in Washington. The incident set off a furor throughout the country as consumer safety groups urged the government to improve its meat inspection system.

The Washington outbreak was followed within months by more outbreaks of food-borne illness caused by *E. coli,* forcing the closing of two other restaurants and sickening 60 more consumers. Annually, the CDC estimates that *E. coli* alone is responsible for 20,000 cases of food poisoning, although these estimates may not be accurate, since physicians are not required to report these poisonings.

A study by the Western States Meats Association found the common bacteria *Escherichia coli (E. coli)* was present in 1.5 percent of ground pork and also in poultry, and 3.7 percent in beef. In the past, people got *E. coli* food poisoning by drinking tap water in foreign countries. In the wake of the reported mass poisonings and deaths from *E. coli,* the Clinton administration vowed to revamp the federal meat inspection system, which currently relies on visual inspections. In related action, the USDA decided to issue new labels for raw meat and poultry that discuss safe handling and cooking methods.

The Shiga gene has continued to spread, and has now been found in other strains of *E. coli,* as well as other bacteria common to the human intestine (such as *Enterobacter*).

Figures from the Centers for Disease Control suggest there may be 20,000 illnesses a year in this country, with 250 to 500 deaths from *E. coli* 0157:H7 alone. According to experts at the Food-borne Diseases Epidemiology Section of the federal centers, an additional 10,000 to 20,000 cases of food poisoning may be caused by Shiga toxin from other strains of bacteria for a total of perhaps 40,000 cases in the United States. This is part of an estimated total of about 7 million cases of food-borne illness in general.

Recent epidemics have included the November 1996 cases involving a 15-month-old Colorado child who died after drinking tainted unpasteurized Odwalla apple juice; another 50 people became sick. In the summer of 1996, a similar epidemic swept Japan, killing 7 people and infecting almost 9,000 Japanese during its four-month reign. In the biggest outbreak, 6,500 people came down with *E. coli* infection in Sakai; the infection was traced to city-supplied school lunches. See also DIARRHEA AND INFECTIOUS DISEASE; ANTIDIARRHEAL DRUGS.

Cause Outbreaks have been traced to many different types of food. It has been found to survive in dry fermented meat despite production standards that meet federal and industry food processing requirements, scientists say. It has been found in salami, where the bacteria may have been present on raw meat that was brought into a plant and subsequently survived the fermentation and drying steps involved in salami production.

Primarily, the organism is found in a small number of cattle farms, living in the intestines of healthy cattle. Meat becomes contaminated during slaughter, and organisms can be mixed with beef when it is ground in huge vats. Alternatively, bacteria on a cow's udders or on milking equipment can find its way into raw milk.

Since contaminated meat looks and smells normal, it is possible to eat tainted meat unknowingly. Although the number of organisms needed to cause disease isn't known, it is believed to be very small.

The problem is not with steak; a bit of bacterial contamination on the surface of a steak is not much of a threat because it is quickly killed when the surface of the meat is cooked. It is the practice of grinding the meat that gives bacteria its chance. When a contaminated steak is minced up and mixed with other beef from other animals, the bacteria become widely distributed—not just on the surface, but throughout the meat. Contaminated and undercooked hamburger is suspected of causing more than half of all outbreaks of bloody diarrhea. Many outbreaks have begun in fast-food restaurants, but since the large chains have begun to sample their meat, the real problem today lies in grocery store hamburger, according to experts. The meat in grocery stores, the experts say, goes largely untested.

The toxin-making bacteria are killed only if the hamburger is cooked to an inside temperature of 155 degrees F, hot enough to eliminate all meat pinkness.

Drinking unpasteurized milk or swimming in or drinking sewage-contaminated water can also cause infection. In July 1991, 80 people were infected while swimming in an Oregon lake. In July 1993, 35,000 New Yorkers had to boil their water because the specific *E. coli* strain eluded chlorination and appeared in New York's tap water.

The disease can also be transmitted from person to person through contact with contaminated stool, if hygiene or handwashing is not adequate. This is especially common in day care centers and among toddlers who are not yet toilet trained.

Symptoms The *E. coli* 0157:H7 bacterium produces toxins that cause severe cramps and then watery or bloody diarrhea, lasting for several days. Other symptoms include nausea and vomiting appearing within hours to a week after eating; there is usually no fever. Most people recover quickly and completely, but the complications are what make this a serious disease.

In certain people at risk (such as among the very young or old), the bacteria may cause HEMOLYTIC UREMIC SYNDROME (HUS), in which the red blood cells are destroyed and the kidneys fail. Between 2 and 7 percent of infections lead to this complication. In the United States, HUS is the main cause of kidney failure in children; most cases are caused by infection with this type of *E. coli*.

Patients are infectious for about six days while bacteria are being excreted in the stool. There is no solid evidence, but it appears that victims can get this infection more than once.

Diagnosis   The infection is diagnosed by identifying the bacterium in stool. Most labs that culture stool don't test for *E. coli* 0157:H7, so it is important to request that the stool be tested for this organism. Everyone with sudden diarrhea and bleeding should have the stool checked for this bacterium.

Treatment   Most patients recover within 10 days without need of specific treatment. There is no evidence that antibiotics help, and there is some evidence to suggest it may set off kidney problems. Antidiarrhea medicine should also be avoided.

HUS, on the other hand, is a life-threatening condition that is treated in a hospital intensive care unit, with blood transfusions and kidney dialysis. With intensive care, the death rate from this complication is between 3 and 5 percent. There is no cure for HUS.

Complications   Patients who have had only mild infection, with diarrhea, usually recover completely. Of those who develop HUS, one third have abnormal kidney function years later and a few need long-term dialysis. Another 8 percent suffer with other complications, including high blood pressure, seizures, blindness, and paralysis for the rest of their lives.

Adults may get an extremely serious bleeding disorder called thrombotic thrombocytopenic purpura, in which blood stops clotting; small red spots and large bruises appear all over the body, and blood oozes through the mouth. The outlook is not promising for patients with this complication.

Prevention   To protect against this type of food poisoning, travelers should not drink untreated water and ice or eat salads, raw fruits and vegetables that can't be peeled, and uncooked milk products. Diners should always make sure hamburgers are well done.

Consumers can prevent infection by thoroughly cooking ground beef, avoiding unpasteurized milk and washing hands carefully. Undercooked beef shouldn't be served to young children, the elderly, or anyone with an impaired immune system.

When caring for an infected patient, hand washing is crucial to avoid person-to-person spread of the disease. About 38 states now ask doctors to report outbreaks of the disease but none regularly test for other strains of *E. coli* that produce the toxin.

European swamp fever   See LEPTOSPIROSIS.

exanthem subitum   See ROSEOLA.

exogenous infection   An infection that develops from bacteria normally found outside the body, which is not usually part of the normal human bacterial population.

eye infections   The most common infection of the eye is CONJUNCTIVITIS, also known as pinkeye. Most of these infections are caused by bacteria (such as staphylococci) or by viruses associated with a cold, sore throat, or illness such as MEASLES. Viral conjunctivitis is the version that often appears in schools, sweeping through classrooms in massive epidemics. Newborns may contract a type of conjunctivitis from their mothers during birth. This type of infection may be caused by common bacteria, organisms responsible for GONORRHEA or genital HERPES, or by a chlamydial infection and may cause blindness in the newborn infant unless treated.

Keratoconjunctivitis is an inflammation of both the conjunctiva and the cornea; it is often caused by a virus. Corneal infections are more serious and can lead to blurry vision or perforation if not treated.

Infection within the eye (endophthalmitis) may make it necessary to remove the eyeball. This can occur after a penetrating injury to the eye, or from infections elsewhere in the body.

See also CHLAMYDIA.

F

Fasciola hepatica The name of the type of liver fluke that causes FASCIOLIASIS.

fascioliasis Infection with a liver fluke (also called the giant intestinal fluke) is found throughout the world, especially the southern and western United States. It is also a common parasite in humans and pigs in central and south China, Taiwan, Southeast Asia, Indonesia, India, and Bangladesh.

Cause The disease is caused by the liver fluke *Fasciola hepatica*, acquired by ingesting encysted forms of the fluke in water plants (such as raw watercress, water chestnuts, or bamboo shoots). The eggs of the infective fluke are shed in fecal material into water; when they hatch, they produce larvae that penetrate and develop in the flesh of snails. These organisms then escape and develop cysts on various water plants. Humans are infected by eating these plants uncooked; the immature flukes are released from the cysts and develop into adult worms in the small intestine.

Symptoms Epigastric pain, fever, jaundice, hives, and diarrhea. Prolonged infection may be related to fibrosis of the liver.

Treatment Oral bithionol is the usual treatment. Most infected people don't have any symptoms, but severe infections occur in very small numbers of people who are infected with large numbers of flukes.

fever An abnormal internal temperature of the body above "normal" due to disease, although the normal range depends on when and how the temperature is taken. Right after activity, for example, the temperature may rise to 99 degrees F. Rectal temperatures are up to a degree higher and under-the-arm temperatures are usually up to a degree lower than 98.6 degrees F. In addition, normal body temperature is lower in the morning and higher in the late afternoon and evening.

The thermal regulatory center in the brain is responsible for controlling the body's temperature. This setting rises during an infection, resulting in a fever when white blood cells release certain proteins as part of the immune response that trigger the brain to release a chemical called prostaglandin. This causes the nerve cells to produce a feeling of coldness, which is why a patient experiences chills during the development of fever.

In response to infection, the brain increases the body's temperature, speeding up the activities of the immune system against the invading germs. What this means is that a fever is actually not a bad thing—it can actually help the body fight disease.

However, a very high fever can be uncomfortable and eventually—if it goes high enough—can lead to seizures and death.

A temperature may be taken with an oral, digital, or rectal thermometer. Those who find a mercury thermometer hard to read may find a digital readout thermometer easier. While some doctors rely on this type of instrument, others insist that digital thermometers are not as accurate. A rectal thermometer is used for infants and young children who can't hold an oral thermometer in their mouths. An oral thermometer should not be used to take a rectal temperature. After each use, the thermometer should be cleaned using lukewarm soapy water and rinsed well with cold water or the thermometer may be rinsed with alcohol followed by cold water. Hot water will break a mercury thermometer.

The course of a fever depends on its cause. The degree of the fever does not really indicate how serious the illness is, however, since severe infections may only cause a low fever, and some mild infections can cause a high fever.

Treatment Medicines called antipyretics will bring down a fever; aspirin and acetaminophen work by slowing the production of prostaglandins. Because fevers are beneficial, however, one should only take antipyretics for fevers over 101 degrees F. Anything lower than this is considered to be a low-grade fever. In an infant younger than three months of age, however, any fever over 100.4 F requires medical evaluation. Treating a fever in children lessens the risk of seizures, which tend to run in families and occur in less than 3 percent of normal children up to six years.

WARNING SIGNS FOR FEVER

Any child under age three months with a rectal temperature higher than 100.4 degrees F must see a health care practitioner as soon as possible. Call a doctor if older infants and children have a fever above 102 degrees F that lasts longer than three days, increases after two days, or if any of the following warning signs develop:

- unusual irritability, screaming, tense or stiff arms or legs
- extreme drowsiness (child hard to wake)
- confusion, delirium, hallucinations
- breathing problems (wheezing, crackling, high-pitched sounds)
- neck pain, stiff neck, holding neck in odd way
- seizures
- sunken or bulging soft spot on head (especially in front)
- vomiting after attempt to give fluids
- dry lips, tongue, and mouth
- no wet diaper or urination in six hours

Arrange appointment for fever accompanied by any of the following symptoms:

- stomach pain
- sore throat, difficulty swallowing
- ear pain; pulling, tugging, or rubbing ear

Febrile seizures last less than 15 minutes and don't cause brain damage or epilepsy.

Aspirin should not be given to anyone under age 18 because it has been associated with Reye's syndrome in children who have the flu or CHICKEN POX. (Reye's syndrome is a very serious condition affecting the brain and liver.)

If the fever is very high, a cooling tub bath, wet sheet, or ice packs may be ordered.

Children should not be rubbed with alcohol, since the fumes can be dangerous and there is evidence that the alcohol can be absorbed through the skin. A child should not be immersed in cold water, which will reduce the body temperature too quickly.

fever blisters Another name for COLD SORE.

fifth disease A viral infection that often affects red blood cells. Fifth disease is also known as "slapped cheeks" disease because of its dramatic herald symptoms of a bright red rash across the cheeks. Named in 1899 as the fifth of six common childhood illnesses that cause a rash (after MEASLES, MUMPS, CHICKENPOX, and GERMAN MEASLES), it is the least well known of them all.

Among healthy children the disease is mild; once the rash appears they are not contagious and may return to school.

Cause The disease is caused by the parvovirus B19, usually occurring in small outbreaks among young children in the spring. The virus itself was discovered in England in 1975, but it was not until 1983 that scientists realized it caused fifth disease.

In much the same way as a cold spreads, fifth disease is passed on via mouth and nose secretions or from contact with contaminated objects. It may also travel through the air in small droplets. It is also found in the blood of infected people, so that a blood transfusion could pass on the disease. Outbreaks occur from late winter through spring among school-age children. Adults who have already been infected with the virus are now immune, but nonimmune adults can catch the disease.

People with fifth disease appear to be contagious during the week before the rash appears; by the time the rash occurs, the person is probably beyond the contagious period. It is believed that people who have been previously infected acquire lifelong immunity. Studies have shown that more than fifty percent of adults are immune.

Symptoms In children, the illness begins with a headache, slight tiredness, or muscle pain followed in two or three days by a rash of rosy red spots on the cheeks, which join into a red rash. Within a few days, the rash has spread over the body, buttocks, and arms and legs. There is often a mild fever in addition to the skin rash. About half the time, the rash will be itchy.

Adults will notice fever and joint pain (especially in the knees) that mimics arthritis and may be severe, flaring up in wet weather and in the morning.

Most babies born to mothers with the disease are normal and healthy, although the virus is able to cross the placenta and infect the fetus. Studies suggest that about 2.5 percent of pregnant women infected with parvovirus have spontaneous abortions or stillbirths.

Those who have sickle-cell disease don't get fifth disease, but when infected with the virus they come down with a more serious infection called aplastic crisis (their bone marrow stops making red blood cells). They require hospitalization and blood transfusions.

Diagnosis Pregnant women can have a test for immunity to parvovirus. These antibody tests are available through state health departments.

In most cases, the disease is diagnosed based on the appearance of typical symptoms. A specific blood test to confirm the diagnosis has recently become available but is not necessary in healthy children.

Treatment There is no treatment for fifth disease. With bed rest, clear fluids, and acetaminophen to lower fever, the rash usually clears within 10 days. Red blood cells are given to sickle-cell patients. Treat fevers over 101 degrees F; calamine lotion will ease the itch of the rash. Adults may take ibuprofen or another nonsteroidal anti-inflammatory drug (NSAID) for the joint pain.

Complications Those in high-risk groups who contract fifth disease may experience chronic anemic conditions afterward. Those at high risk include anyone with sickle-cell anemia, red blood cell abnormalities, undergoing immunosuppressive treatment for cancer, an organ recipient, or HIV patients.

While there is no evidence that parvovirus B19 is a significant cause of birth defects, some studies have shown that infection may increase the risk of miscarriage or spontaneous abortion.

Prevention As yet there is no way to control the spread of fifth disease.

filariasis A group of tropical diseases caused by a range of parasitic roundworms and larvae that transmit disease to humans. About 200 million people are affected by filariasis, which occurs in tropic and subtropic areas of southeast Asia, South America, Africa, and the Pacific. Mosquitoes inject the worm larvae when they bite, which migrate to the lymph nodes where they develop into mature worms in about a year.

Some of the species live in the lymphatic vessels and block them, causing ELEPHANTIASIS (swelling of limbs with thickened, coarse skin). Another type of worm can be seen and felt just underneath the skin, which produces irritating and painful swellings called calabar swellings.

Bancroftian filariasis (*Wuchereria bancrofti filarial nematode*) is spread widely throughout Africa, southern and southeastern Asia, the Pacific, and the tropical and subtropical regions of South America. Malayan filariasis

(*Brugia malayi filarial nematode*) is found only in southern and southeastern Asia. Imported cases of the filariases may be found in the United States, especially among immigrants from the Caribbean and Pacific islands.

Cause Bancroftian and Malayan filariases are transmitted to humans by the bite of an infected mosquito. The infective larvae that are transmitted into humans via the bite pass into the human lymph system, where they develop to maturity during a 6- to 12-month period. Fertilized mature female worms release embryos that develop into moving larvae (microfilariae), which appear in the human blood system at night only.

Symptoms Initial inflammatory symptoms occur between three months to a year after the mosquito bite, with episodes of chills, headache, and fever. The fever is often associated with inflammation of the lymphatic system. There is swelling, redness, and pain in arms, legs, or scrotum.

An ABSCESS may occur as a result of dying worms and secondary bacterial infection. Repeated episodes of inflammation lead to obstruction of the lymphatic system, especially in the genital and leg areas. Chronic swelling stimulates the growth of connective tissue in the skin, causing massive permanent enlargement and deformity (elephantiasis). In Bancroftian filariasis the legs and genitalia are most often involved; in the Malayan variety the portion of the legs below the knees are affected, but genitals are usually spared.

Diagnosis Blood specimen examination for filaria antigen, patient history, and appearance of the patient.

Treatment The prognosis is good in early or mild cases, and if the patient can avoid reinfection. Three weeks of diethylcarbamazine cures the infection. However, reactions to large numbers of dying parasites are common (fever, malaise, nausea, and vomiting), so doses are usually low at first. Oral antihistamines may help control hives, and elastic stockings may help control swelling.

However, no treatment can reverse elephantiasis. Surgery may ease massive enlargement of the scrotum.

Prevention In infested areas, filariasis can be controlled by taking diethylcarbamazine or ivermectin preventively, and by using insecticides, repellents, nets, and protective clothing.

fish and infectious disease The danger of fish contamination is not just with the contaminants they ingest. Because bacteria that live on fish are adapted to withstand the cool and cold waters of lakes and oceans, they can thrive in temperatures cold enough to normally preserve food. These microbes will quickly spoil the fish, unless it is kept at temperatures close to freezing. Even under the best conditions, fish lasts only 7 to 12 days; but it often takes seven days for fish to get from the water to the supermarket, where it may sit for several more days. Bacterial decomposition of tuna, mackerel, mahimahi, bluefish, or albacore can cause immediate gastrointestinal problems, rash, and abdominal pain, although symptoms subside after a day or two.

At the first counter, the word *fresh* is supposed to mean never frozen or heated. In many cases, however, *fresh* means anything the store wants it to mean.

How to protect against contamination Seafood should look and smell fresh, with vivid skin and bright eyes and no fishy or ammonia odor. It is best to select fish from the bottom of the refrigerator case where it is coldest. At home, it should be kept very cold and eaten within one or two days. Although it is important to cook fish thoroughly, no amount of cooking will destroy contaminants.

To best protect yourself, scrape off the fatty skin before cooking. Pregnant women, nursing mothers, and young children should limit consumption of fish that might have high levels of mercury and PCBs.

After weeks, months, or years of eating contaminated fish, methyl mercury poisoning affects the central nervous system, causing numbness or tingling of mouth, lips, tongue, and extremities; visual disturbances; hearing problems; speech disorders; difficulty swallowing; weakness; fatigue; concentration problems; emotional changes and instability; inability to write, read, or remember simple things; stumbling gait. In severe cases, stupor, coma, and death.

flatworms   Any species of worm that has a flat shape (as opposed to a roundworm or nematode, which is shaped cylindrically). There are two types of flatworms that affect humans—cestodes (TAPEWORMS) and trematodes (FLUKES and schistosomes). See also SCHISTOSOMIASIS.

fleas   Throughout history, the bite of the flea is notorious for causing disease. These wingless bloodsucking insects may transmit ARBOVIRUSES to humans. Certain species of fleas can transmit PLAGUE, murine TYPHUS, and possibly TULAREMIA.

flesh-eating bacteria   The popular name for "necrotizing fasciitis," a severe but rare invasive group A strep infection of the skin that can destroy deep muscle in a matter of hours. This type of severe skin infection spreads with an invasive speed that is truly incredible.

Several cases of the disease occurred in 1994 in parts of the northeastern United States, the United Kingdom, and Ontario, Canada. It is more likely to attack adults than children, as well as patients who have just undergone surgery. The cases in Great Britain set off a wave of hysteria about this so-called new disease, and drew massive media attention—even the venerable London *Times* trumpeted that the public should not panic as "death toll rises to 12."

In fact, the country was *not* being gripped by some deadly, new and unknown infection; necrotizing fasciitis appears in about 1,500 to 2,000 cases each year in the United States, killing about 30 percent of those affected.

Cause   The bacterium releases a toxin that tunnels beneath the skin, destroying fat and muscle. Scientists believe that the toxin is able to trick the body's immune system so that instead of attacking the bacteria, the cells of the immune system join forces with the toxin to destroy fat and muscle.

Certain strains of group A strep are more likely to cause this invasive disease. In children, the most common risk factor for developing this disease is CHICKEN POX.

Symptoms   Onset of symptoms is typically rapid; symptoms often begin at the site of a minor wound (or no obvious wound at all) or with breathing problems. There may be swelling of an arm or leg, and the skin is very painful, red, and hot. This may be followed by the appearance of blisters filled with clear fluid, which quickly turn deep red or red-violet, followed by tissue death. The toxins can produce shock and infection throughout the body, with rapid heartbeat and organ failure; onset of illness to hospitalization may take only a day or two. In the most serious cases, death may occur within hours. Reduced blood flow may lead to gangrene. Severe pain at the site of infection is an early, and striking, symptom.

Diagnosis   The infection is diagnosed with blood cultures or aspiration of pus; surgical exploration may be needed. The clinical appearance is unmistakable as tissue dies and liquefies so quickly.

Treatment   Prompt medical attention is critical to survival. Penicillin is the drug of choice. Surgery (removal of infected tissue and limb amputation) is essential to stop the spread of bacteria. Even with treatment, about one third of patients stricken with this lethal bacteria will die, and many are significantly disfigured.

flies and infection   Flies are capable of transmitting at least 65 different diseases, including TYPHOID FEVER, DYSENTERY, CHOLERA, and TUBERCULOSIS. They feed on fecal matter, discharge from wounds and sores, and decayed matter such as spoiled food, spreading the disease organisms they pick up by regurgitating and excreting wherever they land. Because the fly's mouth parts are adapted for sponging up liquids, they are able to feed on solid food only by vomiting on it; the saliva liquefies the solid food, which the fly then soaks up.

Houseflies live only about two and a half weeks during the summer, but they can survive up to three months at lower temperatures. Female flies deposit from 100 to 150 eggs in decaying matter (like grass clippings, garbage, or human/animal waste). Depending on the temperature, the eggs hatch into maggots between eight hours and two days later. Mature maggots burrow for protection into dry surrounding areas, where they eventually mature into adult houseflies. Within two days of maturity, adult flies mate again, and the cycle begins anew.

To control the spread of houseflies, it is important to limit their food sources by controlling sanitation. Homeowners should not allow garbage, grass clippings, weed piles, or other decaying organic matter to build up. (Compost piles are not usually a fly-breeding site unless the compost is wet.) Trash cans should be clean and covered tightly. Window and door screens can keep flies outside. Since flies can enter buildings through ventilation holes, screening should keep them out. Ultraviolet light traps, fly traps, fly swatters, baited fly traps, and other devices can eliminate flies within the home. Chemical control should be the last resort and used only for severe infestations.

flu See INFLUENZA.

fluke A parasitic flatworm of the class Trematoda, including the genus *Schistosoma*. See also SCHISTOSOMIASIS.

folliculitis Inflammation of at least one hair follicle by *Staphylococcus* bacteria. Although this condition can occur anywhere on the skin, it is most often found on bearded areas of the face, neck, armpits, thighs, or buttocks. Folliculitis on the face may lead to pustules; in the armpits, it may cause a BOIL.

Treatment Antibiotics, drainage, and clean linen help cure the infection.

Prevention Because the infection may be spread from one person to the next in the same household, each family member should use separate towels and washcloths, bathe often, and wash clothing well.

fomites Nonliving material (like bed linens) that may convey disease-causing organisms.

Food and Drug Administration, U.S. (USFDA) A federal agency responsible for the enforcement of federal regulations regarding the manufacture and distribution of food, drugs, cosmetics, and vitamins. The agency is the consumers' protection against the sale of harmful products.

food poisoning Food poisoning and food-borne infections include a large group of toxic processes caused by eating food contaminated by toxic substances, by bacteria, or by bacteria-containing toxins. Usually, a person has to eat food contaminated with large amounts of certain germs—bacteria or parasites. Food poisoning is one of the most common causes of acute illness. The most common food-borne diseases are infections caused by bacteria such as *CAMPYLOBACTER* and *SALMONELLA*, which enters the body within contaminated foods such as poultry and eggs.

More than 250 different diseases caused by contaminated food or drink have been identified. Most food items that carry disease are raw or undercooked foods of animal origin, such as meat, milk, eggs, cheese, fish, or shellfish. About 400 to 500 food-borne disease outbreaks are reported each year; not all diseases are likely to be reported, and many cases are sporadic.

SYMPTOMS OF FOOD POISONING

If you have	It could be
Abdominal pain, fever, nausea, vomiting, and diarrhea one week after poisoning	Anisakiasis
Diarrhea, nausea/vomiting appearing 1–6 hours after eating	*Bacillus cereus*
Slurred speech, double vision, muscle paralysis 4–36 hours after meal	Botulism
Cramps, fever, diarrhea, nausea/vomiting appearing 1–5 days after eating and lasting up to 10 days	Campylobacteriosis
Explosive watery diarrhea, abdominal cramps, dehydration; symptoms begin suddenly 1–5 days after infection	Cholera
Nausea, vomiting, and diarrhea within 6–12 hours after eating fish, followed by low blood pressure and heart rate, severe itching, temperature reversal, numbness/tingling of extremities (may last months)	Ciguatera
Watery diarrhea, nausea/vomiting appearing within hours to a week after eating; severe cases include blood diarrhea; enterhemorrhagic infection includes bloody diarrhea and kidney failure	*E. coli*
Mild abdominal pain and diarrhea, nausea/vomiting 6–16 hours after eating	Food poisoning
Explosive diarrhea; foul-smelling, greasy feces; stomach pain; gas; appetite loss; nausea; and vomiting; incubation period 1–2 weeks	Giardiasis
Fever, headache, diarrhea, meningitis, conjunctivitis, miscarriage appearing within days to weeks after ingestion	Listeriosis
Burning mouth/extremities, nausea, vomiting, and diarrhea *within hours* after ingestion	Neurotoxic shellfish poisoning
Burning mouth/extremities, nausea/vomiting, diarrhea, muscle weakness, paralysis, breathing problems *within minutes* after ingestion	Paralytic shellfish poisoning
Diarrhea, rumbling bowels, fever, vomiting, cramps 6–72 hours after ingestion	Salmonellosis
Gastroenteritis, diarrhea, nausea/vomiting 1–7 days after eating	Shigellosis
Explosive diarrhea, cramps, vomiting not longer than a day, between 30 minutes–6 hours after eating	*Staphylococcal* food poisoning
Diarrhea, nausea/vomiting, fever followed by muscle pain and stiffness 2–3 weeks after ingestion	Trichinosis
Gastroenteritis, explosive diarrhea, nausea/vomiting, cramps (*V. vulnificus* can lead to fatal blood infection) 8–30 hours after eating	Vibrio food poisoning (*V. parahaemolyticus, V. vulnificus*)

Any illness that appears suddenly and causes stomach pain, vomiting, and diarrhea should be a suspected case of food poisoning. Estimates of the number of food-borne illnesses vary between a low of 6 million to a high of 81 million cases yearly, with 9,100 deaths, according to the Centers for Disease Control and Prevention. At least one third of the cases have been traced to poultry and meat. According to the Food and Drug Administration, just about everyone experiences a food-borne illness at least once a year, whether it is realized or not. Between 21 and 81 million cases of diarrhea related to food-bore illness are treated in the United States each year. Some food-borne diseases such as BOTULISM or TRICHINOSIS are becoming less common, whereas others such as SALMONELLOSIS or ESCHERICHIA COLI are becoming more common.

The greatest danger from food poisoning is not the toxin itself but the body's natural response to poison—vomiting and diarrhea—that robs the body of vital fluids. If dehydration becomes serious, food poisoning victims need to be hospitalized and given fluids intravenously. However, poisoning from *E.* *coli* bacteria can lead to severe enterohemorrhagic infection that can include bloody diarrhea, leading to kidney failure. It is this type of food poisoning from improperly cooked hamburgers that killed several young children in 1993.

Symptoms   While the time between ingestion and onset of symptoms varies according to the cause of poisoning, symptoms usually develop with some types of shellfish poisoning between 1 and 12 hours for bacterial toxins and between 12 and 48 hours for viral and *Salmonella* infections. Symptoms also vary

---

HOW TO PREVENT FOOD POISONING

Meat, poultry, and eggs are most vulnerable to contamination during storage, preparation, cooking, and serving. To stay healthy, try to observe proper food handling and kitchen safety tips:

- *Proper refrigeration* Temperature in the refrigerator must be 40 degrees F or below (0 degrees F in the freezer). Cooling doesn't kill bacteria, but it stops their growth. Allow air to circulate around refrigerated items. Always wrap food in refrigerator to keep off bacteria in the air.
- *Wash hands* To avoid contamination by bacteria or other organisms when preparing food, wash hands thoroughly with soap and water *before* and *after* handling food.
- *Wash utensils* Wash cutting board and utensils with hot soapy water before touching any other food with them.
- *Thawing* Don't thaw meat at room temperature; thaw meat or poultry in a microwave oven or in the refrigerator and then cook immediately.
- *Marinades* If you marinate meat or poultry, don't serve the marinade unless it has been cooked at a roiling boil for several minutes.
- *Serving* Serve meat and poultry on a clean plate with a clean utensil to avoid contaminating the cooked food with its raw juices.
- *Leftovers* Cool poultry and meat quickly when refrigerating leftovers; do not let stuffed poultry stand for long periods. Remove the stuffing after cooking and promptly refrigerate it.
- *Eggs* Never use cracked eggs, because they may contain *Salmonella* bacteria. Because even an uncracked egg may contain bacteria, cook eggs

thoroughly. Avoid raw eggs (such as in Caesar salad dressing, homemade eggnog, hollandaise sauce, etc.). Keep eggs refrigerated in their cartons in the coldest part of the refrigerator (*not* on the refrigerator door).
- *Mold* Throw out any food with mold (except for cheese, which may be eaten after the mold is trimmed off).
- *Microwave* A turntable should be used to rotate dishes as they cook; because microwave ovens heat food unevenly, cold spots in a food may harbor dangerous bacteria.
- *Cleaning* Don't season wooden salad bowls with oil; it can become rancid. Keep can opener and blender free from food. Always scrub down the sink after working with poultry or meat. Sponges in the kitchen for wiping dishes or countertops should be discarded after one week. (They should never sit in water, which encourages bacterial growth.) Clean sink and counters with detergent containing bleach to kill harmful bacteria.

For more information about food safety, call the U.S. Department of Agriculture's Meat and Poultry Hot Line at 1-800-535-4555 (in Washington, D.C., call 1-202-477-3333 between 10:00 A..M. and 4:00 P.M. For questions about storing or handling fish, call the help line of the Rhode Island Seafood Council at 1-800-EAT-FISH between 8:00 A.M. and 5:00 P.M. ET.

depending on how badly the food was contaminated, but there will often be similar symptoms regardless of the cause: nausea and vomiting, diarrhea, stomach pain, and—in severe cases—shock and collapse.

A doctor should be called if severe vomiting or diarrhea appear suddenly, if the victim collapses, or if there is a suspicion of food poisoning and the victim is a child, an elderly person, or someone with a chronic illness or otherwise compromised immune system.

Treatment   In all cases of food poisoning, symptoms should be treated much like a bout of flu, including drinking fluids (water, tea, bouillon, and ginger ale) to replace fluid loss. Mild cases may be treated at home, with clear liquids, including some salt and sugar. If the person cannot retain fluids because of vomiting, IV fluids are needed. Most cases of food poisoning are not serious (except for botulism), and recovery is usually within three days. If possible, samples of any food left from recent meals should be saved for testing.

Governmental overview began in 1906 with the passage of the Pure Food and Drug Act and the Meat Inspection Act, designed to make American food as safe as possible. In addition, three different governmental agencies are responsible for regulating and monitoring the safety of the U.S. food supply. The Food and Drug Administration is responsible for ensuring the safety and wholesomeness of all food except meat, poultry, and eggs. The Department of Agriculture monitors the safety of poultry, meat, eggs, and egg products and conducts inspections nationwide.

Because of a range of regulatory loopholes, the governmental safety net doesn't always work effectively.

Prevention   To prevent the spread of foodborne diseases, the consumer should do the following:

- Make sure food from animal sources is thoroughly cooked or pasteurized; avoid eating such foods raw or undercooked.

SAFE FOOD STORAGE

Food	Where	How Long
Poultry		
Raw	Refrigerator	1–2 days
	Freezer	9 months
Cooked	Refrigerator	3–4 days
	Freezer	4–6 months
Seafood		
Lean, fish, raw	Refrigerator	1–2 days
	Freezer	6–8 months
Fatty fish, raw	Refrigerator	1–2 days
	Freezer	4 months
Raw shrimp	Refrigerator	1–2 days
	Freezer	9 months
Cooked seafood	Refrigerator	3 days
	Freezer	2 months
Meat		
Ground meat	Refrigerator	1–2 days
	Freezer	3–4 months
Chops (all)	Refrigerator	3–5 days
Frozen lamb chops	Freezer	6–9 months
Frozen pork chops	Freezer	4–6 months
Roasts (all)	Refrigerator	3–5 days
Frozen beef roasts	Freezer	6–12 months
Frozen veal/ pork roast	Freezer	4–6 months
Frozen lamb roast	Freezer	6–9 months
Steak	Refrigerator	3–5 days
Cooked leftovers	Refrigerator	3–4 days
	Freezer	2–3 months
Vacuum-sealed packages		
(unopened)	Refrigerator	2 weeks
(opened)	Refrigerator	3–5 days
	Freezer	1–2 months
Ham		
country dry-cure	Cupboard	1 year
soaked/cooked	Refrigerator	7 days
Dairy		
Raw eggs in shell	Refrigerator	3 weeks
Hard-boiled (in shell)	Refrigerator	1 week
Milk	Refrigerator	5 days
	Freezer	1 month
Mayonnaise (opened)	Refrigerator	1 year

Guidelines provided by the USDA and the Food Marketing Institute

KEEPING HOT FOODS SAFE

To keep hot foods safe, follow these guidelines from the U.S. Department of Agriculture:

- Use a meat thermometer to make sure meats and poultry are cooked completely. Put the thermometer into the thickest part (avoiding fat and bone). Bacteria are killed at 160 degrees F minimum.
- Cook poultry until it reaches 180 to 185 degrees F or higher (or until the juices run clear or the leg moves easily in the socket). Do not cook poultry at a low temperature for a long period of time.
- Don't partially heat food, then finish cooking later; half-cooked food may be warm enough to encourage bacterial growth but not hot enough to kill it. Subsequent cooking might not kill the bacteria.
- Allow at least one and a half times longer than usual to cook frozen foods that have not been pre-thawed.
- Keep hot foods at 140 to 160 degrees F until serving time, especially those served in chafing dishes or warmers. Food should never be kept between 40 degrees and 140 degrees for more than two hours, as this encourages bacterial growth.
- Thoroughly reheat leftovers, and make sure food is evenly heated. Gravies should be brought to a roiling boil.
- The healthiest way to cook a steak is to pre-cook it in a microwave just before broiling or barbecuing. Precook the steak on high for 30 to 90 seconds. Make sure to discard the juice.

GUARD AGAINST SPOILAGE AT THE FOOD STORE

Look for these signs of potential problems at the grocery store:

- Frozen meat: white or bleached color
- Lamb: brown color
- Pork: darkened lean meat and discolored or rancid rind products
- Fish: gray, brown, or greenish gills that feel dry to the touch; cloudy, reddish, sunken, or depressed eyes; soft, easily torn flesh; noticeably strong fishy or ammonia odor
- Clams, oysters, and mussels: should be tightly closed (i.e., still alive); if slightly open, tap—if the shell doesn't close, don't buy it
- Poultry: soft flabby flesh, purplish or greenish color, abnormal odor, stickiness under wings and joints, darkened wing tips
- Thermometer in meat/fish case should be below 45 degrees F
- Check "sell by" date, but realize that if the product is not spoiled, the meat market can legally repackage the product with a new "sell by" date

Packaged Foods
- The package should not be torn, damaged, opened, or contain spoiled or moldy food
- Product must originate from government-inspected, approved source
- Check for common product name; company/brand name; address of produce or distributor; list of ingredients in descending order of amount present, net weight, or volume

Canned Foods
- Canned food with rust or corrosion, or those exposed to temperature extremes, *will spoil*
- Don't buy dented cans, especially if dent affects seal
- Check for leaking, bulging, swollen cans, food with foul odor, or any container which spurts liquid when you open it, or contains milky liquids

- Keep juices or drippings from raw meat, poultry, shellfish, or eggs from contaminating other food.
- Don't leave potentially contaminated food for extended periods of time at temperatures that allow bacteria to grow.
- Promptly refrigerate leftovers and food prepared in advance.

The single most important way to prevent food-borne illness is thorough cooking, which kills most food-borne bacteria, toxins, viruses, and parasites. In addition, proper food preparation—washing hands, cutting board, and knife with soap and water before and right after handling raw meat, poultry, seafood, or

IS YOUR TEMPORARY FOOD FACILITY/PICNIC AREA SAFE?

- Booth covering temporary food facility must be wood, canvas, plastic, tarp, or similar material
- During food preparation, most (if not all) of booth must be completely enclosed using fine mesh fly screen
- All food must be prepared in approved, licensed food establishment or on premises of temporary food facility; no food or beverage stored or prepared in private home can be offered for sale, sold, or given away from a temporary food facility (except for nonperishable home-prepared bakery products, which can be sold from nonprofit food stands only)

HOW TO REPORT CASES OF SUSPECTED FOOD POISONING

According to the U.S. Department of Agriculture's Safety and Inspection Service, consumers should report possible food poisoning in three situations:

- If the food was eaten at a large gathering
- If the food was from a restaurant, deli, sidewalk vendor, or other kitchen that serves more than a few people
- If the food is a commercial product (such as canned goods or frozen food), since contaminants may have affected an entire batch

When making a report, officials need to know the following:

- Your name, address, telephone number
- A detailed explanation of the problem
- When and where the food was eaten
- Who ate it
- Name and address of the place where the food was obtained

If the food is a commercial product:

- Provide the manufacturer's name and address
- Product's lot or batch number
- If the tainted food is meat or poultry, look for the USDA inspection stamp on the wrapper, which will identify the plant where the food was made or packaged

FOOD SAFETY AT PICNICS

- Use an insulated cooler with an ice or frozen gel-pack on top, with foods that need to be kept coldest on the bottom
- Pack food right from the refrigerator
- Wrap food separately in plastic, and don't place directly on ice that's not drinking-water quality. Separate raw fish, meat, or poultry so drippings don't contaminate other food
- Keep cooler in the shade, not the trunk; keep the lid on
- Keep utensils and food covered when not in use
- Keep hot foods hot in an insulated dish or vacuum bottle
- Take along disposal wipes to clean hands before and after food preparation
- Don't leave your food unrefrigerated longer than two hours (one hour if temperature is above 85 degrees F)

eggs will help stop the spread of contamination. Anyone who is sick with diarrhea or vomiting shouldn't prepare food for others.

It's also important to monitor the food supply. In the United States, conditions under which food animals are raised have changed. But we now import 30 billion tons of food a year, including fruit, vegetables, seafood, and canned goods, which often come from developing countries where food hygiene and basic sanitation is poor.

The centralization of the food industry means that a single contaminated product may appear in different foods and different forms, potentially infecting a great number of people. In addition, new and emerging foodborne pathogens are constantly being identified, which cause diseases that weren't recognized 50 years ago. These include bacteria, parasites, viruses, and toxins.

Information on food-borne disease outbreaks can be obtained as follows: Public Inquiries, Centers for Disease Control, 1600 Clifton Road, Atlanta, GA 30333.

Fort Bragg fever Another name for LEP-
TOSPIROSIS, an infection caused by the organism of the genus *Leptospira,* associated with
the urine of a variety of wild and domestic
animals. The disease was first identified in
recruits at Fort Bragg, North Carolina, during
the summer of 1942, when army personnel
came down with high fevers, headaches,
rashes, and other symptoms. They had caught
the disease by swimming in freshwater ponds
and streams contaminated by livestock urine.
See also WEIL'S SYNDROME.

Francisella tularensis The name of the bacteria that causes TULAREMIA, an infectious disease of wild animals occasionally found in
humans. The bacterium was formerly known
as *Pasteurella tularensis.*

fungal infection A disease of the skin (also
called mycoses) caused by the spread of
FUNGI. This type of disease may range from a
mild condition to fatal symptoms. Fungal skin
infections are either considered "superficial"
(affecting skin, hair, nails) or "subcutaneous"
(beneath the skin).

The *superficial* fungal infections include
THRUSH (candidiasis) and TINEA (including
RINGWORM and ATHLETE'S FOOT). *Subcutaneous
infections* are rare; the most common is
SPOROTRICHOSIS, occurring after a scratch becomes contaminated with a certain species of
fungus. Examples of this type of condition
occur in tropical climates.

Causes Harmless fungi are present all the
time on the skin, but they do not multiply
there because of bacterial competition or
because the body's immune system fights
them off. Fungal infections of the skin are
most common in those taking long-term
antibiotics or those taking corticosteroid or
immunosuppressant drugs, or in patients with
an immune system disorder (such as AIDS).

Treatment Physicians use three classes of
drugs to fight fungal disease, but in the past
five years disease-causing fungi have begun

to grow resistant to common drugs, just like
some types of bacteria. Strains of fungi resistant to each of the three types of drugs are
now common in hospitals that care for the
sickest patients—especially patients with cancer and AIDS. This growing resistance
appears to have developed for the same reasons that bacteria have grown impervious: the
use of drugs to combat fungal infections.

High use of antifungal medications occurred because of the large number of people
with impaired immune systems due to AIDS
and chemotherapy. Between 5 to 10 percent of
AIDS patients now have resistant fungi that
cause oral CANDIDIASIS, a common mouth
infection.

fungi A phylum of plants (including yeasts,
rusts, slime molds, smuts, mushrooms, etc.)
characterized by the absence of chlorophyll
and the presence of a rigid cell wall. There are
more than 100,000 different species of fungi
around the world, most of which are harmless
or beneficial to human health (such as molds
used to produce antibiotics, yeasts used in
baking and brewing, edible mushrooms and
truffles, etc.).

However, some fungi can invade and form
colonies in the skin or underneath the skin,
leading to disorders ranging from a mild skin
irritation and inflammation to severe or fatal
systemic infections. See also FUNGAL INFEC-
TION.

Fungi reproduce by sending out spores
(cells that resemble plant seeds). When a
spore lands in a moist place, it sends out
small threads from which the fungus feeds.
These moist places that support fungi include
dead plant and animal matter and BACTERIA.

fungicide A drug that kills FUNGI.

furuncle Another name for a BOIL, this is a
skin infection caused by bacteria that enter
through the hair follicle, forming a painful
pus-filled nodule.

Cause The boil is most often caused by a *Staphylococcus*, which multiplies in a skin gland or hair follicle. Patients must not irritate or squeeze the lesion or they will spread the infection into adjacent tissue.

Symptoms Pain, redness, and swelling, with tissue death deep in the center of the inflamed area, which forms a core of dead tissue.

Treatment Local care, moist heat, and incision and drainage.

G

gangrene Death of tissue generally associated with loss of blood supply, followed by bacterial invasion and putrefaction. It may affect either a fairly small area of skin or an entire limb. It can also occur in the intestines or gallbladder. Internally, gangrene may be a complication of strangulated hernia, appendicitis, or cholecystitis, or impaired blood supply.

Cause In *dry gangrene,* an area of the skin dies because of blocked blood supply, without bacterial infection; this type does not spread to other tissue. It may be caused by arteriosclerosis, diabetes mellitus, a stroke, blood clot, or frostbite. *Wet (or moist) gangrene* follows bacterial infection of dry gangrene or the obstruction of blood flow following a wound. This form of gangrene has an offensive odor, spreads rapidly, and may be fatal in a few days.

Gas gangrene is a particularly virulent form of wet gangrene caused by a deadly type of bacteria (such as various species of CLOSTRID-*IUM,* particularly *C. perfringens*) that destroy muscle while producing a foul odor. Gas gangrene is responsible for millions of deaths during war and is also known as anaerobic myositis and necrotizing fasciitis (FLESH-EAT-ING BACTERIA).

Symptoms Pain in the dying skin tissue that becomes numb and black once the tissue dies. If bacterial infection occurs, the gangrene will spread, giving off a noxious odor with redness, swelling, and oozing pus around the blackened area. Gas gangrene causes pain, swelling, and tenderness of the wound area, with moderate fever, rapid heartbeat, and low blood pressure. The skin around the wound begins to die and rupture, revealing muscle. The patient may also experience toxic delirium. Untreated, gas gangrene is usually fatal.

Treatment In all types of gangrene, surgical debridement is necessary to remove the dead tissue before healing can begin. Improving circulation to the affected area can improve dry gangrene if it is begun early enough. Once the tissue becomes infected, antibiotics are given to prevent the spread of infection. Once wet gangrene is diagnosed, amputation of the affected part is required, along with neighboring healthy tissue, in order to save the patient.

Prevention Gangrene of an extremity with no blood supply (such as vascular disease of toes and feet) can't be prevented once the tissue has lost its oxygen supply.

If possible, wound gangrene is best avoided by meticulous wound care, removal of dead tissue, and maintaining blood supply and cleanliness. Gangrene is a natural process that occurs in the presence of dead tissue; therefore, removing dead tissue helps prevent gangrene. It can be quickly fatal in certain conditions where the infection itself corrodes and destroys healthy skin in a rapid, catastrophic way.

Emergency surgery to remove all of the affected tissue must be done to save the patient's life. This surgery is often radical and deforming.

Gardnerella vaginalis See VAGINITIS.

gas bacillus One of several species of bacillus that produce a gas as a byproduct of metabolism. Examples of gas bacilli include *E. coli* and the clostridial species that produce gas gangrene. See *ESCHERICHIA COLI.*

gastroenteritis, bacterial Inflammation of the stomach and intestines as a result of bacterial infection. See also DIARRHEA AND INFECTIOUS

DISEASE; TRAVELER'S DIARRHEA; ANTIDIARRHEAL DRUGS.

Cause It can be caused by bacterial ENTEROTOXINS.

Symptoms Between two to five days after eating, victims experience fever, headache, nausea, diarrhea, and a sickness often mistaken for the flu. It is common in children but also appears in adults.

Treatment Mild cases can be treated at home. Bed rest, sedation, and IV fluids if the patient is severely dehydrated. If the precise enterotoxin is known, medication and treatment with the appropriate antitoxin may bring relief. After the symptoms subside, water may be given by mouth; if this is not followed by nausea, clear fluids may be added followed by a bland diet. In most cases, the illness subsides slowly without any special treatment; recovery is usually complete.

Prevention Preparing food carefully with attention to hygiene can reduce the chances of gastroenteritis. Those who care for patients with this condition must be meticulous about their own hygiene in order not to spread the infection further.

gastroenteritis, viral Inflammation of the stomach and intestines caused by viral infection. See also DIARRHEA AND INFECTIOUS DISEASE; ANTIDIARRHEAL DRUGS; TRAVELER'S DIARRHEA.

Symptoms Lack of appetite and sudden and violent onset of vomiting and nausea, abdominal discomfort, and diarrhea.

Treatment Bed rest, sedation, and IV fluids if the patient is severely dehydrated. After the symptoms subside, water may be given by mouth; if this is not followed by nausea, clear fluids may be added, followed by a bland diet.

genital herpes See HERPES, GENITAL.

genital papilloma virus See PAPILLOMAVIRUS, HUMAN.

genital warts See WARTS, GENITAL.

genitourinary tract infection See URINARY TRACT INFECTION.

germ The popular term for any microorganism that causes disease. Either a virus or a bacterium is an example of a germ.

German measles The common name for rubella, this is a viral infection that is not very similar to MEASLES, although it also causes a rash on the face, trunk, and limbs. Rubella, which causes a mild illness in children and a slightly more problematic one in adults, is really serious only when contracted by pregnant women in the early months of gestation. During this time, there is a chance the virus will infect the fetus, which can lead to a range of serious birth defects known as rubella syndrome.

Although rubella was once found throughout the world, it is now much less common in most developed countries because of successful vaccination programs. The United States has tried to eradicate the disease by vaccinating all school-age children; in 1969 when the vaccine became available, at least 60,000 Americans had rubella. By 1993, the number dropped to 192.

Cause Rubella is caused by the rubella virus, which is transmitted by particles in the air when an infected person coughs or sneezes. It can also be transmitted on contaminated objects, where the virus can survive for a short period of time on tissues, doorknobs, phones, and so on. It infects only humans.

Before the development of the vaccine, rubella was common in spring and winter, and peaked every six to nine years. There were huge rubella epidemics in the United States in 1935, 1943, and 1964.

Symptoms The infection usually affects youngsters between the ages of 6 and 12 with the rash that starts on the face and spreads downward and out to arms and legs. The rash may run together to make large patches, but it does not itch. It lasts for a few days, with a slight fever and enlarged lymph nodes; some children may have a mild cough, sore throat, or runny nose before the rash appears. Sometimes the entire infection comes and goes without notice; at least 30 percent of children with rubella have no symptoms at all, although they are infectious to others.

Adolescents and adults may have slightly more pronounced symptoms, including headaches, fever, body aches, eye infections, or a runny nose about one to five days before the rash. Swollen glands in the neck and behind the ear typically appear 7 to 10 days before the rash. The virus may be transmitted from a few days before the symptoms appear until a day after symptoms fade.

Incubation period ranges from 14 to 23 days; the average is 16 to 18 days.

Rubella may be confused with other conditions characterized by rashes, such as SCARLET FEVER or drug allergy.

Diagnosis   A lab test to confirm rubella is important, since the symptoms can be so mild they may be overlooked or mistaken for something else. This is especially true during an outbreak where pregnant women may be exposed.

Blood tests are available that reveal rubella immunity or an active rubella infection. If a person has been vaccinated, the blood test will show that the person is immune. Pregnant women need a rubella immunity test at the first prenatal visit; if not immune, the woman will receive rubella vaccine in the hospital after delivery.

If a pregnant woman gets an infection resembling rubella during pregnancy, and she is not immune, blood tests must be done to determine whether rubella is the cause of the illness.

Treatment   There is no specific treatment for rubella, although acetaminophen may reduce the fever.

Complications   Congenital rubella is the most serious complication of rubella infection, since it can cause fetal death or miscarriage. The risk is highest when the pregnant woman is infected in the first 12 weeks of pregnancy (miscarriage rate is as high as 85 percent during this time). At 14 to 16 weeks, the risk drops to just 10 to 24 percent, and after 20 weeks the risk is almost nonexistent.

Infants who survive infection in the womb may be born with a variety of birth defects, including deafness, eye problems (including blindness), heart defects, mental retardation, growth retardation, and bleeding disorders.

Rare complications in adults include bleeding disorders or ENCEPHALITIS.

Prevention   Any child with rubella must be kept at home until well past the infectious stage; babies born with rubella have the infection virus in their nose, throat, and urine for as long as a year.

Vaccination can provide long-lasting immunity. It is given in the United States to all infants as part of the measles and mumps vaccine at about 15 months of age. There is not usually any reaction to the vaccine. The vaccine is a live attenuated virus that provides complete protection to more than 95 percent of those who receive it. Rubella infection itself also provides immunity.

The recommended vaccine, MMR (measles, mumps, rubella), is not effective when given earlier than 12 months because the baby may have maternal antibodies that will interfere with the vaccine's action. A first dose is given at 12 to 15 months; a second booster is given at age four to six, before the child starts school. Older children who missed these shots should receive one dose of MMR.

Women of childbearing age can be given the vaccine if they are not already immune. Anyone who is not sure of having received the vaccine or having rubella should be vaccinated. There is no risk to receiving the vaccine if a person is already immune.

Rubella is common in many countries; anyone who travels abroad should be sure they are immune to rubella or receive the vaccine before leaving. The national recommendations for rubella elimination are as follows:

- vaccination for all children
- premarital screening, vaccination for those who need it
- prenatal screening and postpartum vaccination if needed
- routine vaccination in a medical setting
- proof of immunity for hospital workers and college students

There are some people who should not receive the vaccine. These include pregnant women or women who plan to become pregnant within the next three months; anyone with a high fever or a severe allergy to neomycin. There is no penicillin in rubella vaccine, and it is safe for those allergic to eggs.

germicide   A drug that kills microorganisms.

Giardia lamblia   A type of protozoa (found in the intestinal tract and in feces of humans, sheep, cattle, and beaver) that causes foul-smelling, explosive diarrhea called GIARDIASIS. The protozoa was named for the 19th-century French biologist Alfred Giard, who discovered it. It is most often found in tropical areas and in those who travel to the tropics. Recently, it has become more common in the developed countries, where it is especially common in preschools and among people living in institutions. See also DIARRHEA AND INFECTIOUS DISEASE; ANTIDIARRHEAL DRUGS.

giardiasis   The most common cause of waterborne intestinal infection in the United States, giardiasis is an infection of the small intestine caused by the GIARDIA LAMBLIA protozoa, which is found in the human intestinal tract and in feces. In recent years, outbreaks of giardiasis have been common among people in institutions, preschool children, at catered affairs, and large public picnic areas. Recent tests have revealed the parasite in 7 percent of all stool samples tested in a nationwide study. See also DIARRHEA AND INFECTIOUS DISEASE; ANTIDIARRHEAL DRUGS; TRAVELER'S DIARRHEA.

Cause   Giardiasis is spread by contaminated food or water or by direct personal hand-to-mouth contact. Children can spread the infection by touching contaminated toys, changing tables, utensils, or their own feces. For this reason, the infection spreads quickly through a day care center or institution for the developmentally disabled. Unfiltered streams or lakes that may be contaminated by human or animal feces are a common source of infection to campers.

Symptoms   Giardiasis is not fatal, and about two thirds of infected people have no symptoms. When they do occur, symptoms appear about one to three days after infection and are uncomfortable. The infection interferes with the body's ability to absorb fats in the intestinal tract, so the stool is filled with fat. Symptoms include explosive diarrhea, foul-smelling and greasy feces, stomach pains, gas, loss of appetite, nausea, and vomiting. In some cases, the infection can become chronic.

Diagnosis   Giardiasis is diagnosed by examining three stool samples for the presence of the parasites. Because the parasite is shed intermittently, half of the infections will be missed if only one specimen gets checked. Stool collection kits are available for this purpose.

A different test looks for the proteins of *Giardia* in the stool sample.

Treatment   Acute giardiasis usually runs its course and then clears up, but antibiotics will help relieve symptoms and prevent the spread of infection. Medications include metronidazole, furazolidone, and paromomycin. Occasionally, treatment fails; in this case, the patient should wait two weeks and repeat the medication. Anyone with an impaired immune system may need to combine medications. Healthy carriers do not need to be treated.

Complications Some children get chronic infection and suffer with diarrhea and cramps for long periods of time, losing weight and growing poorly. Those most at risk for an infection are people with impaired immune function, malnourished children, people with low stomach acid, and older people.

Prevention The best way to avoid giardiasis is to stay away from drinking untreated surface water. While chlorine in water treatment will not kill the cysts, filtered public water supplies eliminate it. Also

- maintain good personal hygiene
- don't eat unwashed fruit or vegetables unless they can be peeled
- boil water if in doubt; campers should boil stream water for three minutes before drinking
- if an outbreak occurs in a child care center, the director should notify the local health department. Children with severe diarrhea must stay at home until the stool returns to normal

gingivitis See GUM DISEASE.

glanders An endemic infection (found in Asia, Africa, and South America) that afflicts horses and donkeys and may occasionally be transmitted to humans. The disease has been eradicated in Europe and North America.

Cause The infection is caused by the bacterium *Pseudomonas mallei* transmitted to humans from horses or other domestic animals.

Symptoms Glanders causes an ulcer or abscess where it enters a wound in the skin. If untreated, it may spread to the bones, liver, central nervous system, and other tissues and may be fatal.

Treatment Early treatment with an antibiotic clears the infection.

gonorrhea The most commonly reported communicable disease in the United States, most often affecting the genitourinary tract and (sometimes) the pharynx, eyes, or rectum. Since 1980 the number of people with gonorrhea has been declining; still, in 1993, 440,000 Americans were infected. Many more cases go unreported. People are at risk if they have more than one sex partner or don't use condoms. Most victims (75 percent) are between the ages of 15 and 24. Gonorrheal infections must be reported to local health departments in the United States.

Cause The disease is caused by a spherical bacterium, NEISSERIA GONORRHOEAE, that is always grouped in pairs. It is passed from one person to the next during sex. It is not possible to get gonorrhea from toilet seats or swimming pools.

A woman who has unprotected sex with an infected man has an 80 to 90 percent chance of being infected herself—a much higher rate than with other STDs. But a man who has unprotected sex with an infected woman has only a 20 to 25 percent chance of becoming infected. Men have less risk because it's harder for bacteria to enter the body through the penis than through the vaginal walls.

Symptoms Between three to five days after exposure, symptoms will appear in the genital or rectal area, or in the throat (depending on the sexual practice). Up to 80 percent of infected men experience painful urination, frequent urge to urinate, and white or yellow thick pus from the penis. About half of infected women have swelling of the vagina, abnormal green-yellow vaginal discharge, vaginal bleeding between periods, pelvic discomfort (itching and burning), and pain when urinating. Very few pregnant women have symptoms.

As the infection spreads—which is more common in women than in men—there may be nausea and vomiting, fever, and rapid heartbeat, or peritonitis. Inflammation of the tissues surrounding the liver also may occur, causing pain in the upper abdomen. Severe cases of gonorrhea are also more common in women and are characterized by signs of blood poisoning, with tender lesions on the skin of the hands and feet and inflammation of the tendons of the wrists, knees, and ankles. If the disease spreads to the conjunctiva of the eyes, there may be scarring and blindness.

In both men and women, infection in the throat causes a mild, red, sore throat.

Diagnosis   Culture of the organism from body fluids.

Treatment   For many years, penicillin was the drug of choice, but in the late 1970s the bacteria became resistant. The most resistant strains are found in New York, California, and Florida, but resistance is seen in all states and most of Canada.

Today, treatment involves two antibiotics: a shot of ceftriaxone and doxycycline pills. The pills will also cure CHLAMYDIA, which has similar symptoms to gonorrhea (many people have both infections). Alternatively, instead of a shot a doctor may give a single dose of cefixime, ciprofloxacin, or ofloxacin. Pregnant women get a shot of ceftriazone and erythromycin pills.

An infant born with the symptoms of gonorrhea must be hospitalized and given ceftriaxone.

Complications   PELVIC INFLAMMATORY DISEASE develops in almost 40 percent of untreated women and causes scars in the tubes, infertility, and tubal pregnancies. Untreated pregnant women may experience an infection in the amniotic fluid, smaller babies, or premature birth. Babies born to infected mothers may have gonorrhea conjunctivitis during delivery; untreated infants can become blind. For this reason, drops are placed in all babies' eyes at birth to prevent gonorrhea and chlamydia conjunctivitis.

In men, untreated gonorrhea can lead to infections of the testicles or scar the urethra, which can lead to sterility.

Gonyaulax catanella   A (species of) plankton protozoa that produce a toxin ingested by shellfish along the North American coasts. Eating these toxic shellfish can lead to SHELLFISH POISONING. These protozoa also cause so-called RED TIDE because large numbers of the protozoa color the sea red.

Treatment   There is no known antidote for shellfish poisoning caused by toxin-producing plankton. Administration of prostigmine may be effective, together with artificial respiration and oxygen as needed.

gram-negative shock   See SEPTIC SHOCK.

granuloma   Grouping of cells associated with chronic inflammation, which can occur in any part of the body. Granulomas are usually a reaction to certain infectious agents, although they may occur with no known cause.

Certain infections, such as LEPROSY and SYPHILIS can lead to infective granulomas in many different organs of the body. A pyogenic granuloma is a common benign skin tumor that develops after a minor injury. Pyogenic granulomas can be surgically removed or treated with cryosurgery. See GRANULOMA, INFECTIOUS; GRANULOMA INGUINALE.

granuloma, infectious   A lumpy lesion of GRANULOMA tissue that may develop in diseases such as TUBERCULOSIS, SYPHILIS, ACTINOMYCOSIS, LEPROSY, or other tissue-invading organisms.

granuloma inguinale   A chronic bacterial infection of the genital region, usually assumed to be a sexually transmitted disease. This relatively rare disease occurs most frequently in men living in tropical and subtropical areas.

In the United States, homosexuals are at greater risk; it is relatively rare in heterosexual partners of those affected. Past infection does not confer immunity, and there is no evidence of natural resistance.

Cause   The disease is caused by the bacteria *Calymmatobacterium granulomatis,* a small gram-negative rod-shaped bacillus. It is spread by sexual contact with an infected individual. Granuloma inguinale is communicable as long as the infected person remains untreated and bacteria from the lesions are present.

Symptoms   Within 8 to 80 days after infection, lumps or blisters in the genital area appear, becoming a slowly widening sore. Untreated, the lesions will spread, deepen, multiply, and may become infected.

Diagnosis   Microscopic examination and identification of a smear taken from a lesion and stained.

Treatment   Several antibiotics, including streptomycin, will cure the disease; the sores usually will completely heal within five weeks. All patients who are suspected of having this disease are also tested for SYPHILIS, since infection with both diseases is common.

Complications   If left untreated, granuloma inguinale can cause extensive destruction of the genitals and may spread to other parts of the body.

group A strep   See STREPTOCOCCUS, GROUP A.

group B strep   See STREPTOCOCCUS, GROUP B.

Gulf War syndrome, bacterial cause   Some experts suggest that bacteria may cause at least some of the cases of Gulf War syndrome, a constellation of symptoms including joint and muscle pain, memory loss, depression, skin rashes, and chronic fatigue suffered by veterans of the 1991 Gulf War. The U.S. government insists there is no single Gulf War syndrome. A number of causes have been given for the problems, ranging from chemical weapons exposure to interaction between medications and vaccines.

gum disease   Infection at the roots of the teeth that cause bleeding and receding gums that—if unchecked—can lead to tooth loss. *Gingivitis* is an early, reversible stage of gum disease characterized by inflammation of the gums. Mild gum disease is very common in young adults; it is especially common among pregnant women and diabetics because of their changing hormone levels.

Cause   Gingivitis occurs when plaque (which contains bacteria) is allowed to collect around the base of the teeth. Experts believe that toxins produced by bacteria within the plaque irritate the gums, causing them to become infected, tender, and swollen.

Symptoms   Bleeding gums are nearly always a symptom of gingivitis. Other symptoms include a reddish purple color of the gums, and a soft, shiny, swollen appearance.

Treatment   Good oral hygiene is the main way to both treat and prevent gum disease. In severe cases of gum disease (periodontitis), the dentist will surgically remove part of the gum margin (a technique called gingivectomy) as a way of removing the pockets of infected gums. It is performed in the dentist's office using local anesthetics.

Complications   Untreated gum disease may lead to periodontitis, the advanced stage of gum disease, in which infected pockets form between the gums and the teeth. As the infection spreads, the supporting tissues of the teeth and the surrounding bone erode, loosening the teeth.

Acute necrotizing ulcerative gingivitis (trench mouth) may develop following infection with anaerobic bacteria in those with chronic gingivitis, especially those with lowered resistance to infection. This is a serious condition that can destroy gum tissue; it requires antibiotics. (See VINCENT'S DISEASE.)

New research   Scientists at the University of Michigan School of Dentistry have discovered that it is possible to treat severe root-level bacterial infections with antibiotics, not surgery. The new treatment being studied at the school includes drug capsules to be taken for two to four weeks, depending on the severity of the problem, followed by as many as three rounds of topical antibiotics. These topical drugs are administered by temporarily gluing on experimental drug-impregnated cellulose film into the root surface.

Using this regimen, researchers avoided surgery or extraction for 88 percent of their subjects, including 67 percent of those with teeth identified by other dentists as too infected to save.

Haemophilus   A genus of gram-negative bacteria often found in the respiratory tract of humans and animals. The genus includes *H. influenzae,* which causes respiratory tract infections and one form of MENINGITIS; *H. haemolyticus* affecting upper respiratory tracts; and *H. ducreyi,* which causes CHANCROID.

The *Haemophilus* genus can usually be treated with cephalosporins, tetracyclines, sulfonamides, quinalones, and monobactanes as well as penicillinase-resistant penicillins.

Haemophilus B   See HAEMOPHILUS INFLUENZAE TYPE B (HIB).

Haemophilus ducreyi   A type of bacteria that causes CHANCROID.

Haemophilus influenzae type b (Hib)   A type of rod-shaped bacterium that can cause serious diseases. It is the leading cause of bacterial MENINGITIS in children. *H. flu* meningitis is a serious infection characterized by inflammation of the brain and spinal cord that may be fatal. More than two thirds of all bacterial meningitis victims are children younger than age five; until 1992, most of them were infected with *Haemophilus influenzae* type b (usually shortened to *H. flu* or "Hib"). It's serious because nearly 1 child in every 20 who gets meningitis dies, and up to 35 percent develop permanent brain damage.

According to the Centers for Disease Control, from the 1980s more than half of the estimated 20,000 Americans aged 5 years or younger who became infected with the Hib bacterium each year developed bacterial meningitis. This disorder was the leading cause of acquired mental retardation in the United States, leaving many youngsters blind, deaf, or paralyzed.

However, widespread use of a Hib vaccine licensed for infants in 1990 has dramatically reduced the incidence of a deadly disease that only 10 years ago killed 800 infants each year in the United States. According to the Centers for Disease Control and Prevention, the incidence of invasive Hib infection has dropped by almost 98 percent among infants and children since the introduction of the vaccine. Although Hib meningitis is not yet completely eradicated, the vaccine has been stunningly effective.

Cause   The *Haemophilus influenzae* type B bacterium has several different strains, each with a different capsule around the bacterium. Type b was the most common cause of meningitis in children before the vaccine; the other types are rare. However, the bacteria causes other diseases besides meningitis; one strain (nontypeable) is a common cause of ear infections in children. Other illnesses caused by *H. influenzae* type B bacteria include EPIGLOTTITIS, septic arthritis, CELLULITIS, BACTEREMIA, and PNEUMONIA.

The bacteria enter a person's body through the nose; meningitis results if the bacteria travel through the blood into the membrane covering the brain (the meninges). Healthy children can carry the bacteria in their nose and throat secretions; the infection is spread by kissing or sharing possessions, drinks, food, etc. Child care workers can also spread the bacteria.

Symptoms   If a child is going to develop symptoms, they will appear within two weeks after exposure. All types of meningitis may appear in children either gradually or suddenly. The gradual type is harder to diagnose because the symptoms (at least at first) are vague. Much more common is the abrupt onset variety of meningitis, in which symptoms appear in less than 24 hours, with a sudden high fever (100 degrees F to 106 degrees F) chills, vomiting, stiff neck, intense headache in the front of the head, or a seizure. The neck hurts when the child tries to touch his chin to the chest. There may be muscle spasms and photophobia (eye pain from light).

Some children exhibit unusual behavior as the infection begins, including aggressiveness, irritability, agitation, delirium, or screaming, followed by lethargy or coma. Some may experience a cold or an ear infection before the onset of meningitis.

A baby from age three months to two years may exhibit fever, vomiting, irritability, seizures, and a high-pitched cry. The baby may suddenly become rigid, and the soft spot on the front of the head may become hard or bulging.

Diagnosis A lumbar puncture (spinal tap) is necessary to sample the fluid around the spinal cord and check for bacteria, white cells, sugar, and protein. This will help determine what sort of virus or bacteria is causing the meningitis. Bacterial meningitis causes cloudy fluid, with a high amount of certain types of white blood cells, low sugar, and high protein. Bacteria will grow in blood culture or spinal fluid culture in 24 to 48 hours; rapid tests on fluid or blood give results in just a few hours and are often helpful in identifying the type of bacteria.

Recent antibiotic treatment prior to getting meningitis may make diagnosis more difficult. Lumbar puncture is a safe procedure when done in a large emergency room or in an experienced pediatrician's office and is imperative in correctly diagnosing meningitis.

Treatment Without treatment, a child can die from Hib meningitis; with antibiotics, about 95 percent of children recover. Any child with possible *H. flu* meningitis will be admitted to the hospital for IV antibiotics. A baby or child would also receive dexamethasone with the antibiotic and continue to take it for two to four days to prevent swelling of the brain and subsequent hearing problems. Children should rest in a darkened, quiet room; any fever higher than 101 degrees F should be treated with acetaminophen and sponge baths.

A child with *H. flu* meningitis is considered to be infectious until after receiving 24 hours of antibiotics; however, even after recovery some children will carry bacteria in nose and mouth. Rifampin is given to eliminate this bacteria. Healthy carriers are infectious for a few weeks to a few months.

Children who recover from this type of meningitis, as well as those who are vaccinated, are immune.

Complications Increased pressure on the brain from fluid buildup is a serious complication; signs of this include changes in head measurement, activity, vision, breathing, pupils' response to light, or decrease in urine.

The most common long-lasting complication is hearing impairment. Recent studies suggest that children over six weeks of age who received dexamethasone immediately had less hearing loss than those who did not receive the steroid.

Other, less common, complications include blindness, hydrocephalus, arthritis, seizures, and permanent developmental delays.

Prevention The best prevention for Hib is vaccination for all infants; in late 1990 the FDA approved two new vaccines for use in children two months of age and older. The Hib vaccine is one of the safest of all vaccine products and cannot cause meningitis. About one in every eight children who receive the vaccine may have some slight redness, swelling, or tenderness at the injection site. About 1 in every 140 children will develop a fever higher than 102 degrees F. The reactions begin within 24 hours of the shot and quickly pass.

Before the vaccine, as many as 5 percent of healthy preschoolers carried *H. flu* type b but did not get sick. Vaccinated children cannot become carriers.

An antibiotic called rifampin is used to prevent cases of Hib after exposure; if all babies and young children in a home or child care group are vaccinated, preventive medicine after an exposure is not necessary. Rifampin will temporarily get rid of *H. flu* from the noses and throats of healthy carriers about 95 percent of the time. It helps prevent any exposed child in a day care center or a family from getting *H. flu* meningitis.

hand, foot, and mouth disease   A common infectious disease of toddlers that produces blistering of palms, soles, and the inside of the mouth. The condition often sweeps through day care centers in the summer. There is no connection between this condition and the hoof-and-mouth disease found in cattle.

An infected child can pass on the disease wherever she has the rash or sores; the virus will be present in the stools and the digestive tract for several weeks. Infected children don't need to be isolated, however, because most adults are immune and the illness is not severe. Many children are infected but do not exhibit symptoms; they develop immunity without experiencing the illness. It is possible, however, to get this disease again from a different strain of the virus. The mild illness usually lasts only a few days.

Cause   The disease is caused by the COX-SACKIEVIRUS which is spread by contact with nose and mouth secretions.

Symptoms   Symptoms usually appear within four to six days after infection, and include ulcers inside the cheeks, gums, or tongue, together with a fever, achiness, sore throat, headache, and poor appetite. Two days later, a rash on palms, fingers, soles, and diaper area appear; this is the signal that the virus is abating.

Diagnosis   Tests are unnecessary. If the child is very ill, and the diagnosis is not clear, samples can be taken for culture from the lesions or stool.

Treatment   There is no treatment other than painkillers to relieve blister discomfort.

Acetaminophen is given for fevers above 101 degrees F or for headaches. Small sips of soothing foods and fluids will ease mouth sores, including frozen or diluted juice, lukewarm broth, soft noodles, or gelatin desserts.

Complications   Complications are extremely rare.

Prevention   Hand washing is the only way to prevent this disease. This is especially important in a day care or nursery school. Family members can be protected by washing the towels, washcloths, and bedding used by a sick child.

Hansen's disease   See LEPROSY.

hantavirus   A group of viruses carried by rodents (mice, rats, and voles) responsible for a variety of diseases, including HANTAVIRUS PULMONARY SYNDROME and hemorrhagic fever. The virus is transmitted when humans breathe air contaminated by affected rodents' droppings, urine, or saliva and is not passed directly from human to human.

All of the viruses in this group trigger the leakage of blood from a victim's capillaries, causing rapid organ failure before the immune system can react. Each hantavirus infects primarily one type of rodent. The Hantaan, Seoul, Puumala, Prospect Hill, and Porogia strains are five viruses within the hantavirus genus, the newly added fifth genus within the Bunyaviridae family. The newest strain is the SIN NOMBRE (no-name) VIRUS, which first appeared in the Four Corners area of the western United States. (It was originally called Muerto Canyon [Valley of Death] virus for the spot on a New Mexico Navajo reservation where it was isolated. Because this name offended the Navajo, the virus was renamed Sin Nombre.) Deer mice were the rodents responsible in this outbreak.

The *Hantaan* virus was the first of the group to be identified in a Korean lab in 1976 from the lungs of a striped field mouse. This variety causes a bleeding disease called

Korean hemorrhagic fever, a problem during the Korean War. Named for the Hantaan River in South Korea, the virus infected 2,500 U.S. troops and killed between 5 and 10 percent of its victims. The related *Seoul virus* infects domestic rats, and causes a similar (but less deadly) type of fever. Because it is carried by rats, it is more common. *Puumala virus* affects the bank vole and is found most often in Scandinavia and western Europe.

Deer mice carry the United States strains.

hantavirus pulmonary syndrome   A respiratory illness caused by a new strain of HANTAVIRUS (a group of viruses carried by rodents) that causes its victims to gasp for air as their lungs fill with fluid. It kills about half the people it infects, usually within a week. The syndrome was first diagnosed in this country in 1993 at a Navajo reservation in the Four Corners area of New Mexico, Colorado, Utah, and Arizona.

Hantaviruses can be found throughout the world, where more than 170 names have been given to the hantavirus infections, including the often-fatal hemorrhagic fever. Until 1993, hantaviruses had been linked to the development of hemorrhagic fever. But the strain that was discovered in Four Corners caused a new disease, with debilitating flulike symptoms and respiratory failure.

Today, the number of infections with the hantavirus in the United States is rising, reaching 131; almost half have been fatal, according to the Centers for Disease Control and Prevention. More than 50 of the 131 cases occurred before the Navajo reservation outbreak. Since the Navajo outbreak, more than 100 cases of hantavirus pulmonary syndrome have been reported in 21 states (including New York), with more than half of them fatal. In addition, seven cases have been diagnosed in Canada and four in Brazil.

Cause   HPS is caused by a hantavirus first named Muerto Canyon (Valley of Death) virus for the spot on a New Mexico Navajo

reservation where it was isolated. Because this name offended the Navajo, the virus was renamed SIN NOMBRE (or "no name") virus. The disease can be spread by several common rodent species (deer mice, white-footed mice, and cotton rats) and has been found in 23 states; it is most common in New Mexico, which has had 28 cases; in Arizona, with 21 cases; and in California, with 13 cases. Doctors believe victims become infected by breathing in the dried urine or feces of infected deer mice; about 30 percent of the deer mice in the Four Corners area carry the Sin Nombre agent. Infected rodents have been found in other parts of the country as well.

Oddly enough, some victims have contracted the illness after little or no contact with rodents. Studies have also shown that the virus does not trigger infection in everyone it infects. In fact, the CDC acknowledges that the link between rodents and victims is unclear. Scientists don't know why some people become infected and others don't.

Even more worrying, some people have exhibited symptoms of hantavirus pulmonary syndrome but don't have the virus. In fact, there were half a dozen recent incidents in California where young and healthy people died suddenly of acute respiratory failure, yet did not test positive for hantavirus or any other microbe.

Scientists believe the U.S. outbreak was triggered by climate irregularities associated with the most recent El Niño (the occasional warming of waters in the tropical Pacific). While it is believed that the mice who carry the virus were probably infected for years, the climate-induced explosion in the deer mouse population may have fueled the spread of the disease in humans.

In addition to contact with contaminated urine or droppings, people can become infected with the virus after being bitten by rodents. Many people who have developed the disease live in mice-infested homes. One woman who developed the disease was exposed to rodents her cat dragged into the house, and another died after cleaning a rodent-infested barn.

Researchers don't know why some people are susceptible to the infection while others are not. The hantavirus does not appear to be highly infectious, and it is almost always found in isolated cases. There were only four instances in which more than one case occurred at the same time and place.

Symptoms Hantavirus pulmonary syndrome begins as a flulike illness with fever and chills, muscle aches, and cough; it can be easily misdiagnosed as HEPATITIS or an inflamed pancreas. The virus goes on to damage the kidneys and lungs, causing an accumulation of fluid that can drown the victim. The disease is fatal in almost half of all cases.

Treatment There is no treatment approved specifically for hantavirus, but researchers are currently studying the effectiveness of the antiviral drug Virazole (ribavirin) for HPS.

Prevention Army scientists developed a vaccine against hantavirus infection in 1995. While it is experimental, it is available to protect military personnel in South Korea and other areas of the world where the infection is common, according to the army's Medical Research Institute of Infectious Diseases in Ft. Detrick, Maryland. Such a vaccine does not need the approval of the Food and Drug Administration to be used among military personnel, if they give informed consent.

The CDC cautions homeowners to be cautious around rodent excretion, even though hantavirus is a rare disease. People should assume that all rodent excretions are infected, and should handle the droppings only after spraying them with disinfectant and wearing gloves.

Haverhill fever   A febrile disease transmitted by rat bite, first diagnosed in Haverhill, Massachusetts, in 1925.

Cause The disease is caused by the bacterium STREPTOBACILLUS MONILIFORMIS. This spirochete-like bacterium is normally found in rat saliva.

Symptoms Within 10 days of a rat bite, the patient experiences fever, chills, vomiting, headache, muscle and joint pain, and a rash appears.

Diagnosis Lab analysis of blood or pus can reveal the bacteria that cause the disease.

Treatment Antibiotics are effective against Haverhill fever.

head lice   See LICE.

hearing loss and infectious disease   Hearing loss affects about three and a half percent of children up to age 17. Although ear infections are the most common cause of hearing loss in the United States, there are other infectious causes—many of which can be treated successfully. The most common of these are bacterial MENINGITIS and CYTOMEGALOVIRUS INFECTION, but there is a long list of other infectious agents—viruses, bacteria, and parasites—that can lead to hearing problems. Hearing loss can also be a side effect of antibiotics (such as the aminoglycosides).

Bacterial meningitis Hearing loss related to this disease can be caused by STREPTOCOCCUS PNEUMONIAE (18 to 30 percent), *Neisseria meningitidis* (10 percent), and *Haemophilus influenzae* (6 percent). In pneumococcal meningitis, the incidence and severity of hearing loss is strongly linked to the length of time the disease lasts. Because of vaccination, *H. influenzae* is no longer a major cause of meningitis in the United States, although it remains a serious problem in other parts of the world.

The hearing loss with this disease is related either because of direct damage to the eighth cranial nerve (the hearing nerve) or to inflammation of the interior parts of the hearing mechanism itself.

Recent studies have shown that steroids can prevent hearing loss related to *H. influenzae,* but steroids do not help prevent hearing loss in meningitis caused by *S. pneumoniae* or *N. meningitidis*.

Syphilis   Scientists have known for a long time that congenital syphilis is a cause of hearing loss, but only recently has it been understood that syphilis acquired at any time can lead to hearing problems. There are no controlled studies on treatment, but benzathine penicillin in combination with steroids offers the best hope for improvement.

Borrelia burgdorferi   The agent that causes LYME DISEASE has been linked to hearing loss in about 2 percent of patients with the disease, usually involving low-frequency sound waves. The reason behind the deafness is not clear, but researchers suspect the loss occurs as a result of damage to the auditory center or the hearing nerve. Doxycycline or amoxicillin can be given to patients over age nine; younger children should receive amoxicillin or penicillin V. Those with hearing loss in the high frequencies are more likely to see improvement with antibiotic treatment.

Mycobacterium tuberculosis   While it is uncommon to find TB infecting the middle ear, it may sometimes be the first symptom of the disease. Such infection causes multiple perforations of the eardrum and chronic ear inflammation Anti-TB drugs should be given to treat this condition.

Cytomegalovirus   Of all children born with CMV, 95 percent do not show any symptoms. Among those who do, 60 percent will develop hearing loss. Those who don't have the symptoms rarely develop neurologic problems, but 10 percent of these infants remain at risk for hearing loss. Each year in the United States, about 4,000 children acquire hearing loss linked to CMV. It is suggested that the virus may interfere with the fetal development of the ear. The hearing loss usually centers in the high-frequency sounds, with equal loss in both ears. There is no known treatment.

Measles   About 1 in every 1,000 cases of measles leads to hearing loss. Sensorineural hearing loss associated with measles is usually sudden and occurs in both ears, primarily of the higher frequencies; there may also be vertigo and ringing in the ears. This hearing loss tends to be permanent.

Mumps   Hearing loss as a result of mumps occurs in about 5 of every 10,000 cases; there have been a few cases in the United States since vaccination was introduced in 1967. While scientists don't fully understand the link between mumps and deafness, they suspect the virus may cause the atrophy of the organ of Corti (part of the hearing mechanism) as well as a loss of hair cells within the hearing mechanism.

The onset of hearing loss is quick and occurs in only one ear in 80 percent of the cases; the deafness is usually profound and permanent and usually occurs in the higher frequencies. There may also be ringing of the ears, sensation of fullness in the ear, vertigo, nausea, and vomiting.

Rubella   In the United States, rubella among pregnant women is rare; when it does occur it often leads to deafness (between 25 percent and 51 percent of the time). Hearing loss related to rubella is profound in 55 percent of the cases; severe in 30 percent; and mild to moderate in 15 percent. The hearing loss affects all frequencies, but the middle frequencies cause the most problems.

Recent research suggests that congenital rubella is progressive and continues to damage the ears even after infancy.

Varicella-zoster   Infection with this virus can lead to a syndrome involving facial palsy, herpes of the ear, and hearing loss, first described in 1907. This Ramsay-Hunt syndrome (also called herpes zoster oticus) can produce several patterns of hearing loss, together with ringing of the ears in 48 percent of cases. A patient who also experiences vertigo is not likely to recover from the hearing loss. Prompt treatment with acyclovir seems to be effective.

HIV Studies have reported up to 49 percent of HIV-infected patients have some degree of sensorineural hearing loss, as a possible result of infection of the cochlea, hearing center in the brain, or both. Patients with HIV-associated hearing loss also may experience vertigo and facial nerve palsy. Drug treatment does not seem to affect the hearing loss.

Fungal infections Fungal infections of the ear can cause either a conductive or sensorineural hearing loss. The most common organisms responsible for the loss include the *Candida* and *Aspergillus* species. Among those with impaired immune systems, *Cryptococcus neoformans* and *Zygomycetes* are a particular problem. A variety of antifungal drugs can be used to treat the problem, but there are no studies that prove their efficacy.

Toxoplasma gondii Congenital infection with this organism has been related to hearing loss, although the reason behind the problem is not well understood. Treatment with pyrimethamine, sulfadiazine, or spiramycin is effective.

Visceral leishmaniasis While this is not common in the United States, it is endemic in many other areas of the world, where it causes a type of hearing loss, probably by affecting the covering (myelin) of the hearing nerve. Treatment with stibogluconate sodium is effective and can frequently cure the hearing loss.

Flukes Infestation with the intestinal FLUKE *Fasciola hepatica* can produce hearing loss. While rarely seen in the United States, it is more common in Latin America, Asia, and Africa. A patient is infected by eating raw aquatic plants contained with the flukes. Bithionol is the treatment of choice.

Helicobacter pylori The bacterium that may cause most stomach ulcers and almost all duodenal ulcers and one of the most common chronic infections in humans. The bacteria infect people around the world, ranging up to 40 percent in developed countries and up to 80 percent in developing countries.

Since the 1950s doctors knew that family members of ulcer patients were three times more likely than the general population to have ulcers as well. But the link wasn't firmly established until 1983, when Australian gastroenterologist Barry J. Marshall identified the bacterium in stomach tissue of ulcer patients, when it was first called *Campylobacter pylori*. In an attempt to prove the link between bacteria and ulcers, he swallowed the bacteria and developed an ulcer. Before that time, physicians had believed that ulcers were a noninfectious disease.

In 1994, a conference sponsored by the National Institutes of Health declared that ulcer is an infectious disease and recommended that doctors stop treating symptoms with antacids and, instead, utilize antibiotics to cure the infection.

Ulcers are found in 1 out of every 10 Americans, and *H. pylori* is implicated in 90 percent of those cases. Virtually everyone with the bacteria has chronic gastritis (a mild inflammation of the stomach lining).

Cause Despite that the human stomach is filled with acids, this bacterium manages to thrive there. The bacteria can survive the hostile environment of the stomach by nestling into the stomach's mucous lining. How the bacteria spread is unclear, but groups living in close quarters are particularly vulnerable.

Studies suggest the bacteria are passed via person-to-person contact but are probably not sexually transmitted. If one family member is infected, it is likely that the rest of the family also harbor the bacteria. It is also common in areas of poor sanitation and crowded living conditions and in families with multiple children (especially where children share beds). Scientists suspect the infection may be spread by swallowing infected food or water in addition to person-to-person contact. *H. pylori* is not naturally found in animals.

Symptoms Following infection, patients experience nausea and stomach pain, vomiting and fever, which lasts between 3 and 14 days. If not treated, patients will develop chronic gastritis that can last for decades. While half the world's populations are believed to be infected (including an estimated 40 million Americans), for some reason it only causes ulcers in between 10 to 20 percent of its hosts. It does not always cause ulcers to form, but it almost always produces inflammation of the stomach lining. Some people with the infection don't have ulcers but do experience nausea, gas, bloating, and burning stomach pain. These symptoms occur twice as often in people with *H. pylori* compared to those without the bacteria.

Diagnosis Blood tests can determine the presence of antibodies to the bacteria. This test tells if a patient has ever had the infection, but can't determine if the infection is active. It is not 100 percent accurate, however. A punch biopsy of the stomach can be examined under a microscope for the presence of *H. pylori.*

The newest diagnostic method, breath tests that can detect the bacteria, were cleared for marketing in the fall of 1996 by the U.S. Food and Drug Administration. The simple new breath test—the first of its kind cleared by the FDA—is as good as biopsy in detecting the bacterium and can be administered in a doctor's office. In the 30-minute test, the patient drinks a new, nonradioactive diagnostic drug solution, then exhales into a collection kit. The solution contains the drug Pranactin, which determines the presence or absence of active *H. pylori*. The kit is then sent to the manufacturer, Meretek Diagnostics, Inc., in Nashville, Tennessee. Results are available within two days. In studies of 499 U.S. and Canadian patients with duodenal ulcer, the breath test detected the bacteria 95 percent of the time.

Treatment About 90 percent of *H. pylori* infections can be cured with a combination of anti-ulcer medication and specific antibiotics (Pepto Bismol, Biaxin, metronidazole, clarithromycin and omeprazole, tetracycline, or amoxicillin). Because the treatment may not be completely successful, follow-up testing at least four weeks after completing treatment may be needed to make sure the bacteria are no longer present. If tests reveal no bacteria, the patient is not likely to be reinfected ever again. Persistent infection may require a different medication for longer period of time.

The National Institutes of Health has recommended that all patients with stomach or duodenal ulcers who also have *H. pylori* be treated for both the ulcer and the infection. While there appears to be a relationship between the bacteria and stomach cancer, these cancers are becoming less common in the United States, and therapy for *H. pylori* has not been recommended as a preventive measure.

There is no solid evidence that diet affects *H. pylori* or ulcer healing. With proper medical treatment, ulcers heal as well on a regular diet as with a bland diet. Still, it is wise to avoid smoking, nonsteroidal antiinflammatory drugs (NSAIDs), aspirin, excessive alcohol, and caffeine.

Complications The organism has also been found in a disproportionately large number of patients with certain kinds of stomach cancer. Some scientists suggest the infection may triple the risk of this rare cancer.

Prevention In 1996, the National Institutes of Health has urged U.S. doctors to test all ulcer patients for the bacterium and to treat the infected with antibiotics for two weeks. However, the treatment is not easy; it involves taking 12 to 16 pills for two weeks and carries the risk of some side effects, such as fatigue and dizziness.

Careful personal hygiene (thorough handwashing, using separate personal items such as glasses and toothbrushes) is probably the best way to prevent person-to-person spread.

Since scientists have succeeded in immunizing mice, a human vaccine may be developed in the future.

For more information about *Helicobacter pylori*, contact the International Research Foundation for Helicobacter and Intestinal Immunology, P.O. Box 7965, Charlottesville, VA 22906.

helminth A suffix meaning "worm."

helminthiasis An infestation by any species of parasitic worms. Ascariasis, FILARIASIS, HOOKWORM DISEASE, and TRICHINOSIS are all common types of worm disease.

hemolytic uremic syndrome (HUS) This serious disorder—once considered to be a rare form of kidney disease—has in recent years become more common as a complication of food-borne infection of ESCHERICHIA COLI 0157:H7, characterized by the destruction of red blood cells and failing kidneys.

Between 2 and 7 percent of ESCHERICHIA COLI 0157:H7 infections lead to this complication in certain high-risk people (such as the very young or old). In the United States, HUS is the main cause of kidney failure in children. Most cases are caused by infection with this type of *E. coli*.

Symptoms As the bacteria enter the kidneys, causing bleeding and destroying red blood cells, the victim becomes pale and tired, with a fever and rising blood pressure. The kidneys shut down and urine is no longer produced.

Treatment This is a life-threatening condition that must be treated in a hospital intensive care unit, where the patient receives blood transfusions and is placed on kidney dialysis to maintain life until the organs recover. Most patients do recover at this point, but a small percentage (about 15 percent) do not, and require permanent dialysis or a kidney transplant.

Prognosis With intensive care, the death rate from this syndrome is still between 3 and 5 percent. One third of the survivors will have abnormal kidney function years later and a few need long-term dialysis. Another 8 percent suffer with other complications, including high blood pressure, seizures, blindness, and paralysis, for the rest of their lives. See also *ESCHERICHIA COLI*.

hepatitis The description for any inflammation of the liver. It is generally caused by a virus, but alcoholism or certain drugs can also damage the liver and lead to hepatitis. When the liver is damaged, it can't excrete the blood breakdown substance called bilirubin, which then builds up in the blood. This causes a yellow tinge to skin and eyes (called jaundice). The appearance of jaundice is more or less a warning sign that the liver is no longer able to cleanse the blood. In severe cases of hepatitis, the liver fails altogether, resulting in death unless a liver transplant is done.

Hippocrates was the first to mention epidemics of jaundice, and the disease went on to become a factor in many large military campaigns. During the Civil War, for example, hepatitis struck more than 70,000 soldiers. By the time World War II began, scientists were able to differentiate between two types of hepatitis—"infectious" hepatitis, spread by contaminated food or water, and "serum," spread by infected blood.

By the 1960s, scientists were beginning to learn that the disease was caused by specific unrelated viruses and gave them alphabetical names to distinguish them. The alphabet of hepatitis viruses all belong to different genuses. An international team has reported finding a hepatitis F virus recently, although others have not yet confirmed the finding. Now, a cluster of viruses dubbed HEPATITIS G has recently been found.

The various hepatitis viruses differ in their likelihood of producing chronic infection. Almost everyone, for example, who is infected with HEPATITIS C becomes a carrier of the virus. HEPATITIS A causes only temporary liver damage, which is reversed as the body produces antibodies. HEPATITIS B or HEPATITIS C, however, can cause long-term complications. Delta, or D, virus, is always a coinfection with hepatitis B; HEPATITIS E does not occur in North America. Although the viruses are unrelated to each other, they act in similar ways, attacking and damaging only the liver.

For some reason, hepatitis B and C may quickly develop into fulminant hepatitis, in which the liver cells are completely destroyed. As the liver function stops, toxic substances build up and affect the brain, causing lethargy, confusion, combativeness, stupor, and coma. This can often lead to death, although with aggressive treatment the patient may live. If the victim does not die, the liver is often able to regenerate and resume function, and the brain recovers.

hepatitis A   The most common and least dangerous type of hepatitis, this is the first virus that scientists were able to identify. A foodborne virus, it looks much like a poliovirus with just one bare strand of RNA within a 20-sided shell that can replicate only in the liver. It infects only humans and a few primates, primarily via contaminated feces. Formerly known as "infectious hepatitis," hepatitis A is fairly common; in 1994, 22,000 Americans were reported to have hepatitis A, but thousands of cases go unreported; about 100 people die each year.

While there is not a typical "season" for hepatitis A, it occurs in cycles. In the United States, cases peaked from 1961 to 1971, declined, and then peaked again from 1983 to 1991; numbers dropped again after 1992. Foods have been implicated in more than 30 outbreaks since 1983. The most recent include imported lettuce in Louisville in 1987; ice-slush beverages in Alaska, restaurant iced-tea in North Carolina, and raw oysters in Florida—all during 1988; unidentified food in a Washington restaurant chain in 1989; north

Georgia frozen strawberries, Montana frozen strawberries, and Baltimore shellfish—all in 1990.

The illness is a disease of filth and occurs most often among school-age children and young adults. In overcrowded areas in developed countries and many developing countries, it is so common that 90 percent or more of 10 year olds are healthy carriers and immune as adults. It is estimated that 40 percent of healthy adults in the United States are immune to hepatitis A as a result of previous infection and have lifelong immunity.

The virus dates from 400 B.C., when it afflicted armies in every war; it is believed to have played a role in Napoleon's defeat.

Other former names for hepatitis A include epidemic hepatitis, epidemic jaundice, catarrhal jaundice, infectious icterus, Botkins disease, and MS-1 hepatitis.

Cause   Hepatitis A belongs to the ENTEROVIRUS GROUP of the picornaviruses, which include poliovirus, COXSACKIEVIRUS, ECHOVIRUS, and RHINOVIRUS. Hepatitis A is spread by eating food or drinking water contaminated with the hepatitis A virus (HAV), which is shed in the stool.

The virus enters through the mouth, multiplies in the body, and is passed in the feces; it can then be carried on an infected person's hands and spread by direct contact, or by eating food or drink handled by that person. Anyone can get hepatitis A, but it occurs most often among children. Most people get it either from close personal contact between family members, sex partners (especially homosexual men), and in nursery schools or child care centers.

The virus is hardy and spread easily. Unlike many other viruses, it can live for more than a month at room temperature on kitchen countertops, children's toys, and other surfaces. It can be maintained indefinitely in frozen foods and ice. To inactivate the virus, food must be heated at 185 degrees F for one minute.

A food handler with hepatitis A can spread the disease if he or she touches food that isn't cooked before it is eaten (usually sandwiches or salads). Well water contaminated by improperly treated sewage has also been implicated, since hepatitis A can live for a long time in water. It is difficult to test water for hepatitis A. People who drink treated municipal or county water supplies are not at risk.

It's possible to get hepatitis A from eating raw or undercooked foods, such as shellfish (especially oysters). When they eat, shellfish filter large amounts of water and if it is contaminated with hepatitis A, it will be concentrated in the shellfish. In Florida in 1988, 61 people caught hepatitis A after eating raw oysters illegally taken from contaminated waters. Even though federal regulations and posting of contaminated waters offer some protection, there is still a risk of contracting viruses when eating raw shellfish. In 1990, an infected Missouri dish washer who prepared lettuce infected 110 people who had eaten at the restaurant; two died.

Symptoms   One quarter of all people with hepatitis A won't have any symptoms. Infants and young children tend to have very mild cases; three quarters of children have no symptoms and the rest have low fever and achiness, but rarely jaundice. However, children do serve as the primary source of contagion for adults.

The disease in older patients can be more serious, characterized by fever (100 to 104 degrees F), extreme tiredness, weakness, nausea, stomach upset, pain in the upper right side of the stomach, and loss of appetite. Within a few days, a yellowish tinge appears in the skin and the whites of the eyes. Urine will be darker than usual, and the stool is light colored. Anyone over age 12 may become quite sick for a week or two. Once the jaundice appears, patients begin to feel better. The disease is rarely fatal, and most people recover in a few weeks without any complications.

The incubation period ranges from 15 to 50 days. Patients are most infectious in the two weeks before symptoms develop. Food handlers who know they are infected should not work until they are past the infectious stages, which ends one week after first becoming jaundiced.

Diagnosis   Blood tests showing antibodies to hepatitis A are the best diagnosis. Symptoms of hepatitis A are so similar to other diseases that a doctor needs a test to make the correct diagnosis.

Treatment   There is no drug treatment for hepatitis A. While symptoms appear, patients should rest and eat well—low-fat, high-carbohydrate, easily digested foods in small amounts are good choices. These could include crackers, noodles, rice, or soup. Anti-nausea medicine can be prescribed for severe nausea. Headaches or body aches may respond to acetaminophen. Normal activities may be resumed when the acute illness is over.

Complications   Very rarely, hepatitis A can also develop into fulminant hepatitis in which the liver cells are completely destroyed. As the liver function stops, toxic substances build up and affect the brain, causing lethargy, confusion, combativeness, stupor, and coma. This can often lead to death, although the patient may live with aggressive treatment. If the victim does not die, the liver is able to regenerate and resume function, and the brain recovers.

Prevention   A new vaccine said to be 100 percent effective after a single primary dose became available in 1996 in the United States. In earlier vaccines, more than 99 percent of people in the vaccine studies became immune after two doses; a booster is recommended for this vaccine between 6 and 12 months after the first dose.

In addition, workers in child care centers where there are diapered children must maintain strict rules about frequent hand washing and procedures for diaper changing.

Cooking tainted food kills the virus. Shellfish from contaminated areas must be cooked (boiled) for at least eight minutes to be considered safe for eating.

Those who are exposed to hepatitis A can prevent infection by getting a shot of immune globulin (IG), which is pooled human blood plasma that contains protective antibodies against the disease. People who need a shot of IG include the following:

- all household members and sex partners of hepatitis A patients
- close friends of an infected school-age child
- restaurant staffers where one food handler has hepatitis A; patrons of the restaurant need IG within two weeks of exposure only if the infected food handler handles uncooked food and has poor hygienic practices, or has diarrhea
- staff and residents of prisons, institutions, homes, when two or more residents have hepatitis A
- all staff in child care centers or homes where one ore more children or employees have hepatitis A; if three or more children or their families have hepatitis A, family members of the other children need IG as well
- unimmunized travelers to developing countries

hepatitis B Formerly known as serum hepatitis, this is the most common preventable infectious disease in the United States. The virus, which is far more complex than HEPATITIS A, can destroy the liver and is 100 times more transmissible than the AIDS virus. It is believed that there are 300,000 cases a year in the United States, of which only about 15,000 are reported; about 1.25 million Americans are carriers, which means they are infectious for all their lives.

Almost 6,000 Americans each year die from acute hepatitis B or complications of the infection; around the world, the fatality rate is 2 million per year. It can be prevented by vaccine, but of the group who accounts for most infections—those aged 15 to 39—only about 5 percent ever get vaccinated.

Cause The hepatitis B virus (HBV) is carried in the blood and is also found in saliva, semen, and other bodily fluids. It is transmitted much the same as the AIDS virus, but hepatitis B is even easier to catch: One drop of blood infected with hepatitis B contains millions of viral particles. Still, hepatitis B is not spread by casual contact. The virus must get into a person's blood to cause infection; it enters the blood via sexual contact, blood transfusions, dirty needles, or by sharing toothbrushes, razors, or utensils. Unfortunately, the virus is very stable and can survive on dried surfaces (even thorns or stones) for days. More than half of all cases are linked to sexual intercourse with infected partners.

Many health care workers have become infected from needle sticks, lab accidents, or splashing blood; dentists have caught the infection from patients and gone on to infect other patients. A health care worker with a needle stick from a patient with hepatitis B has between a 6 percent and 30 percent chance of becoming infected. By comparison, the chance of contracting AIDS this way is only about 0.5 percent.

It is possible for infected mothers to pass the virus to their babies during the final three months of pregnancy, during delivery, or during nursing. There is less danger of passing on the infection if the mother contracts the disease in the early stages of pregnancy. All pregnant women should be tested for hepatitis B.

Many millions of people around the world are chronically infected with hepatitis B, and can give the virus to others (unlike those who have had hepatitis A). Because the germ can induce liver cancer, it is believed to be the world's most common viral cause of cancer.

Symptoms It can take up to six months after exposure before symptoms of hepatitis B appear, as compared to only six weeks for hepatitis A. Many people have few symptoms. If they do appear, they appear gradually and include tiredness, nausea, joint and muscle aches, mild abdominal pain in upper right side, poor appetite, hives or rash, and mild diarrhea for three to ten days. This may be followed by jaundice in about half of those who become infected. Nausea is usually not associated with hepatitis B (it is more common with hepatitis A). Other symptoms may include light-colored stools, dark urine, and itchy skin. After jaundice appears, symptoms may improve. Infants infected by their mothers may have no symptoms at first, but they are at high risk for developing cirrhosis and liver cancer in the second decade of life.

In about one third of cases, people aren't terribly sick; another third have no symptoms at all. In fact, the chance of becoming a carrier are greater if the symptoms don't develop. About 25 percent of carriers do suffer chronic symptoms and are at greatest risk of developing cirrhosis. A few may be quite ill for several weeks. Those over age 40 may be more severely ill; children have few symptoms.

The virus can be found in blood and body fluids several weeks before symptoms appear and several months after. The appearance of certain antibodies indicate resolution of disease. People who are chronic carriers (about 10 percent of those infected) are always infectious, although they do not appear to be ill. Those who recover are immune for life.

Diagnosis Hepatitis B can be diagnosed by blood tests; other tests (that look for markers) can differentiate hepatitis B from other types of hepatitis. Liver function tests can measure enzymes produced by the liver that will be elevated in all forms of hepatitis.

Treatment Chronic active hepatitis B is treated with alpha-interferons. Many people report short-term side effects from interferon, such as fever, chills, appetite loss, vomiting, muscle aches, and sleep problems that disappear after a few weeks.

For acute hepatitis, there is no treatment beyond bed rest and a high carbohydrate, low-fat diet. After recovery, patients need a blood test to see if they have retained the E antigen. Those who do are extremely infectious and are at higher risk of developing complications. About 10 percent of these chronic carriers lose the antigen each year. A high percentage of patients go on to develop chronic hepatitis, leading to chronically poor liver function.

Complications Most people recover from the infection entirely and are not at risk for long-term complications. On the other hand, babies, children, and the 5 percent of adult carriers are of more concern.

Between 10 and 85 percent of babies born to infected mothers will develop hepatitis themselves; of those, 90 percent develop chronic hepatitis, at high risk for eventually developing cirrhosis or liver cancer as adults. Twenty-five percent of them will die of liver disease as adults.

Prevention While hepatitis B is completely preventable, thousands continue to come down with the disease each year. The vaccine introduced in 1983 was made from blood plasma; a few years later a vaccine from synthetic products was introduced; a third synthetic vaccine was produced in 1991. The last two vaccines are given in three doses. Anyone at risk for the disease, including all medical and nursing personnel, should have the vaccine. As of November 1991, the vaccine was recommended for all infants; boosters are not currently recommended.

Unlike some vaccines, there is no apparent risk of serious side effects from the hepatitis B vaccine. If any, reactions seem to be limited to a sore arm at the site of injection or a slight fever.

Those who are not immunized but have been exposed may receive immune globulin HBIG for 90 percent protection if they receive the dose within seven days of exposure and begin the hepatitis B vaccine series at the same time.

Babies born to infected mothers receive HBIG within 12 hours after birth. The vaccine series must be started at the same time.

Carriers should follow standard hygienic procedures to make sure their close contacts are not directly contaminated. Carriers must not share razors, toothbrushes, or any other object that may become contaminated with blood. In addition, household members (especially sexual partners) should be immunized with hepatitis B vaccine. It is important for carriers to inform their dentist and health care providers of their status.

hepatitis C   A mysterious blood-borne type of hepatitis that can live quietly in the body for years, hepatitis C was identified in 1988 and called non-A, non-B hepatitis.

Until the virus starts to attack the liver, most people don't know they are infected. Many don't know how they got the disease, and even after it is diagnosed, virtually nothing will get rid of it. The disease can be far more deadly than its cousins hepatitis A and B, both of which can be avoided with a vaccine.

In the United States, hepatitis C virus is linked to 20 percent of all clinical hepatitis cases and is the leading cause of chronic hepatitis. It is also the number-one reason for liver transplants in this country. Hepatitis C can lead to liver cancer, killing up to 10,000 Americans a year and causing almost half of all deaths from liver failure, according to the National Center for Infectious Diseases. Mickey Mantle had hepatitis C, as well as liver cancer and liver damage from excessive drinking.

Not everyone with hepatitis C will get sick; however, about a third of those with chronic hepatitis C will develop either cirrhosis or cancer of the liver. More than half of all patients exposed to the virus become carriers, and up to 20 percent of these carriers develop cirrhosis (a severe liver disease).

While the actual number of patients is not known, it is believed to be the most common form of viral hepatitis in the United States and may affect as many as 4 million Americans (1 out of every 60 people). The Centers for Disease Control estimates that 150,000 Americans are newly infected each year; long-term liver damage in chronic patients kills between 8,000 to 10,000 Americans a year.

The number of newly diagnosed patients (those who were infected years ago and are just now being diagnosed) is clearly rising, especially among baby boomers who were IV-drug abusers. Intravenous-drug users make up about 30 percent of the HCV-infected population; experts believe that almost all such users are ultimately infected by the lethal virus.

Cause   Hepatitis C is spread primarily through blood-related sources, such as IV-drug use, transfusions, and kidney dialysis. It is the cause of most cases of post-transfusion hepatitis. The risk of sexual transmission appears to be small. There is no evidence that this type of hepatitis can be spread by casual contact, by eating tainted food, or by coughing or sneezing. In rare cases, an infected mother can pass the disease to a newborn. Some people carry the virus in their bloodstream and may remain contagious for years.

Before 1989, the infection was spread through transfusions; about 300,000 patients may have contracted the disease this way, before the nation's blood banks began testing for the virus in 1990.

Oddly enough, in about half of cases the patients have done nothing that would put themselves at risk, and the source of the infection cannot be identified.

The virus is related to the YELLOW FEVER virus.

Symptoms   About 25 percent of those infected with the virus will become sick with symptoms, including appetite loss, fatigue, nausea and vomiting, stomach pain, and jaundice within two weeks to six months after exposure. Usually, symptoms appear by two months. Fifty percent of these patients may go on to develop chronic liver disease.

Diagnosis People who have no symptoms usually find out they have hepatitis C when they give blood or get a liver function test when applying for life insurance. Many patients are model citizens who had experimented with heroin in the 1960s and 1970s. A variety of liver function tests, plus liver biopsy, can detect the disease.

Treatment There is no known cure for hepatitis C, but the FDA has approved a drug called recombinant alpha-interferon for treating those with chronic hepatitis C. Alpha-interferon eliminates the virus for between 10 and 25 percent of patients. The drug can temporarily reduce the virus levels in about 50 percent, but these patients then experience relapse. Combining interferon with the antiviral drug ribavirin may improve response to treatment.

However, alpha-interferon has serious side effects. It causes flulike symptoms and makes many patients feel depressed. It is also expensive, costing about $6,000 per year.

Research published in October 1996 identified the structure of a protein that the virus needs to reproduce; scientists hope they may be able to design a drug that can disable the protein, rendering the virus unable to destroy liver cells.

Prevention At the present time, there is no hepatitis C vaccine. Hope for such a vaccine faded, according to the National Institute of Allergy and Infectious Diseases, when their studies showed that exposure to the virus does not protect against reinfection.

Since 1990, U.S. blood donation centers have routinely used a blood-donor-screening test for hepatitis C. Widespread use of this test has significantly reduced the number of transfusion-associated cases of hepatitis C. People who have had hepatitis C should understand that their blood and possibly other body fluids are potential sources of infection. They should avoid sharing toothbrushes, razors, needles, and the like.

In addition, infected patients should not donate blood and should inform health care workers. Limits on sexual activity with steady partners may not be needed; however, those with acute illness and multiple sex partners may be at higher risk and should use condoms to reduce the risk of acquiring or transmitting hepatitis C as well as other infections.

hepatitis D An uncommon version of the hepatitis virus in the United States, HDV infects about 15 million people around the world. Because the virus requires the presence of HEPATITIS B virus (HBV) to produce infection, the frequency of hepatitis D closely parallels HBV. In southern Italy, parts of Russia, and Romania, more than 20 percent of HBV carriers with no symptoms and more than 60 percent of those with chronic liver disease due to HBV are also infected with hepatitis D.

Cause The major way hepatitis D is spread is through contaminated needles (primarily IV-drug abuse and exposure to blood products). Sexual transmission of hepatitis D is less efficient than for hepatitis B, but non-IV-drug-using male homosexuals, female prostitutes, and institutionalized mentally retarded people are at higher risk for developing hepatitis D.

Transmission from mother to child has not been documented in the United States.

Symptoms Hepatitis D can't be distinguished from other causes of hepatitis. The development of a new episode of acute hepatitis in a patient with known chronic hepatitis B infection should prompt a search for evidence of a new hepatitis D infection.

Diagnosis In patients with acute hepatitis D infection, anti-HDV antibody may be detected. The disease can be diagnosed by detecting HDV antigen in liver biopsies or antibodies in blood.

Treatment There is no reliable treatment for hepatitis D.

Prevention   The hepatitis B vaccine can prevent hepatitis D, since hepatitis B infection is required for hepatitis D infection to occur.

hepatitis E   A form of hepatitis that is clinically indistinguishable from HEPATITIS A disease and that occurs primarily in underdeveloped countries. The disease exists in both epidemic and sporadic forms and is usually associated with contaminated drinking water. Major waterborne epidemics have occurred in Asia, North Africa, and East Africa. To date, no U.S. outbreaks have been reported, although imported cases were identified in Los Angeles in 1987. There is no evidence for immunity against this virus in the American population, so in theory it could become a problem in this country.

The disease is most often seen in young to middle-aged adults between ages of 15 and 40. Pregnant women appear to be extremely susceptible to severe disease, and high rates of death have been reported in this group.

Also known as enterically transmitted non-A, non-B hepatitis (ET-NANBH), it is also called fecal-oral non-A, non-B hepatitis or A-like non-A non-B hepatitis. It should not be confused with HEPATITIS C, also called parenterally transmitted non-A non-B (PT-NANBH) or B-like non-A non-B hepatitis.

Major outbreaks have occurred in India (1955 and 1975–76), the USSR (1955–56), Nepal (1973), Burma (1976–77), Algeria (1980–81), the Ivory Cost (1983–84), in refugee camps in Eastern Sudan and Somalia (1985–86), and most recently in Borneo (1987).

Cause   The hepatitis E virus is transmitted by the fecal-oral route. The virus has been transmitted via water and person-to-person; the potential exists for transmission via contaminated food.

Symptoms   Between two to nine weeks after infection, symptoms of malaise, anorexia, abdominal pain, and fever appear. The disease is usually mild and fades away within two weeks. The fatality rate is very low; less than one percent of nonpregnant patients progress to fatal fulminant hepatitis, but in pregnant women the fatality rate rises to 20 percent.

Diagnosis   Symptoms and epidemiological characteristics of the disease, and by excluding hepatitis A and B by blood tests. Confirmation requires identification of certain viruslike particles by immune electron microscope in the feces of acutely ill patients.

Treatment   No antiviral treatment has been proven effective against hepatitis E, although preliminary studies suggest ribavirin and alpha-interferon may work.

Prevention   Good sanitation and personal hygiene are the best preventive measures. There is no current vaccine, and it is not yet clear whether infection with hepatitis E confers lifelong immunity. Several recombinant HEV vaccines are being tested, but none are currently available for commercial use.

hepatitis F   The HFV has been described in France in a handful of cases, and scientists have succeeded in transmitting the infection to primates. There is very little else known about this virus.

hepatitis G   One of the "alphabet" hepatitis viruses, hepatitis G was first identified in 1996. It apparently causes a mild acute hepatitis but is not a clinically significant chronic disease. However, the precise effects on the liver and an individual's health over time remain unknown. Very similar to hepatitis C, hepatitis G is also called hepatitis GB virus C or HGBV-C; hepatitis G is a flavivirus. Coinfection with hepatitis B or C—or both—is common. However, hepatitis G infection doesn't seem to worsen coinfection with hepatitis B or C.

Hepatitis G has at least five subtypes, depending on the part of the country where it occurs. It appears to be primarily a monkey virus that was transferred from one monkey to another until it infected humans via contaminated blood. Researchers have found the virus in blood in the United States, Canada, Peru, Egypt, West Africa, and Europe. About 1.5 percent of Japanese hepatitis patients who don't have the A through E varieties are infected with the G virus. About 18 percent of similar West African patients have the same virus in their blood.

Healthy people in the United States may carry the G virus since research suggests it was present in the nation's blood supply 25 years ago. And experts suggests that between 1 and 2 percent of the nation's blood donors have a previously undetected hepatitis G infection—higher than the rate for either hepatitis B or C.

Cause   In 0.3 percent of cases of community-acquired acute viral hepatitis, hepatitis G is the only identified virus. This strain of viral hepatitis was previously thought to be transmitted only through infected blood; now it is known to be transmitted sexually as well. Researchers in Sweden and Honduras found a surprisingly high rate of infection with the virus in healthy individuals without known risk factors (such as injection drug use and treatment for hemophilia). It was the high rates of infection in homosexual men and in healthy volunteers that led the authors to question the possibility of transmission via sexual contacts. It is known that HGV can be transmitted from an infected mother to her infant during childbirth, but now they believe HGV might be transmitted by "other routes yet to be defined."

There is an increased prevalence of hepatitis G genetic material among groups with frequent exposure to blood or blood products (such as people with hemophilia, patients on hemodialysis, and injection drug users). Other modes of transmission are possible but have not been well documented.

About 10 percent to 20 percent of cases of community-acquired hepatitis and transfusion-associated hepatitis are not associated with the known major hepatitis viruses (A, B, C, D, or E). The fairly recent identification from patients with hepatitis G, which is about 25 percent identical to the hepatitis C virus, has implicated it as a cause of non-A-E hepatitis.

Symptoms   After a brief attack, the virus may remain in the body for years, scientists speculate. They believe the virus may replicate in the liver for years, eventually revealing liver damage. Japanese studies suggest that some hepatitis patients whose liver failed were indeed infected with hepatitis G.

Diagnosis   At this time, HGV infection can be identified only through special liver function tests that indicate current infection. An antibody test for HGV is under development and, when available, should explain the origins of infection more fully than HGV RNA testing can.

It appears that once antibodies are found, the virus is usually no longer present in the blood.

Prognosis   The nature and frequency of HGV infection are unclear; there is also uncertainty about risk factors and means of prevention. Although caution and vigilance must be maintained, there is a growing consensus that HGV is "a virus looking for a disease" and may in fact prove not to be a cause of viral hepatitis. Acute HGV infection is generally reported to be clinically and biochemically mild and transient. Although the viral genetic material can be detected for years after infection in perhaps a minority of people who have been infected, there is no compelling evidence that HGV infection can lead to serious consequences. However, the role of HGV in a more virulent form of hepatitis (fulminant hepatitis) is unknown.

Treatment   There is no proven treatment for HGV infection; at this point, guidelines for its investigation and management cannot be developed.

Prevention   Blood banks don't have a way to screen for hepatitis G. The threat that HGV may pose to the nation's blood supply is an important issue. Some healthy blood donors may have hepatitis G, and transmission through transfusion has been documented. However, there is no commercial test available for screening; antibody testing, when it becomes available, may not be of particular value because it will not identify current infection. Donors already infected with hepatitis B or C will largely be excluded already; and the hepatitis G infection seems largely benign.

herpes   Any of a variety of inflammatory skin diseases characterized by spreading or creeping small clustered blisters caused by the herpes simplex virus. Forms of the virus cause COLD SORES and the sexually transmitted disease genital herpes (see HERPES, GENITAL), characterized by blisters on the sex organs. The virus also causes many other conditions affecting the skin.

There are two forms of the herpes simplex virus—type 1 and type 2. Herpes simplex, type 1 (HSV1) is usually associated with infections of the lips, mouth, and face, whereas herpes simplex, type 2 (HSV2) is usually associated with infections of the genitals and in babies, who acquire the disease during birth.

However, there is a certain amount of overlap between the two, and conditions usually caused by HSV2 may be caused by HSV1, and vice versa. Both types are highly infectious, spread by direct contact with the lesions or by the fluid inside the blisters.

Most people have been infected with HSV by the time they reach adulthood. While the first infection with this virus may cause no symptoms at all, there may be a flulike illness in addition to ulcers on the skin around the mouth; afterward, the virus remains in the nerve cells of the face. Many people experience recurrent reactivations of the virus, suffering with repeated attacks of cold sores, especially during a fever or prolonged sun exposure.

Sometimes the virus infects the finger, causing painful blisters called herpes whitlow. In patients with a preexisting skin condi-

tion (such as dermatitis), the virus may cause an extensive rash of blisters called ECZEMA HERPETICUM.

A person suffering an immunodeficiency disorder (such as AIDS) or someone taking immunosuppressant drugs who is exposed to the virus may experience a severe generalized infection that can be fatal.

A close cousin of the herpes simplex virus, the VARICELLA-ZOSTER VIRUS, is responsible for two other skin blistering disorders—CHICKEN POX and SHINGLES (herpes zoster). Like the herpes simplex virus, the varicella-zoster virus can affect the eyes or the brain, in addition to the skin. Herpes gestationis and dermatitis herpetiformis are among other conditions in which herpeslike groups of blisters may appear on the skin, but neither is related to the herpes simplex or varicella-zoster virus infections.

Treatment of HSV varies according to its site and severity. The antiviral drug acyclovir (taken internally or applied topically to the blisters) is effective in shortening the symptoms during a primary attack, and there is some indication the drug taken prophylactically may lessen future attacks.

herpes, genital   Until AIDS appeared, genital herpes was one of the most common sexually transmitted diseases in the country, striking young, single, and usually middle-class men and women. Despite the hysteria, the medical community has always considered genital herpes to be more of a discomfort rather than a dangerous or life-threatening situation. This nonlethal but incurable disease invades the body and remains for a lifetime, appearing often several times a year with painful sores in the genital area. It is estimated that there are more than 700,000 new cases each year and that the disease is responsible for more than 500,000 physician visits annually.

Cause   Herpes simplex, type 2 causes most of the genital herpes cases. HSV1 causes most herpes infections above the waist. The virus can infect any skin or mucous membrane surface on the body. For example, a person with a cold sore who engages in oral sex can transmit herpes to a partner's genitals.

The infection is spread by contact with the genital secretions of a person with an active lesion. It is possible, however, for a person in the latent phase (with no active lesion) to shed virus and infect a sex partner. Genital herpes can also be acquired by infants as they pass through the birth canal of infected mothers. Neonatal herpes simplex infection can cause serious damage to the brain and many other organs; even with therapy, more than 20 percent of the 1,500 infants infected each year in the United States will die, and many of the survivors are seriously impaired. Because of this, thousands of women in the United States with a history of genital herpes are advised to undergo a Cesarean section when prenatal cultures or exams suggest an active infection near the time of delivery.

HSV2 infection can also lead to serious or fatal complications in adults who have a weakened immune system because of AIDS or who are undergoing drug therapy for organ transplants.

Symptoms Many people who are infected have no symptoms at all; only about 40 percent of victims ever have symptoms. When they do, the primary (or first) appearance of herpes lesions is the worst, with severe local symptoms and many painful lesions. These last up to 10 days, and it may take two to three weeks to completely recover from this first attack. When the sores fade away, the virus remains behind. The virus is now *latent.* During the first attack, some people have a generalized sick feeling, with swollen glands in the pelvic area and fever, fatigue, headache, muscle ache, and nausea. People with no antibodies to herpes (cold sores) usually will be sicker during a first attack. Women usually have lesions on the cervix or vulva. Recurrences may appear on the vulva, skin between vagina and anus, upper thighs, anal area, or

buttocks. Men get lesions on the head or shaft of the penis and the anus.

Most people have a recurrence within six months of their first attack. This recurrence begins with a tingling, itching, or prickling sensation in the area where the virus entered the body. This is followed in a few days by a raised cluster of small painful blisters; there may be several groups of blisters. Eventually, the sores will crust over and dry up. Most people don't have the generalized sick feeling with recurrent infections.

Patients are infectious until the sores heal completely, usually up to 12 days; recurrent infections usually remain infectious for up to a week. Recent studies have shown that it is quite possible to shed virus without symptoms, which is how it is possible to infect a partner when no sores are present.

Neonatal herpes can take many different forms. About one third of babies will have skin, eyes, or mouth lesions before any other symptoms; another third will have a brain infection (ENCEPHALITIS), PNEUMONIA, or infection of other organs. The other third will have both. Respiratory distress, fever, skin lesions, or convulsions are common herpes symptoms in newborns.

Diagnosis Doctors may diagnose genital herpes by symptoms alone, but there are also several lab tests that can confirm the infection. A specimen from the base of a lesion can identify the type of cell called giant cells, which usually indicates a herpes virus. Herpes also grows rapidly in tissue culture; specimens from a new lesion can be identified within 48 hours in the lab. Blood tests can look for antibodies to herpes; the newest blood tests can tell the difference between type 1 and 2, but differentiation is not clinically important as they both behave and are treated in the same way.

Complications Rarely, herpes MENINGITIS (infection in the lining of the brain or spinal cord) or herpes encephalitis (infection in the brain) follows an initial infection. In the past, it was believed that there could be a link between herpes and cancer of the cervix; new studies show that genital herpes probably has no role in cervical cancer.

Treatment   The antiviral drug acyclovir (Zovirax) became available in the 1980s to reduce the number and severity of attacks, but it is not a cure, since it does not kill the virus. Available in ointment, capsule, liquid, and IV forms, capsules are usually used to treat primary genital herpes or a severe recurrence, or to suppress frequent recurrences. Taking acyclovir at the first sign of a recurrence—that is, during the tingling phase before lesions begin—can shorten the healing time from four to five days to one day.

People with more than six recurrences in a year can take daily acyclovir to prevent recurrence. Most patients don't take acyclovir for more than three years. Very few people report side effects with this drug.

IV acyclovir is given for severe primary herpes for hospitalized patients. It is also given to babies born with or exposed to herpes during birth.

Frequent sitz baths in lukewarm water following by drying sores with a hair dryer on cool can ease the pain. A small amount of petroleum jelly on the sores can reduce the irritation during urination. Very painful sores may be eased with an anesthetic ointment. While sores are present, women should wear loose cotton underwear, avoiding pantyhose and tight pants.

Prevention   Several vaccines are currently being tested in clinical trials, but no vaccine is currently available to prevent genital herpes. At least two companies are in the final stages of clinical trials for such a vaccine, however.

herpes simplex, type 1 (HSV1)   One member of the herpesvirus family that is usually associated with infections of the lips, mouth, and face. This virus was first described by the Roman doctor Herodotus around A.D. 100 as "herpetic eruptions" around the mouth during fever. Recurrent episodes can be triggered by stress, ultraviolet light, immune system problems, or exertion. HSV1 is very similar to HSV2, with a nearly identical genetic code. Either type can infect the same body sites. See also HERPES.

herpes simplex, type 2 (HSV2)   A member of the herpesvirus family that is usually associated with infections in the genital area. It may also occur in newborns, who acquire the disease during birth. It is believed to infect one out of every five people in the United States, but only one third of those experience symptoms.

Like its close cousin HSV1, recurrent episodes of HSV2 can be triggered by stress, ultraviolet light, immune system problems, or exertion. See also HERPES.

herpes zoster   See SHINGLES.

Histoplasma capsulatum   A fungal organism that causes HISTOPLASMOSIS; it is a single budding yeast at body temperature and a mold at room temperature. The fungus is spread by airborne spores from soil contaminated with bird droppings and is commonly found in the Ohio and Mississippi River Valleys.

histoplasmosis   An infection caused by inhaling the spores of the fungus *Histoplasma capsulatum,* commonly found in the Mississippi River Valley. Infection confers immunity for life. The disease is endemic in the northern and central United States, Argentina, Brazil, Venezuela, and parts of Africa. Most people who inhale the spores aren't affected by them.

Cause   The disease is caused by a type of fungal organism that is a single, budding yeast at body temperature and a mold at room temperature. It is spread by airborne spores from soil contaminated with excreta from infected chickens, pigeons, and bats. In rare cases when infection does occur, it is either because a person has been exposed to large quantities of the spores (such as pigeon handlers) or because the patient's immune system is impaired, such as in AIDS.

Symptoms   The primary form of the disease doesn't usually produce any symptoms; when it does, they include breathlessness, cough, and joint pain. Spontaneous recovery is usual, although small areas of calcification in the lungs and lymph glands may remain.

In a few people (especially those with impaired immune systems), the disease takes a chronic, sometimes-fatal, form and spreads throughout the body. Called *progressive histoplasmosis,* the disease resembles TUBERCULOSIS and is characterized by ulcerating sores in the mouth and nose; enlarged spleen, liver, and lymph nodes; and severe infiltration of the lungs, with fever, malaise, and a cough. Between 50 to 100 people a year die from this form of disease.

Diagnosis   Examination of tissue or sputum and history will help confirm disease.

Treatment   There are antifungal agents of different toxicities available if the illness is severe enough to warrant treatment. The severe form of histoplasmosis is treated with the antifungal drug amphotericin B.

Prevention   In contaminated, enclosed environments (such as chicken coops) people should avoid exposure to the dust and surrounding soil. A protective mask, and spraying areas with water, may help minimize exposure. Avoid caves.

HIV   The acronym for HUMAN IMMUNODEFICIENCY VIRUS.

Hong Kong flu   See INFLUENZA.

hookworm disease   A condition caused by small round blood-sucking worms that penetrate the skin (usually the feet), causing a red itchy rash called ground itch. The worms, which belong to the species *Necator Americanus* (New World hookworm) or *Ancylostoma duodenale* (Old World hookworm), infest 1 billion people in tropical and Third World countries. One recent survey found that 17 percent of the people of China are infected. There is some risk of contracting hookworms in the United States.

Cause   Hookworm larvae live in the soil and infect humans by penetrating the skin. Once inside the body, they travel to the lungs and then inside the small intestine, where they attach themselves and drain blood for nourishment. Heavy hookworm infestation can cause considerable damage to the intestinal wall. While one hookworm extracts only a fraction of a teaspoon of blood from the circulation every day, more severe infestations can be more serious; an infestation of 1,000 worms can drain almost a cup of blood a day. If the victim can't replace the lost blood quickly enough (as in the case of pregnant women or children), this may cause an iron deficiency and malnutrition. In children, chronic infestation with worms can lead to slowed growth and impaired behavioral, cognitive, and motor development. Occasionally, hookworm disease may be fatal (especially to infants). See also DIARRHEA AND INFECTIOUS DISEASE; ANTIDIARRHEAL DRUGS.

Symptoms   In minor infestations, there may be no symptoms; in more severe cases, the worms can cause abdominal pain, anemia, cough, diarrhea, mental inertia, and pneumonia in addition to the itchy rash.

Treatment   Antihelminthic drugs (such as mebendazole) kill the worms; improved diet and blood transfusions may be necessary. Unfortunately, many areas of the world where infestation is a problem do not have access to drug treatment.

Prevention   Scientists are trying to develop vaccines using hookworm-produced proteins that would generate antibodies to neutralize the anticlotting proteins and cut off the worms' food supply. Such a vaccine would be of great help in areas where reinfestation is a problem.

Of course, the best prevention is to improve sanitation so that transmission can't occur, which is how hookworm disease was eradicated from the southeastern United

States. This is more difficult in most Third World countries.

hordeolum   See STYE.

hospital-acquired infections   Bacteria infections transmitted within hospitals pose one of the greatest and most controllable threats in the United States, where more than 5 percent of hospital admissions and about 14 percent of intensive care patients acquire an infection during their stay. According to some estimates, nosocomial (hospital-acquired) infections rank among the 10 leading causes of death in the United States, with the incidence of bloodstream infections doubling during the 1980s. These infections today affect about 2 million patients each year in acute care facilities and cost about $3.5 billion, according to the Hospital Infections Program of the National Center for Infectious Diseases, CDC.

While the disease-causing organisms found in hospitals can be virulent, the main problem in hospital-acquired infection is that hospitalized patients usually have an underlying disease, invasive procedures, or impaired immune function in the first place.

HPV   See PAPILLOMAVIRUS, HUMAN.

HSV   See HERPES.

human granulocytic ehrlichiosis   See EHRLICHIOSIS, HUMAN GRANULOCYTIC.

human immunodeficiency virus (HIV)   A type of retrovirus that causes AIDS (acquired immunodeficiency syndrome). It is transmitted through contact with infected person's blood, semen, cervical secretions, or cerebrospinal fluid.

The HIV infects the T-helper cells of the immune system, causing an infection with a slow onset of symptoms. As the immune system is destroyed, the patient becomes ill with a variety of other infections such as Kaposi's sarcoma, pneumocystis carinii PNEUMONIA, CANDIDIASIS, and TUBERCULOSIS.

The most important tests for detecting the virus is the initial antibody tests that establish the diagnosis of HIV. The screening test is confirmed by a Western Blot test. Doctors now monitor therapies and patients' progress by measuring the number of T4 lymphocytes the patient has left. When the number of T4 lymphocytes nears 200 or fewer, the patient is at high risk for other infections.

Recently, it has become possible to measure the actual number of viruses present in the blood. This test is called the viral load.

human papillomavirus (HPV)   See PAPILLOMAVIRUS, HUMAN.

humidifiers and infectious disease   The use of a humidifier during the winter can help keep mucous membranes moist and healthy—but poorly maintained humidifiers can be the source of infection.

The nose, throat, and lungs work best when the air has a relative humidity of about 40 percent. If the air during the winter falls below that level, moisture will be absorbed into the heated air from the mucous membranes. Since dried mucous membranes can't clean themselves, they become more vulnerable to invasion from cold viruses. A well-maintained humidifier can keep the air moist and nose and throat moist.

But it's imperative that the device is used correctly. If the air becomes too humid, or the machine isn't properly cleaned, mold and dust mites can multiply.

To keep the risk of infection from molds or bacteria to a minimum, don't let the humidity rise above 40 percent and clean the water reservoir in the humidifier *daily* with a vinegar solution.

HUS   See HEMOLYTIC UREMIC SYNDROME.

immune response   The body's defensive reaction to invading organisms that are recognized as foreign to the body. The response triggers the production of antibodies, lymphocytes (white blood cells), and other substances and cells that destroy the invaders. See also IMMUNE SYSTEM; IMMUNITY; IMMUNIZATION.

immune system   The human body protects itself against invasion from a wide variety of infectious diseases by an intricate combination of organs and cells called the immune system. The network works most efficiently when a person is well rested, eats a healthy diet, and is not under too much stress. Of course, genetics plays a part as well; some people are born with stronger immune systems than others.

When a germ enters the body, the immune system goes into action, triggering the white blood cells called lymphocytes to attack. White blood cells move throughout the body via the organs of the immune system, including bone marrow, lymph nodes, tonsils, adenoids, thymus gland, blood, and lymphatic vessels. Lymphocytes come in two varieties: B cells, which are produced in the bone marrow, and T cells, which mature in the thymus gland. Both of these cells produce antibodies that destroy bacteria and viruses. A third type of white blood cell—the large phagocytes—surround invading microbes and swallow them.

This immune response is often the source of all of the symptoms people experience during an infection—chills, fever, aches, appetite loss, fatigue, inflammation, and rash.

People whose immune system is not working well—such as patients with AIDS—have more difficulty in fighting off invading germs. This is why anyone with an impaired immune system gets sick more often, and more seriously, with illnesses that might not even harm someone whose immune system is working properly. See also IMMUNE RESPONSE; IMMUNIZATION.

immunity   The quality of being unaffected by a particular disease or condition.

immunization   A method of producing immunity to disease through artificial means. This is done through a vaccination, which is an injection of treated antigens to stimulate the body to produce its own antibodies to a specific disease. The material in the vaccination may either be live bacteria, viruses treated so that they are harmless, or dead organisms or their products that are altered to produce the same effect.

While the United States has produced many vaccinations to deal with a variety of infectious disease, the only infection that has been eradicated throughout the world is SMALLPOX.

Preschoolers are the most vulnerable to communicable disease, which is why infants soon after birth are started on a U.S. government-required series of immunizations. While at present there are a series of shots that must be given to protect against childhood diseases, within the next five years scientists predict there may be one vaccine to protect against six diseases.

Immunization is not straightforward, however. Some vaccines are perceived by the public as carrying a risk, especially the pertussis part of the DPT (diphtheria-pertussis-tetanus) vaccine, which had been linked to seizures and other serious side effects. In response to these concerns, a safer acellular version of the pertussis vaccine is now in use.

Reports from health departments estimate that less than half of American children are properly immunized by age two; in the inner city, the rate drops to less than a third. Since 1991, most insurance companies cover children's immunizations, and some health departments offer free shots.

While a serious illness precludes a vaccination, minor colds with low fevers do not interfere with immunization. Slight soreness and swelling at the injection site are normal and are not an indication that the child should not finish the series of shots. Antibiotics prescribed for another illness will not interfere with the vaccination except the oral typhoid vaccine.

A child should NOT be vaccinated if she has had a serious allergic reaction to a previous shot. Anyone who has a severe allergy to eggs should not receive the MMR (measles-mumps-rubella), INFLUENZA, or YELLOW FEVER vaccines. A child with serious illness should be not vaccinated until fully recovered.

immunizations for adults   Anyone over age 65 should get several vaccines, including a tetanus diphtheria (Td) every 10 years, an INFLUENZA vaccine each fall, and one dose of pneumococcal polysaccharide vaccine with a booster every six years for transplant recipients, patients without a spleen, or anyone with chronic kidney failure. See also IMMUNIZATION; VACCINE.

immunizations for chronic disease patients   Anyone with chronic heart disease, lung problems, diabetes, kidney disease, or sickle cell disease should have the pneumococcal vaccine and an INFLUENZA vaccine each fall. See also IMMUNIZATION; VACCINE.

immunizations for health care professionals   Several immunizations are suggested for anyone who works in the health care field and comes into contact with patients. These include the HEPATITIS B vaccine (Recombivax or EngerixB) in a three-dose series; INFLUENZA vaccine every fall; MMR (measles-mumps-rubella) vaccine unless there is proof of immunity; and Td. See also IMMUNIZATION; VACCINE.

immunizations for homosexual males/heterosexuals with multiple partners   Anyone with this sexual history should receive the HEPATITIS B vaccine in a three-dose series, plus routine vaccines recommended for adults. See also IMMUNIZATION; VACCINE.

immunizations for institutionalized patients   Developmentally disabled residents of group-living institutions should receive a HEPATITIS B vaccine in a three-dose series, since these patients have a high rate of hepatitis B. They should also receive an INFLUENZA vaccine each fall. See also IMMUNIZATION; VACCINE.

immunizations for kidney disease patients   Anyone undergoing hemodialysis or who has had a kidney transplant should receive the three-dose series of HEPATITIS B, an INFLUENZA vaccine each fall, and the PNEUMOCOCCAL VACCINE. See also IMMUNIZATION; VACCINE.

immunizations for patients with impaired immune systems   Anyone with an impaired immune system should receive an INFLUENZA vaccine each fall, and a one-time PNEUMOCOCCAL VACCINE with a booster in six years. Those with HIV infection should also receive these two vaccines, plus the primary series of the *HAEMOPHILUS INFLUENZAE* TYPE B conjugate vaccine (Hib). Also indicated are two doses of the measles-mumps-rubella (MMR) vaccine and the inactivated poliovirus vaccine if not immune or without previous vaccination.

Patients who have had their spleen removed should have both the pneumococcal and meningococcal vaccine. See also IMMUNIZATION; VACCINE.

immunizations for pregnant women Pregnant women who are not immune to MEASLES, MUMPS, or rubella should receive these live virus VACCINES right after delivery. Otherwise, pregnant women should receive a booster dose of tetanus (Td) if more than 10 years have passed since the last vaccine, together with a HEPATITIS B vaccine if the woman is at risk of exposure because of lifestyle or contact with a carrier. She should receive an INFLUENZA vaccine if she has medical conditions that warrant this. She should only receive YELLOW FEVER and polio vaccines if she is traveling to an area where there is a high risk of exposure, and travel can't be put off until after delivery. See also IMMUNIZATION.

immunizations for public safety workers Several immunizations are suggested for anyone who works in the public safety field. These include the HEPATITIS B vaccine (Recombivax or EngerixB) in a three-dose series; INFLUENZA vaccine every fall; MMR (measles-mumps-rubella) vaccine unless there is proof of immunity. See also IMMUNIZATION; VACCINE.

immunizations for research lab workers For those who work in research labs, anyone who handles specimens that contain poliovirus should receive inactivated poliovirus VACCINE in the absence of three doses of oral polio vaccine. Anyone who works with PLAGUE bacteria should have a plague vaccine (the three-dose primary series, with boosters every one to two years). Scientists who work with ANTHRAX bacteria (*Bacillus anthracis*) should receive the anthrax vaccine. Finally, people who work with RABIES virus should have the rabies preventive vaccine. See also IMMUNIZATION.

immunizations for veterinarians Vets and animal handlers should receive a RABIES vaccine and blood test every two years, with a booster if necessary. Those working in western states should also receive a PLAGUE vaccine in a three-dose primary series, with boosters every one or two years. See also IMMUNIZATION.

immunoglobulin Any of five distinct antibodies present in the blood and bodily secretions. In response to specific antigens, immunoglobulins are formed in the bone marrow, spleen, and all lymphoid tissue of the body (except the thymus). Kinds of immunoglobulins include IgA, IgD, IgE, IgG, and IgM.

impetigo, bullous Also called staphylococcal impetigo, this is a superficial skin infection caused by *Staphylococcus aureus* bacteria.

Symptoms Thin-walled flaccid bullae that rupture easily and contain fluid ranging from clear to pus. After rupture, the base quickly dries to a shiny veneer, which looks different than the thicker crust found in common impetigo. Lesions are usually found in groups in one area.

Treatment As with common impetigo, bullous impetigo is treated with antibiotics. Topical treatment is not helpful. Septic complications are rare but can occur. See also IMPETIGO, COMMON.

impetigo, common A superficial skin infection most commonly found in children caused by streptococcal bacteria. Impetigo should be treated as soon as possible to avoid spreading the infection to other children and to prevent a rare complication—a form of kidney disease called acute glomerulonephritis.

Impetigo is spread by touching and is usually found on exposed body areas such as the legs, face, and arms. Because impetigo is spread quickly through play groups and day care, children with the infection should be kept away from playmates and out of school until the sores disappear.

Symptoms The condition starts as tiny, almost imperceptible blisters on a child's skin, usually at the site of skin abrasion, scratch, or insect bite. Most lesions occur on exposed areas, such as the face, scalp, and extremities. The red and itchy sores blister briefly, then begin to ooze for the next few days, leaving a sticky crust. Untreated, the infection will last from two to three weeks. It is most prevalent during hot, humid weather.

Treatment   Parents shouldn't let impetigo run its course but instead get treatment for children immediately to avoid spreading the infection to other children. Oral antibiotics that kill strep are given for 10 days.

Complications   Rarely, impetigo can lead to possible kidney disease known as acute glomerulonephritis. In this case, the patient's immune system makes antibodies to the strep, which unfortunately are harmful to the patient's own kidneys.

Prevention   Cleanliness and prompt attention to skin injury can help prevent impetigo. Impetigo patients and their families should bathe regularly with antibacterial soaps and apply topical antibiotics to insect bites, cuts, abrasions, and infected lesions immediately. Impetigo in infants is especially contagious and serious. To prevent spreading, pillowcases, towels, and washcloths shouldn't be shared and should be washed with antibacterial soaps and chlorine bleach.

impetigo, staphylococcal   See IMPETIGO, BULLOUS.

impetigo, streptococcal   See IMPETIGO, COMMON.

infant botulism   See BOTULISM.

infection control   The policies and procedures of a health facility aimed at reducing the risk of hospital-acquired or community-acquired infections spreading to others. See also HOSPITAL-ACQUIRED INFECTIONS.

infectious disease   Any illness that is caused by a specific microorganism. Infectious dis-

eases are a large and important group of conditions; they remain the major cause of death throughout the world. According to the World Health Organization, the 1997 "world's deadliest diseases" are all infectious. In order, they are: PNEUMONIA, DIARRHEA, TUBERCULOSIS, MALARIA, HEPATITIS B, AIDS, MEASLES, TETANUS, WHOOPING COUGH, and ROUNDWORM.

Cause   Infectious disease-causing organisms make up a number of well-defined groups: the most important are viruses, bacteria, and fungi, together with three smaller groups (the rickettsiae, chlamydiae, and mycloplasmas). All of these organisms are fairly simple and can quickly multiply in tissue. In addition, the more complicated parasites (PROTOZOA, worms, and FLUKES) spend only part of their life inside human tissue; colonization of a human being by one of these parasites is usually referred to as an infestation, not an infection.

Prevention   Many serious infectious diseases can be avoided by IMMUNIZATION; by using condoms, practicing good hygiene, and avoiding contact with animal feces. For travel outside the developed world, extra immunizations and careful measures to guard against insects can help.

Symptoms   Symptoms of infectious diseases are caused partly by the damage done to cells and tissues by the microorganisms and the toxins (poisons) they release. Symptoms are also caused by the body itself as it tries to fend off the attack. The strength of a patient's immune system can strongly influence how quickly and how well the infection is fought off. One of the most common signs of infection is fever.

One of the problems with infectious diseases is that there is usually a time lapse (the "incubation period") during which the person has the infection but does not experience symptoms. Often, the victim can transmit the infection during this period; some people may never develop symptoms, but can still pass on the disease. This is how an epidemic can begin and become established before preventive measures can be taken. This is particularly devastating if the disease has a long incubation period and fatal outcome, such as in AIDS.

Treatment   Treatment for infectious diseases often involves antibiotics and other antimicrobial drugs. Because some organisms are susceptible only to certain antibiotics, doctors must carefully choose which medication to prescribe. The "miracle drug" antibiotics such as PENICILLIN and tetracycline have been so often prescribed—and often misused by patients—that they have encouraged the microbes to develop resistance and even immunity. The result: infections that are nearly impossible to treat. Today, doctors are seeing infections that are no longer treatable because the bacterium is resistant to every antibiotic ever developed. Drug companies have begun working on new antibiotics, but these new drugs are years away from approval and widespread use.

Over the past 100 years, many of the developed countries believed they were gradually winning the war against infectious diseases due to better sanitation, pest control, personal hygiene, and quarantines. Effective drugs were developed as were vaccines to provide immunity against certain illnesses. The general health and good nutrition of most people in the developed countries bolstered their immune systems and improved survival. Unfortunately, just as scientists were feeling most complacent, the picture began to change.

During the past 20 years, 30 new diseases have emerged to threaten the health of hundreds of millions of people. For many of these diseases there is no treatment, cure, or vaccine. The mortality rate from infectious disease between 1980 and 1992 increased from 41 to 65 deaths per 100,000. Even discounting AIDS, deaths in the United States from infectious diseases has risen 39 percent over these years. Overuse of medicine, human settlement of uninhabited areas, international travel, and poverty have combined to produce a devastating spread of infectious diseases, according to the World Health Organization.

There is still no really effective medicine against viruses, which do not respond to antibiotics. Treatment for the viral diseases remains primarily symptomatic: controlling pain, fever, inflammation, and fluid intake.

As people push farther and farther into the tropical rain forests, they are coming into more frequent contact with deadly microbial diseases that have been circulating among animals for centuries. Diseases have been crossing over from animal to man and back again for years, but only in recent history could germs take advantage of space-age transportation linking countries and continents around the globe. While the deadly yet rare infections are frightening enough, there are diseases today in the United States hospitals that cannot be cured.

Many organizations such as the National Council on International Health and the American Public Health Association are working with governmental agencies like the Centers for Disease Control and the U.S. Agency for International Development to develop a plan to meet the growing threat of infectious diseases. The CDC, calling infectious diseases a "global crisis," notes that new diseases are emerging just as old diseases, such as TB and PLAGUE, are returning to kill again. Many of these older diseases have developed resistance to modern drugs. Experts say today that the world will be lucky to make it through the next 30 years without a new pandemic.

infectious   mononucleosis See   MONONUCLEOSIS.

infectious parotitis   See MUMPS.

influenza (flu) A contagious respiratory infection that often occurs in EPIDEMICS. The disease is most dangerous not in itself, but because it can lead to PNEUMONIA, especially among older people and those with impaired immune systems. When complicated by pneumonia, the flu is the sixth most common cause of death in the United States, killing 20,000 Americans.

Influenza occurs most often in the winter months. Although illnesses like the flu may occur in summer, these are usually caused by other viruses. Every year as winter begins, the flu spreads across the globe; in the United States, up to 50 million people will be infected. The flu is responsible for about three days of lost work per adult, and field studies indicate the attack rate ranges from a low of about 10 percent in people over age 65 to a high of 36 percent in children from ages 1 to 18. At the peak of a typical epidemic, up to 22 percent of all physician visits are for flulike symptoms.

While more than 90 percent of flu-related deaths occur among the elderly, children under age 5 and women in the third trimester of pregnancy are also at higher risk for complications. The word *flu* is a slang term that applies to a variety of types of viral GAS-TROENTERITIS (stomach or intestinal flu), which are not really related to the true respiratory influenza caused by influenza virus.

History   Influenza is as old as human history; the mysterious 430 B.C. deadly plague in Athens may have been caused in part by deadly flu viruses. Historians also suspect that the mighty army of Charlemagne was destroyed by a flu epidemic of A.D. 876. The first true recorded flu pandemic occurred in the 16th century. In 1647, the flu was causing havoc in North America up through New England, where it was known variously as "jolly rant," "grippe," and "the new acquaintance." Its current name was bestowed after the 1732 epidemic in the American colonies, when English doctor John Huxham linked the disease with an old Italian folk word that linked colds, cough, and fever to the "influ-

ence" of the stars. About every 20 to 50 years, another pandemic (worldwide epidemic) sweeps across Earth, with yearly local epidemics in between. Major pandemics occurred in 1627, 1729, 1788, 1830, 1847, 1872, 1890, 1918, 1957, and 1968.

Several times in this century, influenza has appeared as a much more serious pandemic; these major episodes occur when the flu virus undergoes an "antigenic shift" in which one flu subtype is replaced by a different strain for which the population has not developed antibodies. Therefore, everyone is extremely susceptible to infection.

Still, because there were far more deadly diseases to worry about, even in the beginning of this century the flu did not attract much medical attention until the great Spanish flu pandemic of 1918, the worst of the pandemics, killing 10 million more people than did World War I. In the United States alone, 550,000 people died. The Spanish flu of 1918 left about 21 million dead out of about 1 billion cases before it vanished; scientists still don't know where it went and worry that another outbreak could occur. Its name was particularly insulting to Spaniards, since this particular pandemic appeared to have actually begun in the United States.

The 1918 pandemic was not restricted to the big cities, although more than 20,000 New Yorkers were killed in the fall of 1918. Whole Inuit villages in Alaska were decimated, and Samoa lost 20 percent of its people.

Since World War II, vaccines have helped cut the death rate, which was very low in the 1957 pandemic of Asian flu, and in the 1968 pandemic. In 1976, an outbreak of swine flu in Fort Dix, New Jersey, set off alarms throughout the United States, since it was swine flu that was believed to have caused the mass mortality in 1918, although no one knows for sure. Then-president Gerald Ford signed a law providing $135 million for a vaccine campaign that reached about a quarter of the population. The United States and Canada set up a crash mass vaccination program; however, when some people who had been vaccinated developed Guillain-Barre syndrome (a rare type of temporary paralysis) the United States canceled its program. The dreaded pandemic never developed, and the U.S. government eventually paid about $93 million in damages to Guillain-Barre victims.

Cause The influenza virus was first named *Hemophilus bacterium influenzae,* but this was never proved conclusively. In the same year, W. Smith, F. W. Andrewes, and P. P. Laidlaw proved the cause of influenza was a virus that was experimentally transmissible to ferrets. This virus is now identified as influenza A. Influenza B virus was discovered in 1940, and influenza C was identified nine years after that. At the moment, the virus exists as one of these three types. However, types A and B mutate quickly; several strains of each of these types now exist. The three basic flu types have variants that are designated according to where they first strike, such as New Jersey (A), Bangkok (A), and so on. The 1957 and 1968 Asian flu pandemics were caused by strains of type A.

The highly contagious infection is spread by direct contact or via droplets and dust in the air over short distances from patients who are coughing or sneezing. The virus can also survive for hours in dried mucous, so dirty tissues should be carefully disposed of. Anyone can catch the flu, regardless of age, sex, or race, but certain groups are more likely to develop complications of the disease. Deaths occur primarily among those over age 65, or those with certain chronic diseases.

The contagious period varies, but it probably starts the day before symptoms appear and extends for about a week.

An attack will confer immunity to the specific strain only. Because the viruses that cause flu are always changing (mutating), people who have been infected or who have gotten a flu shot in other years may become infected with a new strain.

Symptoms About one or two days after exposure, symptoms of flu develop suddenly, with fever, headache, and body aches. Intestinal symptoms are uncommon. The throat is sore, dry, and red. A cough appears on the second or third day, followed by a drop in fever with drenching sweats by the third to fifth day. As the fever drops, the patient becomes highly susceptible to secondary bacterial invasion. Fatigue and depression may last for weeks afterward.

Although most people are sick for only a few days, some people have a much more serious illness (such as pneumonia) and may need to be hospitalized.

Diagnosis There is no easy way to diagnose influenza. While the virus can be isolated from the throat, and antibodies can be found in the blood, these tests are expensive and slow. Diagnosis is usually made on the basis of the symptoms and the occurrence of other cases in the area.

Treatment There is no specific cure for the flu. No known antibiotic has any effect on any type or strain of virus, although antibiotics may be used to treat a secondary bacterial pneumonia. Treatment is usually aimed at reducing fever and relieving symptoms. Rest and liquids are usually adequate.

In addition to the vaccine, two oral prescription drugs (amantadine and rimantadine) may prevent or reduce the severity of influenza A but are not effective against type B (which accounts for 30 percent of flu cases). Rimantadine (Flumadine) or amantadine (Symmetrel) are designed to shorten illness by preventing the flu virus from reproducing. They work best if taken as soon as the flu strikes. Rimantadine is a closely related product that produces fewer side effects and can be used safely by adults; it is being tested for safety in children.

Side effects, including nausea, insomnia, and impaired concentration affect about 1 in every 30 patients. Amantadine causes similar side effects in 1 of every 10 patients; it's cheaper than rimantadine when bought as a generic. An antiviral may help even if you've been sick for several days, but once you start to get better they probably won't be very effective.

Prevention Routine vaccination against the flu is the most important way to control the disease. Vaccines are available through personal physicians or the local health department. Research has shown that even in years when new strains emerge, people in high-risk groups who get yearly flu shots tend to have milder illnesses and are less likely to be hospitalized with complications due to influenza A.

The first practical vaccination against the flu was developed in 1943 with killed viruses of both types A and B. Because the influenza viruses are constantly evolving, the vaccines must continually be updated; as new strains of the virus appear, they are included in the vaccine.

Each year, scientists at the U.S. Centers for Disease Control and the World Health Organization make an educated guess about which kind of flu will predominate during the next winter season. These two groups maintain a global network that collects data required to select strains for the coming flu season's vaccine, and monitor the occurrence of especially severe epidemics. A similar process is undertaken in Europe by the WHO and various national authorities there.

In this country, for example, when developing the flu vaccine for the winter of 1994–95, CDC scientists studied flu viruses from 1,500 samples around the world. They chose in March 1994 to include vaccine made from three strains, A-Texas, B-Panama, and A-Shangdong; four drug companies then manufactured 70 million doses of vaccine.

The U.S. Public Health Service recommends annual vaccination only for those most likely to develop complications from influenza. This includes anyone over age 65 or anyone with a chronic debilitating disease such as heart disease, chronic respiratory dis-

ease (such as asthma, bronchitis, or emphysema), or a chronic metabolic disorder (such as diabetes). Other people at high risk are residents of nursing homes and other institutions housing patients of any age with serious long-term health problems, people with kidney disease, cystic fibrosis, anemia, asthma, cancer, or immunological disorders. In addition, household contacts of high-risk people, and health care workers who care for those at high risk, should be vaccinated. The shots are 70 to 80 percent effective in preventing flu.

Immunity to the strains of flu in a particular vaccine occurs within about a week or two of getting the shot. Because the vaccine is made from killed virus, you can't get the flu from a shot.

Because the viruses that cause flu are always changing (mutating), people who have been infected or who have gotten a flu shot in other years may become infected with a new strain. Because of this and because immunity from an earlier flu shot can decrease the next year, people in high-risk groups should be vaccinated each year.

People with severe allergies to eggs should avoid the shot.

In the fall of 1997, a limited recall of flu vaccine was necessary for the first time since flu vaccines had been distributed because certain batches did not fully protect against the disease. Those who had been immunized with the weakend vaccine were asked to be revaccinated to protect against disease.

New research California scientists are preparing to conduct human tests of an aspirin-sized pill containing an ingredient that rids lab animals of flu symptoms within a day. The drug works by disrupting an enzyme found on the surface of major strains of flu virus. Scientists at Gilead Sciences in Foster City were expected to try the drug on Europeans in 1997 to see if it has the same effect on humans as it did on mice and ferrets. While ferrets contract the same type of flu that humans get, scientists cautioned that often, drugs that work in animals don't always work in humans. Swiss pharmaceutical giant Hoffmann-La Roche will carry out the trials in collaboration with Gilead. The company is planning on testing the drug in the United States in late 1997.

In other flu-related research, scientists have discovered that continuous high stress could interfere with the efficacy of the flu vaccine by interfering with the body's ability to mount a defense against the flu virus. They suggest that older patients who are under stress should be sure to get a yearly flu shot.

Moreover, recent research suggests that annual fall vaccinations could also keep working-age people healthier and more productive, reducing wintertime sick days by about a third. Up to this time, flu shots for the 87 million younger workers had been considered to be a matter of personal choice. The new study found that while healthy adults face little risk of dying from the flu, preventing it still has advantages. First, those getting shots have fewer bouts of upper respiratory illnesses of any kind, miss less work, and have lower medical bills.

Researchers are also working on a new cold-adapted influenza vaccine, a type of needleless vaccine that would be administered as a nasal spray. Doctors hope such a spray would be as effective as a shot, but far more convenient, since it could be administered by patients themselves with a doctor's prescription.

Scientists are also investigating a better type of vaccine that is genetically engineered, containing a purified recombinant version of a flu virus surface protein. Currently licensed vaccines contain killed flu virus produced using chicken eggs. They protect from 70 to 90 percent of young adults but are much less effective in the elderly. The new vaccine, being developed by MicroGeneSys of Meriden, Connecticut, can be produced faster with fewer side effects (such as arm pain and tenderness at the injection site). Because the experimental vaccine contains fewer impurities, it can be used at higher doses with less chance of toxicity. And since it doesn't contain any egg proteins, it can be given to patients with allergies to eggs. See also AVIAN FLU.

insects and disease   There are at least 1 million known species of insects in the world, and most are either harmless or helpful to humans. The harmful ones, however, are capable of causing sickness in many ways, such as by becoming parasites to humans, living underneath the skin or on the body surface, or spreading disease on their feet and legs. Biting insects can spread infectious organisms, including MALARIA and FILARIASIS, LEISHMANIASIS, ONCHOCERCIASIS, CHAGAS DISEASE (American TRYPANOSOMIASIS), African trypanosomiasis, and so on.

Insects are found everywhere on the planet, from the poles to the equator, from the highest elevations to the level of the sea. At any one time, there are about 10 quintillion individual insects flying or crawling around on the earth, as they've been doing for the past 400 million years. In fact, insects are among the most successful life forms that have ever lived, outnumbering humans one billion to one. More than half of all known species—and three quarters of all known animal species—are insects. But there are plenty of insects out there yet to be classified: anywhere from 3 to 30 or more unknown species for every one that has been identified. Most insect-carried diseases are confined to the tropics and subtropics, but some are beginning to appear in the United States.

To cut down on the chance of mosquito bites, travelers should use mosquito nets and wear clothes that cover the body. The most effective repellent is DEET, which should be used carefully and sparingly and is not recommended for children. High concentrations (over 35 percent) should be avoided. Travelers should also buy a flying-insect killing spray to use in living and sleeping quarters during the night. For even more protection, clothing and bed nets can be sprayed with permethrin, an insect repellant licensed for use on clothing only. If used correctly, permethrin will repel insects from clothing for several weeks. Portable mosquito bed nets, DEET, and permethrin can be bought in hardware or backpacking stores.

interferon   A natural protein produced by cells infected with a virus that has the ability to interfere with viral growth. Interferon is active against many viruses, but specific interferons are effective only against the virus that produced them. There are three types of interferons: alpha, beta, and gamma.

The substances were discovered in 1957 by two researchers at the National Institute for Medical Research in London. The two (Alick Isaacs and Jean Lindenmann) showed that the protein secreted by infected cells did not interact with viruses directly; instead, the substance induces diseased cells and their neighbors to make still other proteins that could prevent invading viruses from replicating.

Researchers have also discovered that interferons are not a single molecule but that there are various forms, all of which are able to interfere with viral infection. These molecules belong to the family of cytokines—small proteins that carry signals from one cell to another.

The important part that interferons play in the immune system cannot be overestimated. Interferons influence the activity of almost every part of the immune system, boosting the body's ability to fight off attacks to most disease-causing microbes, including bacteria and parasites as well as viruses. Interferons can also inhibit cell division, which may explain in part why they can often impair the growth of cancer cells. One type of interferon

has even been found to help maintain early pregnancy in several animal species.

Because this protein is so important to the body's health, scientists have been concentrating on ways to harness its activity to fight disease. While initial hopes that interferon would prove to be a magic cure for all disease has proved to be unfounded, they have been approved by the U.S. Food and Drug Administration to treat seven diseases, including chronic HEPATITIS C, genital WARTS, KAPOSI'S SARCOMA, and multiple sclerosis.

isolation precautions   Procedures (including isolating in a private room) designed to prevent a patient from infecting others or from being infected by them. Complete isolation is used if a patient has a contagious disease, such as TUBERCULOSIS, that can be transmitted to others by direct contact and airborne droplets. All people entering the patient's room must wear masks, gowns, caps, and gloves, which are afterward burned or sterilized. Bed linen, eating utensils, bedpans, and other items that touch the patient also are sterilized. Even though they wear gloves, nurses must wash their hands after each nursing task.

Partial isolation is ordered if a patient's disease is transmitted in a more limited fashion; for example, only by breathing (as in WHOOPING COUGH) or only by contact with infected skin (such as IMPETIGO), blood (as in AIDS), or feces (as in CHOLERA).

Reverse isolation is used to protect a patient whose resistance to infection is very low or nonexistent. Air entering the room is filtered, and visiting is limited; everyone who visits must wear caps, gowns, masks, and gloves. Bed linen and all items used by the patient are sterilized. In severe cases, such as patients who are undergoing bone marrow transplantation, the patient is placed in an isolator or in a room ventilated with special purified air.

jail fever A nickname for TYPHUS.

Japanese encephalitis See ENCEPHALITIS, JAPANESE.

Jarisch-Herxheimer reaction A reaction following treatment for SYPHILIS (and other intracellular infections) caused by the widespread death of antigens. The syndrome is named for the 19th-century Austrian dermatologist Adolph Jarisch, who first described it.

The reaction is often accompanied by headache and fever and is more common in those with early syphilis. There are no proven ways to prevent the reaction.

jock itch The common term for tinea cruris, a common fungal infection of the genital area. It is most common among males and in the tropics.

Cause The infection is caused by certain fungi of the species *Trichophyton, Microsporum,* or *Epidermophyton floccosum.* These fungi live on skin tissue, hair, and nails. The fungi are transmitted by sharing towels, benches, or shower stalls in locker rooms. Since fungi grow best in warm, moist environments, they thrive in hot, humid weather and among men who sweat a lot, wear tight clothing, or who are obese.

Symptoms Jock itch is a mild but annoying infection characterized by reddened, itchy, scaly areas spreading from the genitals outward to the inner thighs. The rash may be dry, crusted, bumpy, or moist; the scrotum is not usually affected. Some people are prone to jock itch and are often reinfected.

Diagnosis A fungal culture from skin scrapings will provide a definite diagnosis. However, it may be difficult to differentiate jock itch from other yeast infections in the groin. It is important to have the condition correctly diagnosed.

Treatment Antifungal drugs (such as miconazole and clotrimazole) are often prescribed as a lotion, cream, or ointment to ease the itchy rash.

The area should be bathed well with soap and water, removing all scabs and crusts, followed by application of antifungal cream on all lesions. Treatment should be continued for some time after the symptoms have passed to make sure the fungi has been eliminated and to prevent recurrence. Mild infections on the skin surface may require treatment for up to six weeks.

In very severe cases, or if there is no improvement with the cream after a few days, some people require oral medication.

Complications Scratching the rash can lead to additional skin infection.

jungle fever The common name for YELLOW FEVER.

K

Kaposi's sarcoma   A condition characterized by malignant skin tumors that is mainly found in patients with AIDS. Before the development of the AIDS epidemic, Kaposi's sarcoma was a fairly rare condition that developed slowly and was seen almost exclusively in elderly Italian and Jewish men. It is also sometimes associated with diabetes, malignant lymphoma, or other disorders. In patients with AIDS, it is highly aggressive with widespread tumors.

Kaposi's sarcoma was named for the 19th-century Austrian dermatologist Moritz Kaposi, who first identified the disease. It also has been called idiopathic multiple pigmented hemorrhagic sarcoma, or multiple idiopathic hemorrhagic sarcoma.

Symptoms   Blue-red to brown nodules usually start on the feet and ankles, spread farther up the legs, and then appear on the hands and arms. In those with AIDS, tumors also often affect the gastrointestinal and respiratory tracts, where they may cause severe internal bleeding.

Treatment   For mild cases, low-dose radiation therapy is usually effective; for more severe cases, anticancer drugs are necessary to slow the development of tumors. There is no cure.

Kaposi's varicelliform eruption   See ECZEMA, HERPETICUM.

Kawasaki disease   A serious yet relatively rare rash found mostly in infants and children under age five. It is known medically as mucocutaneous lymph node syndrome. While it is possible to experience the syndrome more than once, recurrence is extremely rare.

Cause   Little is known how the syndrome is spread or how a person contracts it, although it does not appear to be transmitted from one person to another. Since outbreaks occur, it is suspected to be related to an infectious agent. However, a genetic predisposition has been indicated.

Symptoms   Most patients experience a high fever (lasting more than five days) that does not respond to antibiotics. There may also be irritability, swollen lymph nodes, red eyes, lips, throat, and tongue. The rash may cover the entire body and may be followed by peeling of the skin on hands and fingers.

Treatment   Most patients are treated in the hospital, where they can be watched and given aspirin and immunoglobulins.

Complications   The most common complication is a ballooning of the vessels of the heart (coronary artery aneurysm). Other organs may also be involved. Between 1 and 2 percent of patients die of the disease and its complications.

Prevention   There are no known ways to prevent the disease.

kerion   An inflamed area of the skin that develops as an immune reaction to a fungus (usually scalp RINGWORM).

Symptoms   Kerion is characterized by a red, pustular swelling that lasts for up to two months and may leave a scar and permanent loss of hair from the affected area. See also TINEA.

Treatment   While the swelling may heal without treatment, applications of ichthamnol paste and antifungal agents are used also.

kidney disorders, infectious   Infection of the kidney is called PYELONEPHRITIS. The infection often occurs when there is an obstruction of the flow of urine through the urinary tract, leading to stagnation of urine. The cause of the obstruction may be a kidney defect present at birth, a kidney stone, bladder tumor, or enlarged prostate. Pyelonephritis also can result from spread by the blood stream.

TUBERCULOSIS of the kidney is caused by infection carried by the blood from elsewhere in the body (usually the lungs).

kitchen infections The dirtiest area of the home, teeming with unseen microbes and deadly organisms, is the kitchen. Disease-causing organisms are found everywhere in the average American kitchen—in the sponges, dish towels, sink, and countertops. The diseases they cause kill more than 9,000 Americans every year, primarily the very young, the very old, and those with impaired immune systems. The cost of treating food-borne infections alone range from $5 billion to $22 billion, according to the U.S. General Accounting Office. Food-borne infections occur far more often in food prepared in the home kitchen than in commercial restaurants.

While state and federal agencies compile statistics about widespread infections traced to food and food-preparation areas, many cases of individual illness are never reported. Studies that have looked at this area have discovered that household exposure to food-borne pathogens is the primary source of illness. For example, from 1989 to 1991 in England and Wales, 86 percent of the 2,766 reported outbreaks of SALMONELLA infection involving more than one person appeared to originate in the home.

Bacteria tend to concentrate in the sink, the drain, and kitchen sponges, according to researchers. In one study, most of the 75 dish-cloths and 325 sponges sampled from home kitchens contained large numbers of virulent bacteria, including ESCHERICHIA COLI and strains of *Salmonella*, PSEUDOMONAS AERUGINOSA, and STAPHYLOCOCCUS. If a sponge remains moist, the number of live microbes does not decrease for two weeks. Bacteria can survive for at least two days in a damp sponge that gradually dries in the air. On dry surfaces, however, bacteria can survive for no more than a few hours. They can colonize even stainless steel, which is not really as smooth as it looks.

If they are not removed immediately, microbes produce an organic substance that allows them to survive sprays of water, light rubbing, and even weak detergent solutions. As other types of microbes appear, they form a biofilm that further protects them.

Cutting boards are another source of contamination in the kitchen. While there have been conflicting reports about whether plastic or wooden cutting boards were more likely to contain germs, recent research suggests that the differences between the two depend on how moist they are. A dry wooden board absorbs moisture and draws the bacteria into its pores.

Fortunately, it is possible to remove these germs from kitchen surfaces. A brisk scrubbing with detergent dissolves food and microbes on metal surfaces. A follow-up rinse with dilute bleach will remove even the most tenacious organisms.

Wood, because of its organic building blocks, will react with bleach, neutralizing its ability to kill germs. Instead, it is possible to hand scrub microbes from the surface of new wooden or plastic cutting boards using soap and water. However, it is not possible to decontaminate plastic boards that are scarred by knives, and bacteria below the surface of a wooden board are not removed by hand scrubbing, and can remain alive for several hours. Microwave heating has successfully killed both *E. coli* and *Staph* microbes on cutting boards. After 10 minutes on high heat in an 800-watt home microwave oven in one study, a medium-sized board emerged bone dry and free of live microbes both on and below the surface. Wetting the board first sped up the time it took to kill microbes, suggesting that the microbes probably boiled to death.

The microwave can be used to disinfect other kitchen items, including dry cellulose sponges (30 seconds); wet sponges take longer (1 minute). Dry cotton dishcloths required only 30 seconds, but took three minutes when wet.

No amount of microwaving disinfected plastic boards, since their surfaces never got hot enough to kill the microbes. However, studies have shown that the normal cycle in a dishwasher can sterilize even well-used plastic boards.

In the future, it may be possible to buy self-disinfecting appliances, packaging, and building materials. It is already possible to purchase sponges with bacteria-killing compounds in the cellulose. Antimicrobial cutting boards are already on the market, and the Japanese are marketing plastic bags that claim to emit germ-killing radiation.

Klebsiella   A genus of bacteria named for 19th-century German bacteriologist Theodore A. E. Klebs, who first identified it. The bacteria, which appear first as small plump rods with rounded ends, cause several respiratory diseases including BRONCHITIS, SINUSITIS, and some forms of PNEUMONIA.

La Crosse encephalitis See ENCEPHALITIS.

lassa fever A recently discovered viral infection found in the tropical regions of the world, especially West Africa; epidemics have been recognized in Nigeria, Sierra Leone, and Zaire. The disease is a major public health concern because it is highly contagious and can cause a severe or fatal illness. The rapid spread of the infection has been clearly identified in the case of hospital outbreaks.

Due to the highly contagious nature of this illness and because the mode of transmission is not understood, strict isolation precautions must be followed when this fever is suspected.

Cause The lassa virus has been found in one species of rodent, but the exact mode of transmission to humans is unclear. The virus is found in all body fluids of an infected person and remains in urine for several weeks after recovery.

Symptoms One to three weeks after infection, the symptoms begin with an increasingly high fever, vomiting, cough, and general weakness that lasts for several days.

Diagnosis If a person has traveled to West Africa and has a severe fever within three weeks of the return, the illness should be reported to a physician who would test for lassa fever.

Treatment At the present time there is no known treatment for lassa fever. Symptoms are treated and patients should be made as comfortable as possible. Strict isolation procedures must be maintained.

Legionella pneumophilia A small gram-negative bacterium that causes LEGIONNAIRES' DISEASE.

Legionellosis Another name for LEGIONNAIRES' DISEASE.

Legionnaires' disease A bacterial infection that can take one of two distinct forms: Legionnaires' disease or Pontiac fever. Legionnaires' disease is the more severe form of infection, which includes PNEUMONIA; Pontiac fever is a milder illness.

An estimated 10,000 to 15,000 people are diagnosed with Legionnaire's disease each year; an additional unknown number are infected with the *Legionella* bacterium but rarely have any symptoms. Cases have been identified throughout the United States and in several foreign countries and is believed to occur worldwide.

Outbreaks usually occur in the summer and early fall, but cases may occur year-round. Between 5 and 15 percent of known cases of Legionnaires' disease have been fatal.

Throughout the spring of 1994, about 30 passengers on weekly cruises from New York City to Bermuda came down with the disease; after the cruise ship stopped sailing, the source of infection was discovered to be sand filters used in the whirlpool baths.

People of any age may contract the disease, but it usually affects middle-aged or older people (especially those with chronic lung disease and smokers). Anyone with an impaired immune system or who takes drugs that impair the immune system are at higher risk. Pontiac fever, on the other hand, commonly occurs in healthy individuals and resembles a flulike illness more than pneumonia.

The disease was named for its first identified outbreak, which occurred in 1976 during a Legionnaire convention at the Bellevue-Stratford Hotel in Philadelphia; 182 Legionnaires became ill and 29 died. Most of them had pneumonia, and because doctors didn't know what the men had, they called it "legionnaire's disease." In January 1977, scientists identified the bacterium that causes the disease and realized it had also caused outbreaks before 1976; nevertheless, the name remained.

Cause   Legionnaires' disease (and a separate variety called Pontiac fever) is caused by the bacterium *Legionella pneumophila* transmitted by breathing in bacteria carried in water droplets through the air. The bacteria live in water and get into air-conditioning cooling towers and circulate throughout a building.

Outbreaks have occurred after persons have inhaled spray from a contaminated water source (such as air-conditioning cooling towers, whirlpool spas, or showers) in workplaces, hospitals, or other public places. Infection isn't spread from one person to another, and there is no evidence of people becoming infected from auto air conditioners or household window air conditioners.

Legionella can be found in many different water systems, but the bacteria reproduce best in warm, stagnant water such as is found in some plumbing systems and hot water tanks, cooling towers and condensers of large air-conditioning systems, and whirlpool spas.

Symptoms   Between 2 and 10 days after exposure, symptoms of fever, chills, and cough appear. The cough may be dry or produce sputum; some patients may also experience muscle aches, headache, fatigue, loss of appetite, and diarrhea.

Symptoms in Pontiac fever usually appear within a few hours to two days.

Diagnosis   It is difficult to distinguish Legionnaires' disease from other types of pneumonia by symptoms alone. Other tests are needed for diagnosis. Lab tests may show decreased kidney function; chest X-rays reveal pneumonia.

A diagnosis requires special tests not normally performed on suspected cases of pneumonia: looking for bacteria in sputum, finding antigens in urine, and comparing antibody levels in two blood samples three to six weeks apart. Experienced doctors are the most important diagnostic tool, since lab tests take several days to months.

Treatment   Erythromycin is the recommended antibiotic for Legionnaires' disease; sometimes, rifampin may be used in severe cases. Pontiac fever does not require medication.

Prevention   Outbreaks must be reported to the health department. The disease can be prevented by better design and maintenance of cooling towers and plumbing systems in order to limit the growth and spread of bacteria.

After the 1994 outbreaks on a cruise ship, public health officials met with industry representatives and issued more strict health guidelines. The new rules require changing hot tub filters more often, testing the water hourly, raising the chlorination level, and improving maintenance intervals. Consumers booking a cruise can ask their booking agent whether the cruise ship adheres to the new guidelines. It is also possible to find out how a ship scored on its most recent sanitary inspection by writing to the U.S. Public Health Service, 1015 N. America Way, Ste. 107, Miami, FL 33132. A score of more than 86 is acceptable.

Leishmania   A genus of protozoan parasite transmitted to humans by any of several species of sand flies. Infestation causes one of a variety of diseases called LEISHMANIASIS.

leishmaniasis   A variety of diseases that affect the skin and mucous membranes caused by infection with single-celled parasites. More than 350 million people in 88 countries of the world are presently at risk; 12 million people are already affected by the disease, which is fatal in one form.

At least three types of the disease affect the skin, one is common in the Middle East,

North Africa, and the Mediterranean; the others are found in Central and South America.

Cause The parasites that transmit the infection belong to the genus *Leishmania,* a protozoa transmitted by the bite of a tiny insect called the phlebotomine sand fly. Of 500 known species, only 30 of them carry the disease, and only the female sand fly transmits the protozoan, infecting itself with the parasites contained in the blood it sucks from its host. During a period of 4 to 25 days, the parasite continues its development inside the sand fly, where it is transformed. When the infectious female sand fly feeds on a fresh source of blood, its sting inoculates its new victim with the parasite.

The sand fly is found throughout the tropical and temperate regions of the world. The female lays its eggs in the burrows of rodents, in the bark of old trees, ruined buildings, cracks in house walls, and in rubbish.

Symptoms There are several types of this disease, with a wide range of symptoms. The *visceral* type—also known as kala azar—is characterized by irregular bouts of fever, weight loss, swelling of spleen and liver, and anemia. Untreated, this form of leishmaniasis is fatal almost 100 percent of the time. In *mucocutaneous* leishmaniasis, lesions can partially or completely destroy the mucous membranes of the nose, mouth, and throat and can cause severe disfigurement. The *cutaneous* form of the disease produces skin ulcers on exposed parts of the body such as the arms, legs, and face, causing many lesions (sometimes up to 200) and severe disability. Most of the time the patient is permanently scarred.

Treatment It is essential to understand the different geographic strains of the different parasites in order to properly treat the disease. All forms of this disease can be treated effectively with drugs (such as sodium stibogluconate or glucantime) given by injection. All types of this disorder with secondary bacterial infection should also be treated with antibiotics.

Prevention No effective vaccine currently exists. Insect control is important in the control of the disease.

leprosy A chronic bacterial infection (also called Hansen's disease) that damages nerves in the skin, limbs, face, and mucous membranes. Untreated leprosy can lead to severe complications, which can include blindness and disfigurement, but leprosy can be cured with proper medication. Contrary to popular belief, it is not highly contagious. While the disease still carries a significant stigma, patient care has become integrated with routine health care. Anti-leprosy organizations have fought to repeal stigmatizing laws and practices; patients are no longer referred to as "lepers."

Although leprosy is one of the oldest diseases in human history, it was not until 1873 that Armauer Hansen first identified the bacilli under a microscope. Today there are about 20 million leprosy patients in 87 countries, primarily in Asia, Central and South America, and Africa, but probably fewer than 20 percent have access to treatment. India has the highest prevalence of leprosy, followed by Brazil. In the United States, there are more than 6,000 known cases. Most are found in California, Florida, Hawaii, Louisiana, New York, and Texas. There are about 200 new cases each year in the United States, and 12,000 new cases each week around the world. Approximately 16 percent of the new cases of leprosy are children.

History Ancient religious traditions associated with leprosy continued to influence social policy well into the 20th century. Leprosy was first mentioned as a curse in Shinto prayers of 1250 B.C.; it was also mentioned in some Egyptian legends to explain the exodus of the Hebrews. For hundreds of years, those with leprosy were taken to a priest, not a doctor, and were found "guilty," not sick.

These customs led to the forcible confinement of patients in "leprosaria" or leper colonies; their children, whether infected or not, were denied an education in community schools. In eighth-century France, leprosy was considered grounds for divorce, and the Roman empire enforced banishment. Some countries passed legislation providing for the compulsory sterilization of leprosy patients because of fears that the condition was hereditary. Others would not permit patients to handle the nation's currency. Others "steam treated" patients' letters before allowing them in the mail, and some countries did not allow patients to vote. In medieval Europe, leprosy patients had to carry a "clapper" to warn others that a person with leprosy was approaching. Even as late as 1913, state Senator G. E. Willett of Montana was forced to give up his seat after he was diagnosed with leprosy.

Religious customs also affected many treatments for leprosy. In 250 B.C., Chinese patients pricked their swollen limbs to let out the "foul air." Ramses II of Egypt believed that people with leprosy who used his water wells would be cured. And in medieval Europe, it was believed that leprosy could be cured by the touch of a king.

Historically, topical treatments ranged from turtle soup, whiskey, and various poultices (onion, sea salt, and urine in Egypt; arsenic and powdered snake bones in China; water mixed with blood of dogs and infants under age two in Scotland; elephants' teeth; the flesh of crocodiles, snakes, lions, and bears). Other ingredients ranged from carbolic acid, creosote, phosphorus, mercury, and iodine, and plant extracts included madar, cashew-nut oil, gurjum oil, or chaulmoogra.

The idea of caring for patients with leprosy became popular among missionaries following Biblical directives and the teachings of Jesus; this service became fashionable about A.D. 1100 in Europe, after Crusaders (including a king) returned with the disease. Special hospitals were built, operated, and supported by cathedrals, but when the outbreak of Bubonic Plague in the 1300s wiped out entire populations, patients with leprosy began to be segregated again. Some countries seized the property of those with leprosy before burning them alive.

Leprosy is erroneously associated with the Old Testament, where references to *tsara'ath,* a term that most closely translates to "leprosy," actually refers to a broad spectrum of problems that affected cloth, leather, linen, and house walls as well as humans. Most medical historians doubt that leprosy even existed among the Hebrews in Moses' time. Biblical scholars also have problems with the translation of the Greek term *lepra* partly because the Greeks had a specific term for leprosy. The Greek word *lepra* was most likely used to mean a variety of severe skin diseases. Greek medical writings later than the third century B.C. provide the earliest clinical references to modern leprosy. No mention of leprosy occurs in the New Testament after the Gospels.

Cause Leprosy is caused by a rod-shaped bacterium, MYCOBACTERIUM LEPRAE, that is spread in droplets of nasal mucus. A person is infectious only during the first phase of the disease, and only those living in prolonged close contact with the infected person are at risk. Leprosy is probably spread by droplet infection through sneezing and coughing. In those with untreated leprosy, large amounts of bacteria are found in nasal discharge; the bacteria travel through the air in these droplets. They can survive three weeks or longer outside the human body, in dust or on clothing.

Although relatively infectious, leprosy is still one of the least contagious of all diseases. This—together with the fact that only 3 percent of the population are susceptible to leprosy—means that there is no justification for the practice (still prevalent in some countries) of isolating patients. Only a few people are susceptible because most people acquire a natural immunity when exposed to the disease.

Most of the body's destruction is caused not by bacterial growth but by a reaction of the body's immune system to the organisms as they die. In *lepromatous leprosy,* damage is widespread, progressive, and severe. *Tuberculoid leprosy* is a milder form of the disease.

Symptoms Damage is first confined to the nerves supplying the skin and muscles, destroying nerve endings, sweat glands, hair follicles, and pigment-producing cells. It first causes a lightening (or darkening) of the skin, with a loss of feeling, and sweating. Some types of the disease produce a rash of bumps or nodules on the skin. As the disease progresses, bacilli also attack peripheral nerves; at first patients may feel an occasional "pins and needles" sensation or have a numb patch on the skin. Next, patients become unable to feel sensations such as a light touch or temperature. Gradually, even hands, feet, and facial skin eventually become numb as muscles become paralyzed. Delicate connections between nerve cells and nerve endings are severed, and whole sections of the body become totally numb. For example, if the nerve above the elbow is affected, part of the hand becomes numb and small muscles become paralyzed, leading to curled fingers.

When a patient can no longer sense pain, the body loses the automatic withdrawal reflex that protects against trauma from sharp or hot objects, leading to extensive scarring or even loss of fingers and toes. Muscle paralysis can lead to further deformity, and damage to the facial nerve means eyelids can't close, leading to ulceration and blindness. Direct invasion of bacteria may also lead to inflammation of the eyeball, also leading to blindness.

Treatment Several antibiotic agents are effective against leprosy and are best used in combinations of two or three. This multidrug therapy is the current preferred treatment: it combines dapsone, clofazimine, and rifampin. Multi-drug therapy was developed as leprosy bacilli became resistant to the sulfone drug dapsone alone after decades of constant use.

The most powerful of these three drugs is rifampin, a drug first used against tuberculosis and found to be effective against leprosy in 1968. Particular combinations of these drugs were recommended in 1984 by the World Health Organization as standard treatment for mass campaigns against leprosy.

The three drugs are often distributed in blister packs containing a month's supply of pills; dapsone is taken daily, clofazimine is taken every other day, and rifampin is taken monthly. Now there are more than 1 million people receiving these drugs worldwide, and more than 1 million others who have already completed treatment.

While the medication can usually cure leprosy within six months to two years, patients are no longer contagious within a few days after treatment begins. To prevent a relapse, treatment needs to be administered for at least two years after the last signs of the disease have disappeared. In the United States, patients are eligible for treatment by the Public Health Service at special clinics and hospitals, or at the Gillis W. Long Hansen's Disease Center in Louisiana, the only institution in the United States devoted primarily to treatment, research, training, and education related to leprosy. Eleven regional centers, located primarily in major urban areas, treat those with leprosy on an outpatient basis.

No vaccine for leprosy is available because scientists have not been able to grow cultures in lab environments. However, about 95 percent of the population is immune to leprosy, which occurs naturally in armadillos.

Post-treatment care After leprosy is cured, patients must learn to watch for wounds and injuries they cannot feel and must wear special shoes to protect insensitive feet.

leptospirosis A bacterial disease characterized by a skin rash and flulike symptoms caused by a spirochete bacterium excreted by rodents. Also known as autumn fever, there are about 100 cases and a few deaths reported in the United States each year. Leptospirosis is considered to be a disease that is reemerging in this country and is possibly the most common disease that rats carry and transmit to humans in the United States. There are several strains of the organism; infection with one usually provides immunity to that organism alone, but not to other strains.

Although the disease is not new in the United States, it is hard to diagnose and its prevalence may be unknown. Those especially at risk are urban patients who complain of flulike symptoms (especially during the summer) and who could have been exposed to rat urine or to pools of infected water in alleys and parks of the inner city.

Unrecognized leptospirosis might be common in city dwellers; one 1992 Baltimore study found 16 percent of blood samples taken at an STD clinic were positive for leptospirosis. An earlier study found that about a third of children tested in Detroit also had been exposed. None of the inner-city patients had been diagnosed with leptospirosis.

Cause The infectious disease is caused by the spirochete *Leptospira interrogans* transmitted in the urine of wild or domestic animals, especially rats, livestock, and dogs. People get the disease when broken skin or mucous membranes contact the infected urine or water, soil, or vegetation. The bacteria survive best in warm water (72 degrees F) that is stagnant; most cases have been reported from swimming, wading, or splashing in pools, streams, or puddles that were contaminated with animal urine.

In addition to urban dwellers, leptospirosis is an occupational disease of farmers, sewer workers, or others whose job requires contact with animals (especially rats). Most victims are male teenagers and young adults. Leptospirosis is not usually transmitted from person to person.

Symptoms Leptospirosis has two phases. After an incubation period of up to three weeks, the first phase begins with an acute illness of sudden headache, fever and chills, severe muscle aches, and skin rash appears. Up to 10 percent of infected patients develop a serious systemic form of the illness, called Weil's syndrome. This phase starts a few days after the fever drops; fever will return and bacteria may spread to the brain, causing MENINGITIS. Other serious symptoms include jaundice, confusion, depression, or decreased urine. The kidneys are often affected, and liver damage is common. People infected with this potentially fatal form of leptospirosis are usually very ill and are often hospitalized.

Leptospirosis is often mistaken for viral meningitis or HEPATITIS, but its two distinct phases separate it from those infections.

Diagnosis The disease is diagnosed using specific blood, urine, or fluid tests available through state public health laboratories. If positive, they are sent to the Centers for Disease Control and Prevention lab for confirmation. However, it takes up to a month to get a final determination. A physician must request such testing; it is not routinely done, and local labs do not ordinarily perform these tests. However, researchers have developed an experimental test that can detect within 24 hours tiny amounts of the bacterium's genetic material. The test has not yet been validated.

Treatment Tetracycline and erythromycin are effective, and in about one third of cases patients improve rapidly. Fluid replacement is essential if jaundice or other signs of severe illness occur. Kidney dialysis may be needed in some cases.

Complications Untreated patients may develop Weil's syndrome, a severe form of leptospirosis that can cause permanent kidney and liver damage; most patients recover, but sometimes the disease is fatal.

Prevention The disease can be prevented by good sanitation practices, including using boots and gloves in hazardous places and practicing rodent control. It is common practice to immunize livestock and dogs against the disease, but even vaccinated animals can shed the bacteria in urine for a long time and infect humans.

lice Small wingless insects about the size of a sesame seed, with six legs and claws for grasping the hair; they feed on human blood. Lice are crawling insects that cannot jump or fly. Lice are divided into three species: *Pediculus humanus capitis* (head louse), *Pediculus humanus corporis* (body louse), and *Phthirius pubis* (the crab, or pubic louse). All three have flat bodies that measure up to 3 mm across.

Head lice live on and suck blood from the scalp, leaving red spots that itch intensely and can lead to skin inflammation (dermatitis) and skin infection (impetigo). The females lay a daily batch of pale eggs, called "nits" that attach to hairs close to the scalp; the nits hatch in about a week, and the adults can live for several weeks.

Head lice are not simply a plague of the poor, but are found among people of all walks of life. About 6 million cases of head lice occur each year among U.S. schoolchildren between ages 3 and 12, even among those who shampoo daily. Children are most often affected by contracting the lice through direct contact, usually at school by sharing hats, brushes, combs, or headrests. Pets cannot get head lice.

Because lice move so quickly, it is usually the nits that will be seen on the hair shaft. Nits are the tiny eggs of a louse that are yellow when newly laid, turning to white once they hatch. Nits are small, oval-shaped eggs that are "glued" at an angle to the side of the hair shaft. They hatch within eight days, and the empty eggshells are carried outward as the hair grows. Both head and pubic lice lay eggs at the base of hairs growing on the head or pubic area. Nits can be seen anywhere on the hair, especially behind the ears and at the back of the neck.

Nits should not be confused with hair debris, such as fat plugs or hair casts. Fat plugs are bright white irregularly shaped clumps of fat cells stuck to the hair shaft. Hair casts are thin, long cylinder-shaped segments of dandruff encircling the hair shaft; they are easily dislodged.

Lice infestations are diagnosed by the presence of nits; by calculating the distance from the base of the hair to the farthest nits, it's possible to estimate the duration of the infestation.

All nits must be removed, according to the National Pediculosis Association. Since no lice pesticide kills all nits, any nits left on the hair can be confusing; thorough nit removal will reduce or eliminate the need for more treatments.

Nits can be removed with a special nit removal comb, with baby safety scissors, or with the fingernails.

Head lice and their nits can also be found on eyebrows and eyelashes. If one person in a family has head lice, all family members should be checked. However, only those who are infested should be treated with lice pesticide.

Body lice live and lay eggs on clothing next to the skin, visiting the body only to feed. Body lice affect people who rarely change their clothes.

Crab lice live in pubic hair or (rarely) armpits and beards. Pubic lice are commonly known as "CRABS" because they resemble a crab under the microscope. Crab lice cause incessant itching, are visible to the naked eye, and are easily transmitted during sex. It's also possible to pick them up from sheets or towels. They can live away from the host's body for up to one day, and the eggs can survive for several days. Affected patients who don't wash underwear, sheets, and towels in hot enough water are likely to be reinfected.

Treatment For *head lice*, lotions containing malathion or carbaryl kill lice quickly; the lotion should be washed off 12 hours after application, followed by combing the hair with a fine-toothed comb to remove dead lice and nits. Shampoos containing malathion or carbaryl are also effective if used repeatedly over several days. Combs and brushes should be plunged into very hot water to kill any attached eggs. The National Pediculosis Association discourages the use of lindane products (such as Kwell), because they appear to be potentially more toxic and no more effective than other treatments. Still, no product kills 100 percent of nits. Lice medications are not intended to be used on a routine or preventive basis.

All lice-killing medications are pesticides, and therefore should be used with caution. A pharmacist or physician should be consulted before using or applying pesticides when the person is pregnant, nursing, or has lice or nits in the eyebrows or eyelashes or has other health problems (such as allergies). Head lice pesticides can be absorbed into the bloodstream; therefore, they should not be used on open wounds on the scalp or on the hands of the person applying the medication. These pesticides should not be used on infants and should be used with caution on children under age two. Instead, lice and nits can be removed manually or mechanically.

The product should be used over a sink (not a tub or shower) to minimize pesticide absorption and exposure to the entire body. Eyes of the affected individual must be kept covered while administering the pesticide.

All nits must be removed from the hair shaft. Bedding and recently worn clothing should be washed in hot water and dried in a hot dryer. Combs and brushes should be cleaned and then soaked in hot (not boiling) water for 10 minutes. Lice sprays should not be used, according to the National Pediculosis Association. Vacuuming is the best way to remove lice and attached nits from furniture, mattresses, rugs, stuffed toys, and car seats.

Neighborhood parents and the child's school, camp, or child care provider should be notified of the infestation. Children should be checked once a week for head lice.

Body lice can be killed by placing infested clothing in a hot dryer for five minutes, by washing clothes in very hot water, or by burning.

Pubic lice can be treated with an over-the-counter treatment, including A-200 Pyrinate, Rid, and Nix or with Kwell, a prescription medication (not recommended for use by pregnant women).

For more information about *lice,* contact. The National Pediculosis Association, P.O. Box 149, Newton, MA 02161 or call (800) 446-4NPA. For more information about *head lice treatment,* write for a free brochure to: The Office of Public Affairs, Nonprescription Drug Manufacturers Association, 1150 Connecticut Avenue NW, Washington, DC 20036.

Listeria monocytogenes   A species of bacteria that infect many domestic and wild animals and in humans cause MENINGOENCEPHALITIS and sometimes infections of the womb. See also PREGNANCY AND INFECTIOUS DISEASE; LISTERIOSIS.

listeriosis   A food-borne illness that may cause no symptoms in healthy people but that is particularly dangerous to a fetus or newborn, the elderly, and people with damaged immune systems. The illness is common among cattle, pigs, and poultry.

Listeriosis occurs in about 7.5 cases for every 1 million people. Once thought to be exclusively a veterinary problem, it was identified as a human disease in 1981 when a Canadian outbreak was linked to tainted cole slaw made from cabbage grown in soil fertilized with *Listeria*-infected sheep manure. Four years later, another outbreak was traced to Mexican-style soft cheese in California, which sickened 150 people including many pregnant women, resulting in newborn deaths.

From 1987 to 1992, the government recalled cooked products from 27 firms, including hot dogs, bologna and other luncheon meat, chicken salad, ham salad, sausages, chicken, sliced turkey breast, and sliced roast beef. Cheese, dairy, sandwich, prepared salad, and smoked fish recalls from 1987 to 1992 included 516 products from 105 firms.

Cause Listeriosis is caused by one species in a group of bacteria called *Listeria monocytogenes,* found in cow's milk, animal and human feces, soil, and leafy vegetables. In the past 10 years, there have been several outbreaks that seem to have been linked to the ingestion of soft cheeses (such as feta, some types of Mexican cheeses, Camembert, blue-veined cheeses) and deli-type lunchmeats. One recent study found that 20 percent of hot dogs tested contained the bacterium *L. monocytogenes.* Those with impaired immune systems may catch the disease from undercooked chicken.

The bacteria is remarkably tough, resisting heat, salt, nitrite, and acidity much better than many other organisms. It can survive on cold surfaces and can multiply slowly at temperatures as low as 34 degrees F. (Refrigeration at 40 degrees F or below stops the multiplication of many other food-borne bacteria.) Freezing the food will stop the bacteria from multiplying, and commercial pasteurization will eliminate the organism in dairy products. *Listeria* does not change the taste or smell of food.

When *Listeria* is found in processed products, the contamination probably occurred after processing (rather than due to poor heating or pasteurizing).

Listeriosis also can be spread through sexual contact, although it is not known how common this is.

Babies can be born with listeriosis if their mothers eat contaminated food during pregnancy. Pregnant women are 20 times more likely than other healthy adults to get listeriosis; about one third of all cases happen during pregnancy. However, it is newborns rather than their mothers who suffer the most serious effects of infection during the pregnancy.

Patients with AIDS are 300 times more likely to get listeriosis than healthy people. Others at increased risk include persons with cancer, diabetes, kidney disease, those who take glucocorticosteroid drugs, or the elderly. While healthy adults and children sometimes become infected, they rarely become seriously ill.

Symptoms Healthy adults may not have any symptoms at all or may experience a flu-like illness with fever, muscle aches, and nausea or diarrhea. If infection spreads to the nervous system, it can cause a type of meningitis, leading to symptoms including headache, stiff neck, confusion, loss of balance, or convulsions.

If a pregnant woman develops the infection, she may experience fever, tiredness, headache, sore throat, dry cough, or back pain. After a few days she will feel better but notice that the fetus is not moving; she may miscarry up to the sixth month or go into labor prematurely; some infants may be stillborn.

If the fetus is affected early in the pregnancy, the baby will probably be born prematurely, with low birth weight and very ill, with breathing problems, blue skin, and low body temperature. If the baby survives, there may be a bloodstream infection or MENINGITIS. Half of these babies die, even if treated. Fetuses affected later in the pregnancy may be carried to term with normal birth weight; if infected during delivery, they may develop meningitis; 40 percent may die. Some surviving babies may have permanent brain damage or mental retardation.

Complications Adults with impaired immune systems may develop MENINGITIS with fever, intense headache, nausea, and vomiting. This is followed by delirium, coma, collapse, and shock; sometimes, abscesses and skin rash appears.

Diagnosis There is no routine screening test for susceptibility during pregnancy as there is for rubella and some other infections. A blood or spinal fluid culture will reveal the infection. During pregnancy, a blood test is the most reliable way to diagnose the infection.

Treatment   Antibiotics are most helpful in pregnant women to prevent disease in the fetus. Babies with listeriosis receive the same antibiotics as adults, although a combination of antibiotics may be used until diagnosis is certain. Even with prompt treatment, some infections result in death, especially those with other serious medical problems.

Prevention   While most people don't have to worry about the disease, scientists at the Atlanta-based Centers for Disease Control warn that pregnant women, the very old, and those with damaged immune systems might want to avoid deli-counter foods and soft cheeses (there is no risk for hard cheese, processed slices, cottage cheese, or yogurt). Those at risk are advised to cook hot dogs to a steaming 160 degrees for several minutes to avoid contamination; hot dogs at restaurants, ball parks, etc., should be avoided, since cooking temperatures can't be verified. One study found that garlic inhibits the growth of this harmful bacteria in the intestine, probably because of a sulfur compound found in fresh garlic.

liver fluke   See FLUKE; SCHISTOSOMIASIS.

lockjaw   See TETANUS.

loiasis (loaisis or loaiasis)   A form of the tropical parasitic disease FILARIASIS caused by an infestation of the *Loa loa* worm, which may travel for 10 or 15 years underneath the skin and causes an inflammation known as a *calabar swelling.*

Sometimes the migrating worms can be seen underneath the conjunctiva in the eye. Commonly called the eye worm, the name *loa loa* actually means "worm worm." The disease is limited to the region of the rain forests in the Congo River area in central and western Africa and equatorial Sudan; it is especially common in Cameroon and on the Ogowe River. An estimated 20 million people are infected with the worm; in the Congo River basin, up to 90 percent of villagers in some areas are infected.

Cause   The disease is acquired through the bite of an infected African deer fly. Once inside the body, the infective larvae develop slowly into a mature adult (the process takes about a year). During this period, it lives and moves around underneath the skin. In periods of growth and development, *Loa loa* makes frequent excursions through the connective tissues, where it is often noticed by the victim. Adult worms (which live for up to 15 years) move in the subcutaneous tissues where the female deposits the microfilariae. Microfilariae may become apparent in the victim's blood within five to six months of infection and may remain in the blood for as long as 17 years. They move into peripheral blood during the day and into the lungs at night.

Symptoms   Symptoms of loiasis generally don't appear until several years after the bite of the infected fly, although they have been known to appear within four months. Most of the symptoms observed in victims infected with *Loa loa* occur during periods when the migrating adults appear near the surface of the skin. The worms often appear near the eye, where they can be easily seen and extracted before they damage the conjunctiva.

Allergic reactions to the migrating worms can cause calabar swellings in the arms and legs, triggered by metabolic products from the worm that sensitize the victim. The painful swellings develop quickly and last three to five days, appearing when the worms are still and disappearing when the worms move on. Recurrent swelling can create painful cystlike enlargements of the connective tissues around the tendons.

Occasionally, the adult worm migrates into the conjunctiva and cornea, causing pain and swelling.

Dying worms can cause chronic abscesses.

Diagnosis   Lab diagnosis is based on finding microfilariae during the day, or adults in the subcutaneous tissues.

Treatment   Diethylcarbamazine has been the preferred drug for the past 40 years, and usually cures the disease, and may also be useful as a preventive measure. The drug kills both worms and microfilariae. However, it should be used with caution in patients with heavy infestations of worms, since this can provoke eye problems. Antihistamines and prednisone may be needed to ease allergic reactions due to the disintegration of microfilariae.

Complications   Caucasians may experience a strong allergic response, causing giant hives and swelling of the mucous membranes accompanied with fever. Evidence of heart or kidney problems may be found in up to 20 percent of these cases.

Prevention   Repellents containing DEET or dimethyl phthalate, wearing long pants, and sleeping in well-screened areas are important ways to protect against insects.

lower respiratory tract infections   See RESPI-RATORY TRACT INFECTIONS.

lung fluke   See FLUKE; SCHISTOSOMIASIS.

Lyme disease   A recently identified tick-borne illness whose hallmark symptom is a bull's-eye red rash surrounding the tick bite. Untreated, Lyme disease can cause a host of problems, including arthritis and disorders of the heart and central nervous system. It is most commonly found in the northeast coastal states from Maine to Maryland, in the upper Midwest, and on the Pacific coast. It is most often contracted in the late spring or early summer when ticks are abundant, although it may occur whenever the temperature is above 40° F for several consecutive days.

While the disease has been portrayed in sometimes frightening fashion in the media, most of the time it is easily treated and does not progress to the chronic stage. It probably causes severe long-term effects in less than 10 percent of untreated patients; moreover,

recent studies indicate that many people who think they have Lyme disease actually have other conditions.

In the United States, the disease was first recognized in Lyme, Connecticut, after two mothers were told in 1975 that their children had juvenile rheumatoid arthritis. This type of arthritis is a disabling condition of children in which joints are swollen and painful. When the women discovered many others in the area had the disease—which does not normally occur in clusters—they took their concerns to Yale University.

By the late 1970s, Yale researchers Allen Steere and Stephen Malawista found that many patients they studied were afflicted with a mysterious disease that produced a variety of symptoms, in addition to the joint swelling. They determined the cause was apparently a microorganism transmitted by at least one species of tick found widely in the woods around Lyme. In 1982, it was identified by Willy Burgdorfer of Rocky Mountain Labs in Hamilton, Montana, who discovered the spiral-shaped bacterial species that today bears his name: *Borrelia burgdorferi*.

Now that scientists knew the cause, they could confirm that a group of skin conditions and neurological syndromes identified in Europe were also manifestations of Lyme disease. Since then, researchers have identified the disease throughout the world, including Australia, Africa, and Asia. It also occurs in almost every state in the United States, although it remains concentrated in the northeast, Minnesota, and northern California.

While it was only recently identified in this country, Lyme disease is not a new affliction. German scientists have found evidence of the disease in 19th-century ticks, making these insects the bacterium's earliest known hosts. The ticks came from the Vienna Natural History Museum in Austria, which supplied 21 ticks pickled in alcohol to the scientists. The genetic material in two matched that of *Borrelia garinii*, one of three forms of the bacteria that can induce Lyme disease. The 21 ticks had come from a Hungarian cat in 1884, and from a fox caught in Austria in 1888. Scientists suspect that the disease may have occurred even earlier, but finding even older ticks to study has been difficult.

European victims of Lyme disease suffer slightly different forms of the disease, probably because there are differences in the strains of *B. burgdorferi* active in different parts of the world. Europeans patients experience long-term neurological complications, such as cognitive deficits and dementia; up to 10 percent of untreated Europeans also suffer for many years with a skin condition in which affected areas of the skin become red, thin, and wrinkled. In the United States, these symptoms are rare.

Cause   The disease is caused by BORRELIA BURGDORFERI, a spirochete form of bacteria. It is transmitted primarily by the deer tick, the tiniest of which is about the size of the period at the end of this sentence, which are found on deer, birds, filed mice, and other rodents. The tick must be attached to its victim for between 36 to 48 hours before an infectious dose of *B. burgdorferi* can be transmitted. For this reason, simply by checking themselves often for ticks, most people can avoid becoming infected.

Most people are diagnosed in the spring, summer, or early fall because this reflects the life cycle of the infected tick. In the northeastern United States, about half of all adult *I. scapularis* ticks are infected. In some places (Block Island and Nantucket Island) the numbers are even higher. Even so, in most sections of the northeast, only between 1 and 3 percent of people have contracted Lyme disease.

The tick that transmits Lyme diseases in California relies on intermediate hosts (such as lizards) that are resistant to infection; for this reason, ticks—and consequently humans—in the west are infected much less often than in the northeast. The same is true for species that transmit Lyme in some areas of Europe and Asia.

Symptoms   Most people who do become infected will usually display one or more symptoms. Between three days and a month after becoming infected, about 60 percent of victims will notice a small red spot that expands over a period of days or weeks, forming a circular, triangular, or oval-shaped rash called ERYTHEMA CHRONICUM MIGRANS. The reddened area, which usually appears at the bite site, neither itches nor hurts. Sometimes the rash resembles a red raised bull's-eye rash with a clear center at the site of the bite.

The rash can range in size from a dime to the entire width of a person's body. As the infection spreads, several rashes can appear at different sites on the body. Without treatment, the rash begins to disappear within days or weeks.

As the spirochetes move through the body via the bloodstream, other symptoms affecting other parts of the body may appear. These may include flulike symptoms (such as headache, stiff neck, appetite loss, body aches, and fatigue). Although these symptoms may resemble those of common viral infections, Lyme disease symptoms tend to persist or may occur intermittently.

Early neurological problems may also appear in about 20 percent of patients. Some patients may experience Bell's palsy in one or both sides of the face, which may become paralyzed for weeks or months before returning to normal. Other symptoms may include MENINGITIS, ENCEPHALITIS, or numbness and tingling of other parts of the body.

Complications   After several months of being infected, slightly more than half of those people not treated with antibiotics develop recurrent attacks of painful and swollen joints that last a few days to a few months. The arthritis can shift from one joint to another; most often, the knee is infected. About 10 to 20 percent of untreated patients who experience temporary arthritic symptoms will go on to develop chronic Lyme arthritis. In contrast to many other forms of arthritis, Lyme arthritis typically is not symmetrical.

One out of 10 Lyme patients develop heart problems (such as irregular heartbeat) for a few days or weeks, generally appearing several weeks after infection. Most people won't be aware of this problem unless a physician detects it, although some patients might realize they can't exercise as they once did. This condition usually lasts only for a week to 10 days and almost never requires a pacemaker. Other nervous system complications include subtle changes such as memory loss, difficulty with concentration, and change in mood or sleeping habits. Nervous system abnormalities usually develop several weeks, months, or even years after an untreated infection. These symptoms often last for weeks or months, and may recur. Less often, Lyme disease causes eye inflammation, hepatitis, or severe fatigue. Pregnant women who contract the disease run the risk of miscarriage, stillbirth, or birth defects.

Diagnosis Lyme disease is not easy to diagnose because its symptoms and signs mimic those of many other diseases, such as viral infections or MONONUCLEOSIS. Joint pain can be misdiagnosed as inflammatory arthritis, and neurologic signs may be misidentified as a primary neurologic disease such as MULTIPLE SCLEROSIS.

Diagnosis of Lyme disease includes consideration of exposure to ticks (especially in Lyme disease areas), symptoms, and the result of blood tests to determine whether the patient has antibodies to Lyme bacteria. The tests are most useful in later stages. Lab tests for Lyme disease have not yet been standardized across the country.

Treatment Antibiotics (tetracycline or amoxicillin) usually provide a complete recovery if given early enough. Most patients who are treated in later stages of the disease also respond well. Pregnant women may require hospitalization.

Unfortunately, cases that are not diagnosed soon enough may resist antibiotic therapy. In a few patients, symptoms of persistent infection may continue or the disease may recur, so that physicians prescribe repeated long courses of antibiotic therapy. The value of this approach, which can have serious side effects (such as inducing formation of gallstones) remains controversial.

Patients with late chronic Lyme disease may exhibit varying degrees of permanent damage to joints or the nervous system. In general, this occurs among patients who were not diagnosed in the early stages of the disease, or for whom early treatment was not successful. Deaths from Lyme disease have been reported only very rarely.

Prevention A vaccine has been developed and is being tested in a large number of patients. A vaccine is already available for field dogs at risk for developing the disease because of the area in which they live.

Experts at the Centers for Disease Control don't recommend preventive treatment with antibiotics after a tick bite. It's better to avoid tick bites in the first place; avoiding their habitat is the best way to prevent tick bites, but ticks may also be found in lawns, gardens, and on bushes adjacent to homes.

When walking in the woods, stay on trails and avoid brushing up against low bushes or tall grass. Ticks do not hop, jump, fly, or descend from trees—a person must come in direct contact with them (they may blow in a strong breeze). To prevent bites, wear protective clothing (light-colored, long-sleeve shirts and light-colored pants tucked into boots or socks); this allows ticks to be more easily spotted.

An insect repellent preferably containing no more than 30 percent DEET (N-diethylmetatoluamide) may be used on bare skin and clothing. Duranon can be applied to clothing only, but not to the skin. All insect repellent should be used with caution (especially on children) and should not be applied to the hands or face.

Ticks and hosts (mice, chipmunks, voles, and other small mammals) need moisture, a place hidden from direct sun, and a place to hide. Therefore, the clearer the area around a house, the less chance there will be of getting a tick bite. All leaf litter and brush should be removed as far as possible away from the house. Low-lying bushes should be pruned to let in more sun. Rake up leaves every fall, since ticks prefer to overwinter in fallen leaves. Woodpiles are favorite hiding places for mammals carrying ticks; woodpiles should be neat, off the ground, in a sunny place, and under cover.

Gardens should be cleaned up every fall; foliage left on the ground over the winter provide shelter for mammals that may harbor ticks. Stone walls on the property increase the potential for ticks.

Shady lawns may support ticks in epidemic areas; lawns should be mowed and edged. Entire fields should be mowed in fall, preferably with a rotary mower.

Birdfeeders attract birds that carry infected ticks; don't place feeder too close to the house. Clean up the ground under the feeder regularly. Suspend bird feeding during late spring and summer, when infected ticks are most active. Building eight-foot fences to keep out deer may significantly reduce the abundance of ticks on large land parcels. Examine pets allowed outside on a daily basis; tick collars and/or dips may be needed.

Three pesticides may help: chlorpyrifos (Dursban), carbaryl (Sevin), and cyfluthrin (Tempo). One or two applications a year in late May and September can significantly reduce the tick population.

For more information, contact: The American Lyme Disease Foundation, Inc., Mill Pond Offices, 293 Rte. 100, Ste. 204, Somers, NY 10589; telephone (914) 277-6970 or (800) 876-LYME; fax (914) 277-6974.

lymphangitis   Inflammation of the lymphatic vessels that cause tender red streaks to appear on the skin above the lymphatic vessels. The infection may spread to the bloodstream. This condition is a clear indication of serious infection and requires immediate treatment with antibiotics.

Cause   The infection is caused by a spread of bacteria (usually streptococci) from an infected wound into the lymphatic channels.

Symptoms   The red streaks extend from the site of infection toward the nearest lymph nodes; there is usually a fever, chills, headache, and general feeling of illness.

Treatment   Antibiotics together with warm, moist compresses, usually clear up the infection without complication.

lymphogranuloma venereum (LGV)   A sexually transmitted disease involving the lymph glands in the genital area caused by a specific strain of CHLAMYDIA. The incidence of the disease is highest among sexually active people in the tropical or subtropical climates; it has also been found in some areas of the southern United States.

Cause   The infection is spread by sexual contact.

Symptoms   The first symptom is a small, painless pimple on the penis, female external genitalia, or vagina that appears from 3 to 30 days after exposure; it is so small it often goes unnoticed. The infection then spreads to the lymph nodes in the groin, and from there it moves to surrounding tissue. An individual remains infectious as long as there are active lesions.

Treatment   The disease responds to certain antibiotics such as tetracycline or sulfamethoxazole.

Prevention   There are several ways to prevent the spread of LGV, including using condoms, washing genitals after sex, avoiding sexual contact if infected, notifying all partners in case of infection, and reducing the number of sex partners.

Complications   Inflamed and swollen lymph glands, which may drain and bleed.

mad cow disease The common name for BOVINE SPONGIFORM ENCEPHALOPATHY (BSE), a fatal infectious disease of the brain and spinal cord in cows, causing microscopic holes in brain tissue. Scientists believe there is a link between mad cow disease and a similar fatal brain disease in humans known as Creutzfeldt-Jakob disease.

Mad cow disease, which was identified in British cows in 1986, gets its nickname from the fact that it causes infected animals to be clumsy and nervous. It is one of a group of diseases called transmissible spongiform encephalopathies, which take different forms in different species. Forms of the disease also occur occasionally in mink, deer, and elk. Bovine spongiform encephalopathy was only discovered in 1986.

Creutzfeldt-Jakob disease (CJD) is a human form that is also always fatal and causes severe dementia. Mad cow disease and CJD are assumed to be related because both attack and destroy the brain in the same fatal way.

CJD is believed to be acquired through injection or transplantation of tissue from an infected cadaver. Most cases, however, occur sporadically with no known cause. About 250 cases are diagnosed each year in the United States. CJD usually strikes people in their 50s and 60s and can take a year or two for symptoms to become apparent. But once the disease begins, the course is swift: Damaged brain cells interfere with a person's ability to think, see, speak, and move. Muscles go into spasm, and balance is destroyed. The dementia that develops mimics Alzheimer's disease, a related disorder that is not classified as a spongiform disease. CJD occurs around the world; among its most famous victims was choreographer George Balanchine, who died in New York City in 1983.

When a cluster of 12 cases of CJD were diagnosed in Great Britain in 1996, British health officials said they could have been linked to consumption of BSE-infected beef. Since CJD can take several decades to show up, no one knows whether these cases are an isolated cluster, or the forerunners of a vast epidemic among people who ate beef in England in the 1980s. The incidence of CJD in Britain is still small, but increasing. It nearly doubled between 1990 and 1994, reaching 55 cases in 1994. CJD would be expected to strike one out of every million people.

The BSE epidemic in cattle had peaked in Britain in 1993, and reported cases have been reduced by 70 percent, but the disease has also been found in cattle in Ireland, France, Portugal, and Switzerland. U.S. Department of Agriculture officials maintain that BSE does not exist in the United States, which banned beef imports in 1989. There has been no evidence of BSE after examination of thousands of brain specimens from U.S. cattle in 43 states. The number of cases of Creutzfeldt-Jakob disease in the United States has remained stable at one case per million each year since 1979.

Until now, the best known of the spongiform diseases has been kuru, caused by ritualistic cannibalism among the Fore group in the highlands of Papua–New Guinea. Now that these practices have stopped, the disease has largely disappeared.

Cause An early theory held that BSE might be caused by an infectious agent called a slow virus (or PRION) that can't be destroyed by cooking. Now, scientists suspect an abnormal protein in the cell membrane may be transmitted through consumption of affected tissue, which then sets off a chain reaction, damaging other proteins nearby.

It is believed that the disease in England began when cattle were fed protein derived from infected sheep. There has been no evidence that BSE spreads by direct contact from cattle to cattle, or from cattle to humans. Instead, scientists suspect that the risks of developing CJD may occur from consumption of spinal cord or brain tissue from BSE-infected cows.

Symptoms Symptoms appear about two to eight years after infection and include clumsiness, nervousness, and brain impairment. Death occurs about two weeks to six months after symptoms appear.

Diagnosis There is no test available to test for BSE in a living animal short of brain biopsy. It can be diagnosed only by examination of the dead animal's brain tissue.

Treatment There is no cure for CJD or mad cow disease. Treatment is symptomatic.

malaria   An infectious disease caused by a parasitic protozoa within the red blood cells, now believed to be one of the major reemerging infections of the world. It is so serious that every 30 seconds somewhere in the world a child dies of the disease.

Malaria is one of the oldest known infections. First mentioned in ancient Sanskrit and Chinese documents, malaria was described in detail by Hippocrates who discriminated among different types of malarial fever in the fifth century B.C.; early physicians thought the illness was carried by hot, wet air, which is where it got its name—from the Italian word for "bad air." Long the scourge of the ancient world, it is believed that the army of Alexander the Great was probably wiped out by malaria during its march across India.

Among Africans, it is believed that the never-ending pressure of the illness led to the rise of the sickle-cell trait common in that population. The slight deformity of the red blood cells in sickle cell anemia discourages the infiltration by the malarial parasite.

It is believed that malaria was introduced into the United States by European colonists and African slaves in the 16th and 17th centuries, where it then became endemic in many areas of the country, following the migration of the colonists. It was a particular problem in warm, wet areas of the United States such as the Chesapeake Bay region and the Mississippi Valley. It is believed that Andrew Jackson, Ulysses S. Grant, and George Washington all at various times suffered from malaria.

The first treatment against the disease was begun as early as 1630, when "Jesuit's bark" (the bark of the chinchona tree) was used to ease the fever of a Spanish magistrate in Peru. News of the treatment spread to Europe, where chinchona bark cure was enthusiastically adopted—except by the profoundly anti-Catholic Oliver Cromwell, who refused to take Jesuit's bark for malaria and died of the disease. Eventually, quinine was isolated from the bark, leading to the development of the synthetic version (chloroquine). This cheap, effective drug almost won the world's battle with malaria until resistant strains of the disease began appearing in the 1960s.

The incidence of the disease peaked in 1875, but it is estimated that more than 600,000 cases were reported in 1914. By 1934, the number of cases dropped to 125,556, and by the 1950s, experts concluded that malaria had been eliminated in this country, through the efforts of spraying, removing breeding sites, accurate assessment, and focused control. It was still understood that international travel could reintroduce the disease into this country. Since 1957, nearly all cases diagnosed in the United States have been acquired by mosquito transmission in areas where malaria is known to exist. About half the cases occur among native U.S. citizens, and half occur in foreign-born people.

Environmental changes, the spread of drug resistance, and increased air travel could lead to the reemergence of malaria as a serious public health problem in the United States, according to the U.S. Centers for Disease Control and Prevention. Recent outbreaks of mosquito-transmitted diseases in densely populated areas of New Jersey, New York, Texas, and Michigan are evidence that the risk exists.

Indeed, the parasite that causes malaria has become resistant to the usual antimalarial drugs. Only 10 percent of the world's population was at risk of catching this disease in 1960, but today that number has grown to 40 percent. The number of deaths worldwide is very high, ranging from 1.4 million to 2.4 million a year, according to the World Health Organization. Most of the deaths occur in children under age five, and most occur in Africa.

Cause Malaria is caused by four different species of the *Plasmodium* parasite transmitted by the *Anopheles* mosquito. The deadliest parasite causing the sometimes-fatal version of malaria is *Plasmodium falciparum;* others are *P. vivas, P. malariae,* and *P. ovale.*

Parasites in the blood of an infected person are taken into the stomach of the mosquito as it feeds; when the mosquito bites a person, parasites are injected into the person's bloodstream, migrating to the liver and other organs. After an incubation period from 12 days to 10 months (depending on the variety), parasites return to the bloodstream and invade the red blood cells. At this point, symptoms appear. Rapid multiplication of the parasites destroys the red cells and releases more parasites capable of infecting other red blood cells. This leads to the shivering, fever, and sweating that is the hallmark of the disease; the loss of healthy red cells causes anemia.

The mature parasites remain in the blood and don't reinvade the liver, although a few may remain behind in the liver in a dormant state. These can be released months or years later, causing a relapse of malaria in people who thought they were cured.

Symptoms Symptoms vary and may appear from 8 to 12 days after a bite in falci-

parum malaria to as many as 30 days for other types. Early signs may mimic the flu, causing fever, chills, headache, muscle ache, and malaise. As each new batch of parasites is released, symptoms of shivering and fever reappear. The interval between fever attacks is different in different types of malaria; in quartan malaria caused by *P. malariae* it is three days; in tertian malaria (*P. ovale* or *P. vivax*) it is two days; in malignant tertian (or quotidian) malaria (*P. falciparum*)—the most severe kind—from a few hours to a few days.

In the most serious form of malaria (falciparum malaria), red blood cells become sticky and block the small blood vessels to the brain, kidney, and lungs, damaging these organs. Patients with this variety can die within several days without antibiotics. Irreversible complications can come on suddenly.

Malaria is more severe in children; more than 10 percent of untreated children will die. If infection occurs during pregnancy, there is a risk of premature delivery, abortion, and stillbirth.

Anyone who becomes ill with chills and fever after being in an area where malaria is endemic must see a doctor. Delaying treatment of falciparum malaria can be fatal. Because malaria is often misdiagnosed by North American doctors, travelers to malaria-ridden areas must be tested with a specific blood test for malaria, which requires direct microscopic exam of red blood cells to look for the parasite.

Diagnosis Blood smears are necessary for a diagnosis; the parasite can be specifically identified on blood smears on slides. Antibody tests are not always helpful because many people have antibodies from past infections.

Treatment People who become ill with fever during or after being in a high-risk area should seek prompt medical attention. Malaria can be treated effectively in the early stages, but delaying treatment can have serious consequences. Effective drugs include chloroquine, quinacrine, and chloroguanide.

More recently, scientists in China discovered a drug called artemether (derived from a Chinese herb qinghaosu) appears to be as effective as quinine in preventing malarial deaths. The need for a different drug is imperative, since the parasite is becoming resistant to quinine and chloroquine.

There are side effects with both the standard and the newer treatment. Quinine increases the risk of low blood sugar and ABSCESSES at the injection site. Patients treated with artemether are slower to come out of their malaria-induced coma, and more likely to have convulsions. Other animal studies suggest brain stem damage is related to high doses of artemether.

Falciparum malaria requires hospitalization, with IV fluids, red blood cell transfusions, kidney dialysis (if kidneys fail), and assisted breathing.

Prevention The World Health Organization has been trying to eradicate malaria for the past 30 years by killing mosquitoes that carry the parasite, but as the mosquitoes and parasites became resistant to insecticides, prevention now aims at avoiding bites and taking preventive medicine (such as mefloquine or lariam).

Malaria can often be prevented by the use of antimalarial drugs and use of personal protection measures against mosquito bites. While the risk of malaria is slight in the United States, people traveling to high-risk areas should take precautions. The risk for tourists who stay in air-conditioned hotels on tourist trips in urban or resort areas is lower than that for backpackers, missionaries, and Peace Corps volunteers. Decisions on whether to use antimalarial drugs depends on the traveler's itinerary, duration of travel, and the place where the traveler will spend each night.

Researchers are studying possible vaccines, but the parasite's complex life inside its human host makes a vaccination difficult. Recently, scientists at Walter Reed Army Institute of Research in Washington, D.C., tested vaccine that prevented malaria in six of seven volunteers bitten by infected mosquitoes. Further study is needed to see if the vaccine works against different malaria strains and determine how long immunity lasts.

Anyone who has been diagnosed with *malariae* should not give blood because i possible to transmit the infection to others 40 years.

Before going on a trip, the CDC Travelers Hotline at (404) 332-4559 or the Malaria Hotline at (404) 332-4555 can describe current recommendations.

Mantoux test   See TUBERCULIN TEST.

Marburg virus   One of two exotic filoviruses (the other is EBOLA) found primarily in Africa, that has a 25 percent fatality rate and grotesque symptoms.

The previously unknown virus first appeared in the late summer of 1967, when three employees at a vaccine factory in Marburg, Germany, came down with what doctors thought was the flu. By the next day, symptoms became bizarre, including unusual rashes, severe diarrhea, peeling skin, bloody vomit, and hemorrhaging from every orifice. The number of infected people grew, including household members of patients and the physicians who treated them, until 30 people were ill; 7 died by the end of the year, and others experienced liver failure, impotence, and psychosis. The infections were confined to three cities, but centered in Marburg. Several nearly identical cases were identified in lab workers in Frankfurt at the same time, and in Belgrade in September. Of the 31 patients, 25 had directly handled monkey blood, either while dissecting the animals and working with their organs or cells or while cleaning culture containers.

Spouses and health care providers in contact with the lab workers got sick with exhaustion, weight and hair loss, sweats, and psychiatric problems for weeks afterward. The three outbreaks were traced to several shipments of vervet monkeys from the same area of Uganda, although there was no evidence of that illness among monkey trappers. Experts believe the monkeys became infected while enroute—probably while in London, where they were kept for some hours together with other species of birds and animals; half of these monkeys died before reaching Europe.

In the monkey's tissues, scientists discovered a large new rod-shaped virus, which turned out to be remarkably similar to the Ebola virus.

Nearly a quarter of a million of vervet monkeys had been imported into Europe and the United States by the late 1960s because researchers had found their kidney cells ideal for growing viruses. Although the total number of Marburg virus cases were few, the epidemic created alarm because the mortality rate was so high, the symptoms were horrific, and there was no effective treatment.

Because of the epidemic, labs began to use other species of animals for experiments, and the Marburg virus seemed to disappear. However, in 1975 an Australian tourist died of the disease in a hospital in Johannesburg, South Africa. A traveling companion of the victim and a nurse who had cared for them both became ill as well, but they eventually recovered.

However, nine years after the first Marburg outbreak, a similar illness struck in Zaire and Sudan but with much worse symptoms—the dreaded Ebola virus, close cousin to the Marburg; scientists there discovered that the virus was shaped like a question mark. This virus was named after a river near the epidemic's starting point—Ebola-Zaire.

Ebola reappeared in 1989 in the Washington suburb of Reston, Virginia, when imported Philippine monkeys began to die; workers isolated a virus similar to Ebola, but while several people were infected by the virus, none showed any symptoms. This strain of filovirus was named Ebola-Reston.

mastitis   An infection of the breast that usually occurs during breast-feeding. Acute mastitis is most common during the first two months of nursing.

Cause   The infection is usually caused by either streptococcal or staphylococcal bacteria.

Symptoms   The breast is painful, with swelling and redness and swelling of nearby lymph nodes, together with fever and fatigue. If untreated, an abscess may form.

Treatment   Antibiotics, rest, painkillers, and warm soaks will cure the problem. In most cases, breast-feeding may continue.

mastoiditis   An infection of one of the mastoid bones (the prominent bone behind the ear), usually as a result of otitis media. Mastoiditis usually affects children, sometimes causing hearing loss. This disease has become uncommon since the widespread use of antibiotic drugs to control ear infections.

Cause   The disease occurs when infection spreads from the middle ear to a cavity in the mastoid bone, and from there to a honeycomb of air cells in the bone itself.

Symptoms   Severe earache, headache, and fatigue. Swelling behind the ear is often enough to actually move the external ear. Symptoms also may include fever, a creamy discharge from the ear, and progressive hearing loss.

Complications   The infection may spread to inside the skull, causing MENINGITIS, BRAIN ABSCESS, or a blood clot in veins inside the brain. Or the infection may spread outward, affecting the facial nerve and causing a facial paralysis.

Diagnosis   Mastoiditis can be identified from a physical exam. Early diagnosis is essential because of the potential serious complications.

Treatment   This infection is not easy to treat and often requires intravenous antibiotics for several days. If the infection persists, an operation called a mastoidectomy may be required. In this procedure, the surgeon makes an incision behind the ear to open up the mastoid bone and remove the infected air cells. A drainage tube is left in place and removed several days after the operation.

measles   A childhood viral illness causing a widespread red rash and fever considered to be the most contagious disease in the world. One infected person in a crowded room is able to transmit the illness to almost every unvaccinated person in the room. The medical name for measles is rubeola; It is sometimes called "red measles" to distinguish it from the much milder disease known as rubella (GERMAN MEASLES). While measles was once commonly found throughout the world and was not normally considered dangerous, complications can lead to death.

Doctors have known about measles for centuries; it was first described by the 10th-century Persian physician al-Rhazes, who called the illness by its Arabic name, *hasba* (meaning "eruption"). It was so common that he thought measles was a natural occurrence of childhood, like losing baby teeth, instead of an infectious illness. In fact, its present name did not appear until the 14th century, where it was derived from the Arabic word *miser*, used to describe the unhappiness of lepers.

It spread quickly across North Africa into Europe, where it was introduced by explorers to the New World with tragic results. In central Mexico, the native population was decimated, dropping from about 30 million to 3 million in just 50 years by *pequena* (little leprosy).

In populations that have never been exposed to it, the disease can be a killer; 800 children died of measles during an epidemic in the Charlestown area of Boston in 1772. And a hundred years later, within three months of the arrival of a foreign ship, a quarter of the inhabitants of Fiji—some 30,000 peo-

ple—died from measles. It is so remarkably virulent that in 1951 a single person with measles landed in Greenland and within six weeks, all but five of the 4,300 never-before-exposed Greenland natives came down with the disease.

Although measles was known to be a viral disease since 1911, it wasn't until 1954 that two Harvard researchers isolated the actual measles virus in the lab. When a vaccine was finally licensed in 1963, experts thought the disease would be eradicated by 1982. When this did not occur, the target date was revised to 1990. But instead of disappearing, measles cases began to rise again from only 1,500 cases in 1983 to 28,000 cases in 1990. Half of those reported cases occurred in children under age five. Because many high schools and colleges experienced measles outbreaks in the late 1980s and early 1990s, most schools now require older students to be re-immunized.

Since 1991, measles cases have again been decreasing; there were 963 cases in 1994 and just 301 in 1995—the lowest number for a single year since the disease became reportable in 1912, when, according to the national Centers for Disease Control, 12,000 people died in United States. It is still a killer in developing countries, where more than 1 million deaths a year are recorded—especially among malnourished children with impaired immunity.

One case of measles confers lifelong immunity; the vaccine also confers lifelong immunity. Anyone who received two doses of vaccine during childhood will not get measles.

Cause   The measles virus is spread by airborne droplets from nasal secretions. Symptoms appear after an incubation period of between 9 to 11 days, and the patient is infectious from shortly after the beginning of this period until up to a week after symptoms have developed. Infants under six months of age rarely contract measles because they still harbor some immunity from their mothers.

The virus survives best in low humidity; it can survive in the air for several hours. It is so infectious, it is capable of traveling down a hall on air currents and into other rooms where healthy people are located, infecting them as well. It is also possible to contract the disease from touching bedding or towels touched by an infected person, or by directly touching secretions from a person's nose, mouth, eyes, or cough.

A milder form of the disease can occur among people who don't develop adequate immunity from just one dose of vaccine, who were immunized too early, or who had received an older less effective variety of the vaccine. As their immunity wears off, these people become susceptible to measles, which causes a low fever and rash on face and trunk.

Symptoms   About 10 days after the virus enters the body symptoms of a high fever (up to 105 degrees F) and general sick feeling occur. This is followed the next day by red, sore eyes, a stuffy nose, and cough. On the second day of fever, a rash (Koplik's spots) of tiny white dots on a red base appears inside the mouth. After three or four days, a bright red splotchy rash will begin on the head and neck and spread down to cover the entire body. The spots may be so numerous that they appear together as a large red area. The rash begins to fade within three days and will disappear by six days.

The fever will begin to drop on the second day of the rash, and the runny nose and sore eyes also diminish as the fever falls. The cough, however, may last for up to two weeks.

Everyone with measles feels terrible, but babies and young children usually fare the worst, feeling much sicker than they would with a COLD, the flu, or CHICKEN POX.

Patients are infectious from just before the fever begins to the fifth day after the rash appears. The most infectious period occurs right before the rash begins. Patients during the infectious stage must remain isolated.

Diagnosis   Physicians can diagnose measles from symptoms alone, although blood tests that check for antibodies to the virus are available in large labs.

Treatment   There is no cure for measles. Symptoms are treated with fluids and acetaminophen. Antibiotics will not help the virus, but may be needed to treat a secondary infection. Patients need to rest in a darkened room because their eyes are sensitive to light.

A physician should be called immediately if any of the following signs appear:

- vomiting
- signs of dehydration
- wheezing or breathing problems (which may be a sign the virus has spread to the lungs, causing measles PNEUMONIA)
- fever for more than four days after the rash appears
- fever that subsides and returns
- unusual drowsiness, fussiness, stiff neck (signs of measles ENCEPHALITIS) caused by the spread of virus into the brain
- ear pain, pulling at the ear

Complications   Infants, older people, and those with serious health problems may become severely ill with measles and die. It is a common cause of death and blindness in developing countries.

Infants are the most likely to get complications including secondary ear and chest infections, which usually occur as the fever returns a few days after the rash appears. There may also be diarrhea, vomiting, and abdominal pain. Measles PNEUMONIA in children may trigger serious breathing problems.

About 1 in every 1,000 patients goes on to develop ENCEPHALITIS (brain inflammation), with headache, drowsiness, and vomiting beginning 7 to 10 days after the rash begins. This may be followed by seizures and coma, leading to mental retardation or death. (Note: Febrile seizures are common with measles and don't necessarily indicate the presence of encephalitis.) Very rarely (one in a million cases) a progressive brain disorder called sub-acute sclerosing panencephalitis develops many years after the illness.

Measles during pregnancy causes fetal death in about one fifth of cases, but there is no evidence that measles causes birth defects.

Prevention   In the United States, children are routinely vaccinated first at age 12 months and again at age four or older by an injection usually combined with mumps and rubella that produces immunity in 97 percent of patients. Side effects of the vaccine are reported to be mild, including low fever, slight cold, and a rash about a week after the shot. The vaccine was first licensed for use in 1963 and is very effective; only one injection produces long-lasting (probably lifelong) protection.

The vaccine should not be given to infants under age one or to those with a family history of epilepsy or who have had seizures before. In these cases, simultaneous injection of measles-specific immunoglobulin, which contains antibodies against the virus, should be given.

The booster now recommended at 4 to 6 years of age or at 10 to 12 years, will protect 95 percent of those who may have failed to become immune after their first vaccine dose.

Pregnant women who have never had measles or been immunized should avoid anyone with measles. If the pregnant patient does come in contact with an infected person, she should be passively immunized against measles with immunoglobulin within five days.

Schools require evidence of measles immunity upon enrollment. Some people need to be reimmunized against measles. Everyone immunized before their first birthday or who received the previously available "killed" measles vaccine (or a vaccine of unknown type) between 1963 and 1967 should be reimmunized. It is safe to be reimmunized even if a person is actually already immune. People born before 1957 are probably immune to measles because of exposure to the disease. Thus, people who are now between the ages of 30 and 40 are those most likely to require reimmunization.

meningitis   Any infection or inflammation of the membranes covering the brain and spinal cord, caused by either bacteria, fungi, or virus. Bacterial meningitis is by far the most serious type of meningitis. Most of the time, however, the infectious agent is a virus.

The most common cause of bacterial meningitis in adults are STREPTOCOCCUS PNEU-MONIAE, *Neisseria meningitidis,* or HAEMOPHILUS INFLUENZAE (HIB). Until 1992, most victims younger than age five were infected with *H. flu* (Hib); today, this type of meningitis has almost disappeared in children younger than five because of an effective vaccine. Pneumococcal meningitis (caused by *S. pneumoniae*) and meningococcal meningitis (caused by *N. meningitidis*) are now the most common and serious types of bacterial meningitis. The dread of bacterial meningitis, no matter which bacterium is responsible, is not just on its reputation as a killer but also on the real possibility of lingering neurological complications. These lingering deficits, which occur in between 20 and 30 percent of those surviving bacterial meningitis, can be especially devastating in infants and children. The deficits can include persistent hearing loss, mental retardation, and recurrent convulsions.

Viral meningitis is a less severe version that is rarely fatal, although infections involving arbovirus, herpesviruses, or polio may be more severe. Yeasts such as CANDIDA and CRYPTOCOCCUS may cause a severe—often fatal—meningitis.

Regardless of cause, the onset of meningitis is usually sudden, and characterized by a severe headache, neck stiffness, irritability, malaise, and nausea and vomiting. See also MENINGITIS, BACTERIAL; MENINGITIS, MENINGO-COCCAL; MENINGITIS, PNEUMOCOCCAL; MENINGITIS, VIRAL.

meningitis, bacterial More than two thirds of all victims of bacterial meningitis are children under age five. Until 1992, most of them were infected with HAEMOPHILUS INFLUENZAE TYPE B (called "*H. flu*" or "Hib"). The illness has nothing to do with influenza, however, despite the name of the bacterium. Because of an effective vaccine, Hib meningitis has practically disappeared among young children.

The fears of bacterial meningitis is based not only on its reputation as a killer, but on the possibility of neurological complications—lingering problems that can be devastating in infants and children who are still developing. These complications can include hearing loss, mental retardation, and recurrent convulsions; they occur in 20 to 30 percent of patients who survive.

Cause Today, the two most common causes of bacterial meningitis are pneumococcal meningitis (caused by *Streptococcus pneumoniae*) and meningococcal meningitis (caused by *Neisseria meningitidis*). *H. flu* meningitis has almost disappeared because of childhood vaccines.

Symptoms Classic signs of meningitis include sudden high fever (100 degrees F to 106 degrees F) with chills, vomiting, stiff neck and intense headache in the front of the head, or a seizure. The neck will hurt if the patient tries to touch the chin to the chest. There may be muscle spasms or leg pains, and bright light may irritate the eyes.

All types of bacterial meningitis can appear suddenly or gradually in children. The less-common gradual type is harder to diagnose because symptoms are similar to other mild childhood illnesses: cold symptoms, fever, lethargy, vomiting, loss of appetite. A sudden attack is easier to diagnose, although it may indicate a more serious case.

Abnormal behavior may also announce the onset of meningitis, including aggressiveness, irritability, agitation, delirium, or screaming. This is followed by lethargy and stupor or coma.

Babies between ages three months and two years may have fever, vomiting, irritability, seizures, and a high-pitched cry. Rigidity may appear. The front soft spot on the baby's head may bulge.

Sometimes the illness is preceded by a cold or an ear infection. Any sudden change in consciousness or any unusual behavior in a young child may be a sign of meningitis.

Diagnosis A lumbar puncture (spinal tap) must be done to diagnose meningitis. Normally clear, the fluid is analyzed for the presence of bacteria and other evidence of infection. Bacteria will grow in the fluid within 48 hours; rapid tests on urine or blood can give results in a few hours and are most helpful in determining what type of bacteria are causing the meningitis.

However, since the disease can progress so quickly, treatment with intravenous antibiotics is started even before any test results are available.

Treatment Without treatment, most children would die from Hib meningitis; with antibiotics, 95 percent recover. Current antibiotics used in the treatment of bacterial meningitis include a class of antibiotics called cephalosporins, especially cefotaxime and ceftriaxone, and various members of the penicillin family. At least a week of treatment is needed.

See also MENINGITIS, MENINGOCOCCAL; MENINGITIS, PNEUMOCOCCAL MENINGITIS, VIRAL; MENINGOCOCCUS.

meningitis, meningococcal A severe bacterial infection of the bloodstream and meninges also known popularly as "spinal meningitis." (See MENINGITIS, BACTERIAL.) It is one of the more serious types of MENINGITIS, caused by a specific type of bacteria that can be fatal in some cases.

This type of meningitis is one that usually occurs as an isolated event. It affects about 3,000 Americans a year; half are younger than 2 and two-thirds are younger than 20. The highest rates occur among babies between four months and one year of age, and in young adults living together (as in a college dorm). Epidemics of meningitis have not occurred in the United States or most other industrial countries since World War II. Virulent epidemics still happen in developing countries, however. More than 40,000 cases were diagnosed during a 1989 epidemic in Ethiopia; as many as 3 million cases may have occurred during the 1960s in China.

Before the development of antibiotics, about half of all patients with this type of meningitis died. Today, most recover—except those with massive blood infection caused by the bacteria. Because the bacteria multiply and spread so quickly, it is very difficult to treat and antibiotics can't destroy enough of the bacteria fast enough. In this group of patients, 10 to 12 percent of victims will die.

The fear of this type of meningitis is based not only on its reputation as a killer but also on the possibility of neurological complications—lingering problems that can be devastating in infants and children. These complications can include hearing loss, mental retardation, and recurrent convulsions; they may occur to a greater or lesser degree in 20 to 30 percent of patients who survive.

Cause The bacteria that cause meningococcal meningitis is *Neisseria meningitidis* (or MENINGOCOCCUS), divided into nine separate groups (groups B and C are common in North America). The organism is a close relative of the bacterium responsible for GONORRHEA.

Patients can become infected by inhaling the bacteria, by direct mouth to mouth contact, or by indirect contact. Most patients develop only very mild upper-respiratory symptoms. More serious cases occur when the bacteria enter the bloodstream.

Up to 30 percent of any group of healthy people will have this bacteria in their throats at any one time without having symptoms. This type of meningitis is contagious but requires close personal contact to transmit. It is more commonly found in institutions and schools, such as colleges, child care centers, military barracks, and homes for the developmentally delayed.

In North America the disease usually occurs in isolated cases, although there may be a small outbreak of 5 to 10 cases at a time. It occurs most often in February and March and least often in September. In some parts of the world, meningococcal meningitis has been epidemic; there are also occasional smaller outbreaks. Epidemics are rare in the Western world. In other areas, epidemics last one to three years.

Symptoms Signs of meningococcal meningitis include sudden high fever (100 degrees F to 106 degrees F) with chills, vomiting, stiff neck and intense headache in the front of the head, or a seizure. The neck will hurt if the patient tries to touch the chin to the chest. There may be muscle spasms or leg pains, and bright light may irritate the eyes. Abnormal behavior may also announce the onset of meningitis, including aggressiveness, irritability, agitation, delirium, or screaming. This is followed by lethargy and stupor or coma. Sometimes the illness is preceded by a cold or an ear infection. Any sudden change in consciousness or any unusual behavior in a young child may be a sign of meningitis.

Babies between ages three months to two years may have fever, vomiting, irritability, seizures, and a high-pitched cry. Rigidity may appear. The front soft spot on the baby's head may bulge.

Diagnosis A lumbar puncture (spinal tap) must be done to diagnose meningitis; the procedure samples a small amount of fluid from the spinal cord to check for appearance, bacteria, protein, and sugar. Bacteria will grow in the fluid within 48 hours; rapid tests on spinal fluid or blood can give results in a few hours and are most helpful in determining what type of bacteria are causing the meningitis.

Throat cultures aren't helpful, since so many people have this bacteria in their throats.

Treatment Penicillin G administered intravenously in high doses will cure most patients with this disease. Patients should be carefully nursed with supportive care and maintained in isolation for the first 24 hours.

People diagnosed with this type of meningitis are infectious until they have taken antibiotics for 24 hours. Healthy carriers with the bacteria in nose and throat rarely develop the disease, as the organism is part of the normal bacteria in humans. The carrier state lasts weeks to months. It is the carrier state that predisposes to epidemics.

Complications Signs of the blood infection are fever, unresponsiveness or coma, rapid spreading rash, and shock. If the bacteria penetrate and damage the blood vessel lining, blood seeps out and causes a rash of small flat spots on arms, legs, and trunk. A child with a high fever and this type of rash needs immediate medical attention; in about 10 to 20 percent of patients, the infection quickly overwhelms the body. Called fulminant meningococcemia, it causes large purple bruises all over the skin and leads to fatal shock.

In addition, bacteria in the blood can lead to arthritis, heart problems, and PNEUMONIA. There may be long-term complications due to damaged nerves leading to the brain, such as hearing loss or mental retardation.

Prevention Scientists are trying to develop a vaccine for this disease that works in young children. The very first clinical trials (sponsored by North American Vaccine) for a vaccine for group C meningococcal infection have recently been completed. Researchers found the vaccine was well tolerated with no serious side effects. Until such a vaccine is approved, all people can do is practice good personal hygiene.

Physicians must report cases of meningococcal meningitis to the health department. When someone is diagnosed with meningococcal meningitis, ciprofloxacin or rifampin should be given to household members, close friends at school, and all preschoolers cared for in the same room as soon as possible (within 24 hours) of the diagnosis. "Close contact" would include anyone who has shared glasses, food or utensils, or who has kissed or had sexual contact with the patient.

Casual contact among people in a classroom, office, or factory setting is not usually significant enough to cause concern.

The only available vaccine is effective against groups A,C,Y, and W-135 but not group B. It isn't very effective in children under age two, and it takes up to two weeks to develop immunity. The vaccine is recommended for military recruits, children without spleens, and travelers to areas with epidemics of group A or C.

meningitis, pneumococcal The second most common cause of bacterial meningitis, this version is fatal in one out of every five cases. It occurs sporadically during the cold and flu season, not in epidemics, and is found more often in males. Highest rates are among children under the age of two, elderly people, and alcoholics.

Cause Pneumococcal meningitis is caused by STREPTOCOCCUS PNEUMONIAE, a circular-shaped bacterium found in pairs, a common cause of EAR INFECTIONS, PNEUMONIA, and SINUSITIS, in addition to meningitis. There are more than 80 types of this bacteria.

Most people have this bacteria in their nose and throat and can spread the infection by sneezing, coughing, or direct contact. However, most people don't get sick; it requires another condition to allow the bacteria to get into the bloodstream, such as a weakened immune system, HIV infection, sickle cell disease, or cancer. The bacteria can also invade the brain if there is injury or weakness in the nose cavity or a fracture line in the skull. Cases have been reported as a result of a violent sneezing attack.

Symptoms Classic signs of meningitis include sudden high fever (100 degrees F. to 106 degrees F) with chills, vomiting, stiff neck and intense headache in the front of the head, or a seizure. The neck will hurt if the patient tries to touch the chin to the chest. There may be muscle spasms or leg pains, and bright light may irritate the eyes.

Sometimes, the symptoms are similar to other mild illnesses: cold symptoms, fever, lethargy, vomiting, loss of appetite. A sudden attack is easier to diagnose, although it may indicate a more serious case.

Abnormal behavior may also announce the onset of meningitis, including aggressiveness, irritability, agitation, delirium, or screaming. This is followed by lethargy and stupor or coma.

Babies between ages three months to two years may have fever, vomiting, irritability, seizures, and a high-pitched cry. Rigidity may appear. The front soft spot on the baby's head may bulge. Adults most often experience a headache, fever, and stiff neck.

Sometimes the illness is preceded by a cold or an ear infection. Any sudden change in consciousness or any unusual behavior in someone ill with a respiratory infection may be a sign of meningitis.

Diagnosis A lumbar puncture (spinal tap) must be done to diagnose meningitis. Normally clear, the fluid is analyzed for the presence of bacteria and other evidence of infection. Bacteria will grow in the fluid within 48 hours; rapid tests on spinal fluid can give results in a few hours and are most helpful in determining the presence of bacteria in the usually sterile spinal fluid.

However, since the disease can progress so quickly, treatment with intravenous antibiotics must be started before any test results are available.

Treatment Some types of *S. pneumoniae* are not resistant to penicillin and other common antibiotics. Hospital care and IV drugs will be prescribed. Patients should be kept in darkened, quiet rooms, with painkillers and treatment for fever.

Complications Signs of blood infection are fever, unresponsiveness or coma, rapid-spreading rash, and shock. If the bacteria penetrate and damage the blood vessel lining, blood seeps out and causes a rash of small flat spots on arms, legs, and trunk. A patient with a high fever and this type of rash needs immediate medical attention.

The acute fulminant variety of meningitis occurs most often when *N. meningitidis* is the cause.

meningitis, viral A form of MENINGITIS (inflammation of the brain's lining) caused by a virus, usually less serious than its bacterial form. Viral meningitis is a fairly common and relatively mild illness when compared to its bacterial cousin. It is also called aseptic meningitis because there is no bacteria in the spinal fluid.

Cause ENTEROVIRUSES are the usual cause, a type of virus that affects only humans and is spread by the fecal-oral route. Enteroviruses live in human intestines; the two most common are ECHOVIRUSES and COXSACKIEVIRUS.

The virus is spread by direct contact with infected feces, nose or throat secretions. Most children are carriers without symptoms; the virus spreads most easily among young children in a group situation. Viral meningitis usually strikes young children in the summer and early fall; although anyone can get viral meningitis, most people over age 40 are immune.

Scientists don't know why so few children who are exposed to the disease come down with symptoms; those who are well fed, well rested, and healthy are less likely to become infected.

Symptoms Symptoms usually appear quite suddenly, with a high fever, severe headache, nausea and vomiting, and stiff neck. There may be sensitivity to light and noise, sore throat, or eye infections. There may also be accompanying neurological problems, such as blurred vision.

Most people recover completely within two weeks, although there may be muscle weakness, tiredness, headache, muscle spasms, insomnia, or personality changes (such as an inability to concentrate) for months afterward. These are rarely permanent.

Diagnosis Viral meningitis can be diagnosed by lumbar puncture (spinal tap).

Treatment There is no cure for viral meningitis; eventually the immune system will develop antibodies to destroy the virus. Hospitalization with IV fluids and painkillers may be necessary for the severe headache, dehydration, nausea, and vomiting.

Patients should drink clear fluids, eat a bland diet, and get plenty of rest. Children should be taken for a hearing test several weeks after recovery.

Complications Increased pressure on the brain from a buildup of fluid in the meninges is a serious complication. Some infants who have meningitis early in life have delayed language. Patients with a weakened immune system may have chronic infections with enterovirus.

meningococcus A bacterium of the genus *Neisseria meningitidis,* an organism that can cause MENINGITIS. The bacteria are often found in the nose and throat of healthy carriers. While not highly communicable, crowded conditions (such as in army camps or college dorms) concentrate the number of carriers.

meningoencephalitis An inflammation of both the brain and the meninges, usually caused by a bacterial infection.

meningoencephalitis, primary amebic (PAM) A severe infection of the gray matter of the brain caused by a free-living single-cell ameba that lives in warm freshwater. Most cases have been reported in young boys and teen-age boys and girls. PAM is a relatively rare infection in the United States.

Cause The ameba (*Naegleria fowleri*) found in stagnant or slow-moving water causes amebic meningoencephalitis. It can live in the soil as a cyst that reactivates when placed in water. If water containing the ameba goes up the nose while swimming, the person will be exposed to the disease. The amoeba can survive in warm inland water, unchlorinated or incorrectly chlorinated water, dams, and ponds but not in sea water or salty estuaries. Flowing streams and rivers with cool water have not been associated with the disease. Most patients got the infection after diving into freshwater swimming holes.

Symptoms The disease is characterized by fever, headache, vomiting, and ENCEPHALITIS, followed rapidly by coma and death.

Treatment Early treatment with amphotericin B can successfully treat the disease.

meningomyelitis Inflammation of the spinal cord and its surrounding membranes.

Microban A colorless, odorless antibacterial product registered and approved by the U.S. Food and Drug Administration that can be embedded in toys, hospital equipment, and other items to protect against the growth of mold, fungus, and bacteria (including *ESCHERICHIA COLI, SALMONELLA* BACTERIA, *Staphylococcus,* and STREPTOCOCCUS). The product, which can't be washed off, has recently been introduced in a line of children's toys by Playskool. Microban has existed for 15 years and has undergone extensive testing. It is already used in products for hospitals, labs, and food processors.

Playskool announced it would include Microban in some of its newborn and toddler toys first, including its Roll'n Rattle Ball and Busy Band Walker. It introduced about 15 protected toys in 1997 and expanded its selection in 1998.

microbes Life-forms (also called microorganisms) that are too small to be seen by the human eye. Some of them are so small, they can't be seen with even the most powerful microscope. There are hundreds of thousands of different microbe species that come in all different shapes and sizes, including the PROTOZOANS, algae, FUNGI, slime molds, BACTERIA, RICKETTSIAE, and VIRUSES.

Many scientists believe that microbes were probably the first life-forms on Earth, but they weren't discovered until about 300 years ago, when Dutch scientist Antonie van Leeuwenhoek first saw the tiny moving creatures with a microscope he had made himself. He called these creatures "animalcules."

Microbes are a necessary and useful part of our environment. No area of the body other than the brain is totally free of bacteria. Human feces are made up of 94 percent microbes. They process our digestion and produce most of our antibiotics, maintain our soil and plant environment, and even produce alcoholic beverages by the process of fermentation. All but a few of the millions of microbial life-forms are beneficial to us. The very few that do cause disease are called pathogens.

Microsporum A genus of dermatophytes of the family Moniliaceae. One type (*M. audouinii*) causes TINEA capitis (ringworm) in children. Other types include *M. canis* and *M. gypseum*. The genus was formerly known as *Microsporon*.

Microsporum canis A species of fungi that is found most often among dogs and cats but also occurs among humans and causes in RINGWORM (or dermatophytosis). *Microsporum canis* has specifically adapted itself to cats, which are often carriers without symptoms. The fungi can live in the environment for up to 18 months. Any building or room in which infected animals have been housed could potentially be a source of infection. Brushes, bedding, cages, and other items are all potential sources of infection. These fungi have also been cultured from dust, heating vents, and furnace filters. They can be diagnosed by observing the skin with a special light called a Wood's lamp, where about 50 percent of the time affected hairs may glow green.

middle ear infection See EAR INFECTION.

miliary tuberculosis See TUBERCULOSIS.

molluscum contagiosum A harmless viral infection that causes groups of tiny pearly white lumps on the skin's surface; palms of the hands and soles of the feet are not affected. This virus is the cause of a frequent opportunistic infection in AIDS patients.

Cause The virus is one of two poxviruses that specifically infect humans, causing a skin disease that responds to treatment in most people with healthy immune systems. But in AIDS patients, the virus is often progressive and resists treatment. (Variola, the cause of SMALLPOX, is the other poxvirus specific to humans.) Despite being in the same family, variola and molluscum contagiosum virus have very different ways of infection. Infection with molluscum is easily transmitted by direct skin contact or during intercourse.

The virus is transmitted from person to person by direct or indirect contact and can live in the body for up to three years, although individual lesions persist for only six to eight weeks.

Symptoms Each pimple looks like a shiny small circle with a central depression. The pimples appear primarily on the genitals, thighs, and face.

Diagnosis Diagnosis is made by direct examination of the skin.

Treatment In healthy patients, the infection usually clears up within a few months without treatment. Because they are unattractive, most people want them removed.

moniliasis   Another   name   for   *CANDIDA ALBICANS.*

monkeypox   A genetic cousin of the SMALL-POX virus, monkeypox is native to monkeys but is occasionally able to infect and kill humans. In 1997, monkeypox among humans broke out in Zaire, where it has been responsible for at least 92 cases of sickness (including three deaths in children under age three). The Zaire outbreak may have originated in tree squirrels native to the rain forest; once it crossed into humans, it spread through 12 villages in central Zaire.

Cause   For years, experts understood that it was possible for monkeys to infect humans with monkeypox. But now, according to the CDC, it appears that for the first time humans have infected other humans. Researchers were evacuated from politically troubled Zaire before they were able to pinpoint how the disease is transmitted from animals or between people. So far, the virus has remained in Zaire and is not likely to reach the United States.

Symptoms   A disfiguring rash similar to smallpox, featuring head to toe blisters, with a high fever and respiratory problems.

Prevention   Vaccinia vaccine, which prevents smallpox, also protects against monkeypox. But because vaccination was stopped once smallpox was eradicated from the earth, the generation born after 1980 may be vulnerable to the new disease. Vaccination may need to be revived if the monkeypox continues to spread.

mononucleosis, infectious   An acute herpesvirus infection caused by the EPSTEIN-BARR VIRUS and characterized by sore throat, fever, swollen lymph glands, and bruising. Known as the "kissing disease" because it is transmitted in saliva, young people are most often infected. In childhood the disease is most often mild. The older the patient, however, the more severe the symptoms are likely to be. Infection confers permanent immunity.

Cause   The disease is usually transmitted by droplet EBV virus but is not highly contagious. CYTOMEGALOVIRUS (CMV) INFECTION can cause a similar infection; both EBV and CMV are members of the HERPES family of viruses.

Symptoms   Between four to six weeks after infection, classic mono begins gradually with symptoms of sore throat, fatigue, swollen lymph glands, and occasional bruising. Although the symptoms usually disappear in four to six weeks, the virus remains dormant in the throat and blood for the rest of the patient's life. Periodically the virus can reactivate and be found in the patient's saliva, although it doesn't usually cause symptoms.

Mono may also start abruptly with high fever and severe, swollen sore throat similar to strep throat.

Rarely, about 10 percent of patients have a third type, with a low persistent fever, nausea and vomiting, and stomach problems.

About half of all patients have an enlarged spleen and a few have an enlarged liver or mild jaundice.

Diagnosis   Symptoms   of   fever,   sore throat, and swollen glands, are used to diagnose the disease. Blood tests and blood counts are needed for confirmation. The mono spot is a rapid antibody test that looks for a specific reaction in the blood of infected patients. Liver function tests will reveal abnormal liver function—so-called mono-hepatitis that may occur.

Treatment   There is no specific treatment for the disease other than symptom management. No antiviral or antibiotic drugs are available. Some doctors prescribe steroids to reduce the tonsil inflammation because the patient can't swallow. Enforced bed rest may prevent injury to the swollen spleen. Painkillers and saline gargles may help the sore throat.

Complications   There may be a swollen spleen or liver inflammation; heart problems or involvement of the central nervous system may rarely occur (mono-meningitis), but this disease is almost never fatal. If the spleen ruptures, immediate surgery and blood transfusions will be necessary.

About half the time, the patient will also have a strep throat, which does require antibiotic treatment. Occasionally, patients will have such intense swelling of the lymphatic system of their throat, they require hospitalization for IV fluids to prevent dehydration.

Prevention Most people exposed to patients with mono have already been infected with EBV and aren't at risk for developing disease themselves, since 95 percent of adults over age 35 have antibodies to the virus. Transmission routes are not fully understood, although doctors suspect it is transmitted via saliva.

Morbidity and Mortality Weekly Report A weekly epidemiologic report on the incidence of communicable diseases and deaths in 120 urban areas of the United States. It is published by the Centers for Disease Control and Prevention in Atlanta, Georgia. The publication also includes information on accident rates and important international health data.

morbidity rate The number of cases of a particular disease occurring in a single year per specified population unit. It may be calculated on the basis of age groups, gender, occupation, or other population group.

morbilli See MEASLES.

morbillivirus, equine (EM) See EQUINE MORBILLIVIRUS.

mosquito bites Mosquitoes are found throughout the world; the females bite in order to obtain blood to produce their eggs. Because their eggs are laid and hatched in stagnant water, they are most commonly found in areas near marshes, ponds, reservoirs, and water tanks.

Mosquito bites may cause swelling and itching for several days; the main problem of these bites is the infections that may be transmitted in the insect's saliva.

Because mosquitoes spread so much disease, scientists are continually working to develop new methods to eradicate them. Among the new possibilities include a protozoan, a fungus, and an Argentian nematode that may attack mosquitoes. Some scientists are developing poisoning bacteria and blue-green algae; others are developing new types of repellents.

The problem with eradicating mosquitoes is that they continually become resistant to almost any poison that scientists can develop; in any population of insects, some are likely to have a genetic resistance to any insecticide. Those few survive and reproduce, passing on their genes to offspring; eventually most of the insects in later generations have inherited the ability to survive the insecticide.

Treatment Because mosquitoes can spread disease, mosquito bites should be washed with soap and water followed by an antiseptic. To control itching, a nonprescription antihistamine, calamine lotion, anesthetic gels, or ice pack may help. Or try making a paste of salt and water or baking soda and water to apply to the bite.

Prevention Use insect repellents, such as

DEET (N1N-diethyl-m-toluamide): By far the best repellant that should be applied on all exposed skin. It comes in various strengths, but the more concentrated is more effective; children should use milder versions because there have been a few cases of toxicity with small children

bath oil: Although many consumers swear by Avon's Skin-so-Soft, recent research by the military (and the Avon company) demonstrate that it is not nearly as effective as DEET.

zinc: Some experts recommend daily doses (at least 60 milligrams), although they warn it can take up to four weeks to work; extra supplements should be taken only with approval of physician

mud fever See LEPTOSPIROSIS.

Muerta Canyon virus See SIN NOMBRE VIRUS.

multiple sclerosis and viruses Multiple sclerosis is a chronic disease of the nervous system, affecting young and middle-aged adults in which the sheaths covering nerves in the brain and spinal cord are damaged (called demyelination). The disease affects different parts of the brain and spinal cord, causing a variety of symptoms including paralysis, eye problems, speech defects, and shaky movements. While not normally considered to be an infectious disease, the true cause of the illness is not known.

Some scientists suspect a "slow virus" might trigger the development of MS, which is characterized by recurrent relapses followed by remissions. MS is known to involve a problem with the body's immune reaction. T cells (immune system cells that attack invading viruses and bacteria) for some reason attack instead the nerve covering (myelin sheath). Without its myelin covering, the nerves basically short circuit.

What some scientists suspect is that perhaps a common infection initially triggers the T cells to attack. In fact, T cells from patients with MS react not only against myelin from the brain and spinal cord but also against various common viruses and bacteria. This could mean that for some reason, the T cells could not tell the difference between some infectious organisms and its own myelin. Peptides from viruses that are similar to myelin include EPSTEIN-BARR, HERPES simplex, INFLUENZA, and the bacterium *PSEUDOMONAS AERUGINOSA.*

In research, at the University of Pennsylvania, mouse HEPATITIS virus leads to myelin destruction much like the damage seen in MS. As with many viruses, this one stays in the animal's body long after the initial infection and can cause destruction of myelin later in life. Further damage is caused by the mouse's immune system response to the virus.

mumps An acute viral illness that was at one time a common childhood disease, featuring swollen and inflamed salivary glands on one or both sides of the face or under the jaw. In 1968 there were 152,000 mumps cases; today, only a few thousand people per year get mumps.

Before the mumps vaccine was available, almost every child got mumps sometime in childhood. While the incidence of the disease is much lower today, an unimmunized child remains at high risk for getting mumps. The diseases is still widely found in developing countries, which is why anyone over one year of age should have a vaccine when traveling abroad.

Cause Mumps is spread by airborne droplets of the mumps virus that are expelled by a patient with mumps who is coughing, sneezing, or talking. The virus invades and multiplies in the parotid gland, but it is attracted to all the glands.

Symptoms The disease will appear two to three weeks after exposure, beginning with mild discomfort in the area just inside the angle of the jaw. Many infected children have no symptoms. In more serious cases, however, the child complains of pain and has difficulty chewing; the glands on one or both sides become painful and tender. Fever, headache, and swallowing problems may follow, but the fever falls after two to three days and the swelling fades within 10 days. When only one side is affected, the second gland often swells as the first one subsides.

Diagnosis Mumps is usually diagnosed from symptoms; it can be confirmed by culturing the virus from saliva or urine, or by measuring antibodies to mumps virus in the blood.

The skin test for mumps—considered unreliable—is no longer available.

Treatment   While there is no treatment, a patient may be given painkillers and plenty of fluids. In moderate to severe cases the child may need to stay in bed. Males with testicular involvement may be given a stronger painkiller; corticosteroid drugs may be needed to reduce inflammation.

Complications   While mumps is normally considered to be a mild disease, sometimes it can be more serious, causing a mild inflammation of the coverings of the brain and spinal cord (MENINGITIS) in about one in every 10 children with mumps. More rarely, it can cause an inflammation of the brain itself (ENCEPHALITIS), which usually improves by itself without permanent brain damage.

While serious complications are not common, one out of every teenage and adult males with the disease will have an inflammation and swelling in one or both testes. In extremely rare cases, this can lead to sterility. Mumps can also cause inflammation of the ovaries in older girls and women, inflammation of the pancreas or heart muscle, or auditory nerve damage resulting in deafness.

There is no evidence that mumps in pregnancy has any effect on the fetus.

Prevention   All healthy children who have never had mumps should be immunized on or before their first birthday. If in doubt, it is safe to be immunized or reimmunized against mumps.

The vaccine is available by itself, or in combination with measles and rubella (MMR) or mumps and rubella (MR). Typically, the combination MMR vaccine is given at 15 months of age because it includes a measles vaccine; it protects the child against all three diseases. The vaccination, which has been used since 1967, can also be given to older children and adults. It is highly effective and one injection produces long-lasting (probably lifelong) immunity.

According to the U.S. Centers for Disease Control, in very rare instances the mumps vaccine produces a mild, brief fever. This fever may occur one to two weeks after receiving the vaccine. Occasionally there is some slight swelling of the throat glands. Serious reactions are extremely rare.

Males who have already gone through puberty who have never been immunized against mumps or had the infection should avoid contact with any infected person. If symptoms do develop, passive immunization with antimumps immunoglobulin can provide some protection against the development of swelling in the testes.

Some children anyone who has a severely impaired immune system, a severe allergy to eggs, or anyone with a high fever or who has received blood products or immune globulin in the past three months should not receive the mumps virus vaccine.

mycetoma   A rare tropical skin and bone infection that can be highly disfiguring, producing a hard swelling covered by the openings of multiple drainage channels that discharge pus.

Cause   Mycetoma is caused by FUNGI or actinomycetes (a type of bacteria).

Treatment   Antibiotics are the medications of choice if mycetoma is caused by actinomycetes; fungal disease may be hard to treat with drugs, and it may be necessary to surgically remove affected skin.

Mycobacterium   A genus of rod-shaped bacteria having several significant species. *Mycobacterium leprae* causes LEPROSY; *M. tuberculosis* causes TUBERCULOSIS; *M. avium intracellulare* causes MYCOBACTERIUM AVIUM COMPLEX (MAC), a significant cause of death in AIDS patients. The genus is responsible for more suffering around the world than all other bacterial genera combined. Currently, more than 60 species of mycobacteria have been well defined.

Mycobacterium avium **complex (MAC)**   The most common bacterial opportunistic infection in people with HIV, it consists of two similar organisms—*Mycobacterium avium* and *M. intracellulare*. In one study, 43 percent of people with AIDS surviving two years after diagnosis tested positive for MAC, suggesting that the infection may be an almost inevitable complication of HIV infection. MAC is also sometimes called *Mycobacterium avium intracellulare (MAI)*. Some studies have shown that MAC occurs more often in Caucasians than in Latinos and African Americans; homosexual and bisexual men may have a higher incidence of infection than those in other risk groups.

Cause The MAC organisms are found commonly in water, water mists or vapors, dust, soil, and bird droppings. They usually enter the body via contaminated food and water, although they also can be inhaled into the lungs. Once inside the body, the organisms colonize and grow in the gastrointestinal tract or the lungs, where they don't usually cause any symptoms at first. Eventually, since they are not stopped by the body's normal response to infection, they attack the tissue lining the gut and reproduce tremendously. After a local infection, the MAC organisms usually enter the bloodstream and spread throughout the body.

Symptoms The most common symptoms include fevers, night sweats, weight loss, loss of appetite, fatigue, or progressively severe diarrhea. Other symptoms include abdominal pain, nausea, and vomiting. Respiratory symptoms (cough and breathing problems) are fairly uncommon. However, painful joints, bone, brain, and skin infections can result when MAC bacteria spreads to other parts of the body.

Treatment Since MAC bacteria are closely related to the organism that causes TUBERCULOSIS, some of the drugs used to treat TB are also used against MAC. While it is not clear if treating MAC prolongs survival, treatment definitely reduces symptoms and improves the quality of life. A dozen or more drugs are available to treat MAC; most experts agree that treating an advanced MAC infection requires several drugs because no drug is effective alone. MAC bacteria can quickly become resistant to a particular drug.

Prevention Taking prophylactic drugs (such as rifabutin) can prevent or delay the onset of MAC in people with HIV infection. Since MAC organisms have been found in most city water systems, as well as hospital water supplies and bottled water, boiling drinking water is suggested. AIDS patients also are advised not to eat raw foods (especially salads, root vegetables, and unpasteurized milk or cheese). Conventional cooking (baking, boiling, or steaming) destroys MAC bacteria, which are killed at 176 degrees F. Fruits and vegetables should be peeled and rinsed thoroughly.

Patients should avoid animal contact (especially birds and bird droppings). Pigeons, in particular, can transmit not just MAC but also the organism that causes CRYPTOCOCCOSIS, another opportunistic infection found in people with HIV infection.

Finally, HIV patients should avoid or reduce alcohol consumption, since regularly drinking alcohol can hasten the development of MAC infection in those with HIV.

Mycobacterium avium intracellulare See *MYCOBACTERIUM AVIUM* COMPLEX.

Mycobacterium leprae Also called Hansen's bacillus, this is the organism that causes LEPROSY. The rod-shaped bacterium was identified in 1874 by a Norwegian Armauer Hansen; as a result, both the microbe and the disease were named for him.

Mycobacterium tuberculosis Also known as Koch's bacillus, this slow-growing organism is the cause of TUBERCULOSIS. Often shortened to *M. Tb*, the bacterium was discovered in 1882 by German physician Robert Koch, the father of modern bacteriology and discoverer of the organisms that cause ANTHRAX and CHOLERA.

This slow-growing bacillus (rod-shaped bacterium) belongs to the family Mycobacterium species. Most members of this family live in water or soil and don't infect humans, although *M. bovis* infects cows and can cause TB in those who drink unpasteurized milk from infected cows.

A single bacterium is called a tubercule bacillus. An extremely tough type of bacteria, the TB bug can live for weeks in the dark, where it forms spores. It cannot survive in a clean, well-ventilated sunny environment. It is most often transmitted by respiratory secretions from coughing. The organism can remain airborne and alive in these secretions and on surfaces for days.

mycology   The study of FUNGI and fungoid diseases.

mycoplasma   Free-living bacteria that lack a cell wall. The lack of a cell wall means that the bacteria are resistant to antibiotics such as PENICILLIN, which work by attacking bacterial cell walls.

Mycoplasmas are found everywhere in nature, some living on decaying matter or occupying harmless places within other organisms. But many others are disease-causing bacteria of vertebrates, insects, and plants. Only a limited number of mycoplasma species infect humans; the most important of these is *MYCOPLASMA PNEUMONIAE*, a common cause of respiratory infection (including PNEUMONIA). It is also possible that mycoplasmas could be involved in the progression of AIDS.

Mycoplasmas were first isolated in 1898 in France, as the source of a cattle disease called pleuropneumonia. When similar microbes were found to cause other infections (including a particular form of human pneumonia) they were called pleuropneumonia-like organisms or PPLOs. They were later correctly reclassified as mycoplasmas, and *M. pneumoniae* was identified in the early 1960s.

The term *mycoplasma* is used as a general designation for any member of the class, or as *Mycoplasma,* the name of a particular genus within that class.

mycoplasma pneumonia   A contagious disease of children and young adults caused by *MYCOPLASMA PNEUMONIAE.* The disease is also called Eaton-agent pneumonia, primary atypical pneumonia, or walking pneumonia.

Anyone can get the disease, but it occurs most often in older children and young adults. The infections occur sporadically throughout the year, but they are most common in late summer and in fall; widespread community outbreaks may occur every four to eight years.

Cause   Mycoplasma pneumonia is caused by *M. pneumoniae,* a microscopic organism related to bacteria. It is spread through contact with droplets from the nose and throat of infected people when they cough or sneeze. Scientists believe transmission requires close contact with an infected person. The contagious period is probably less than 10 days.

Symptoms   After an incubation period of between 9 to 25 days, symptoms of dry cough, fever, sore throat, headache, and malaise appear. Ear infections may also occur. Symptoms may last from a few days to a month or more.

Diagnosis   The disease can be diagnosed based on the symptoms; a nonspecific blood test may help in the diagnosis.

Treatment   Antibiotics including erythromycin or tetracycline are effective.

Prevention   There are no vaccines to prevent the spread of mycoplasma infection, and there are no reliable methods for control.

Mycoplasma pneumoniae   The organism that causes the contagious disease MYCOPLASMA PNEUMONIA. While classified as a bacterium, it does not have a cell wall and can't be seen on routine smears or grown on routine culture plates. It does not usually cause anything other than a respiratory disease.

mycosis Any disease caused by a fungus.

mycotic infections, systemic See FUNGAL INFECTION.

mycotoxicosis A type of fungus-derived metabolite found on certain kinds of food capable of causing one type of food poisoning. Ever since the Middle Ages, thousands of people have died from various types of mycotoxins—most notably, ergot poisoning. But it was a 1960 turkey epidemic in England that spurred a worldwide research effort to track down the vast number of toxic compounds derived from fungus that cause these poisonings. While most of the deaths from mycotoxicosis have been among animals eating tainted food, symptoms are still found frequently among humans.

It's estimated that one of the most widespread of these toxins are aflatoxins found in a wide variety of food, including grains, peanuts, tree nuts, and cottonseed meal; meat, eggs, milk, and other products from animals that consume aflatoxin-contaminated feed are additional sources of potential exposure.

Peanuts can develop a toxic mold when not properly stored, which is why consumers should never eat moldy or shriveled food (especially grains or peanuts) and should be cautious about eating unroasted peanuts sold in bulk.

Aflatoxin is a cancer-causing byproduct of the *Aspergillus flavus* mold found in peanuts, corn, wheat, rice, cottonseeds, barley, soybeans, Brazil nuts, and pistachios. The molds that produce aflatoxin grow in warm, humid climates in the southeastern United States, but the mold can also be produced in the field when rain falls on corn and wheat left in the field to dry. Aflatoxin-producing mold can even grow on plants damaged by insects or drought, poor nutrition, or unseasonable temperatures.

Aflatoxin has been called the most potent natural carcinogen known to humans; poor diet also seems to predispose animals to cancer in the wake of aflatoxin ingestion.

Still, scientists know very little about why or how the aflatoxins are produced by the mold, and because it is sometimes difficult to see, all susceptible crops are subject to routine testing in the United States. Unfortunately, it is not possible to detect the mold with 100 percent accuracy.

While the way agricultural products are stored can affect the mold's growth, the length of time of such storage is also important; the longer agricultural products are stored in bins, the greater the chance that environmental conditions favorable to aflatoxin production will be created. Stored nuts or seeds might accidentally get wet or the storage bin might not facilitate drying quickly enough to stop the mold from growing.

Aflatoxins are more common in poor-quality cereals and nuts; while most of these low-grade products don't enter the human food market, they are sold as animal feed, which can go on to contaminate animal products (such as meat and milk). For this reason, cottonseed meal (a product often contaminated with high levels of aflatoxin) is banned for use as an animal feed. Cottonseed oil, however, rarely contains aflatoxin, since the toxin sticks to the hulls of the seed.

Milk is commonly contaminated with aflatoxin, and powdered nonfat milk can contain eight times more than the original liquid product since the aflatoxin adheres to the milk's proteins. In addition, measurable levels of aflatoxin can be found in some baby foods that use dry milk to boost the protein content of the product.

Prevention Pasteurization, sterilization, and dry processing techniques can substantially reduce aflatoxin contamination of dried milk. Meat products are less often contaminated because little aflatoxin is carried over into the meat, except for pig liver and kidneys. Chicken may become contaminated with aflatoxin when the bird appears to be only mildly sick.

Symptoms In humans, aflatoxin is believed to cause liver cancer, according to some East African studies, which seem to show a correlation between the two. Epidemiological evidence also suggests men are more susceptible than women; many scientists believe a poor diet and liver disease also increase susceptibility to liver cancer as a result of aflatoxin exposure. Data from the African studies were strong enough to prompt the FDA and the EPA to develop strict regulations to control levels in food and animal food sold in the United States.

Aflatoxin can also cause acute poisoning; severe liver disease has been detected in those who ingest highly contaminated food, and children around the world exhibit symptoms similar to Reyes syndrome (fever, vomiting, coma, and convulsions) after exposure.

myiasis, cutaneous   A fly larvae infestation of the skin usually found only in the tropics. When the African tumbu fly lays eggs on clothing, the larvae from the eggs penetrate the skin, eventually causing a swelling that looks like a boil. Various other types of flies may lay eggs in open wounds, on the skin, or in the ears or nose.

Prevention Infestation can be avoided by covering open wounds and (in Africa) by thoroughly ironing clothes that have been drying outside.

Treatment Oil drops over the swelling suffocates the larvae, which then come to the surface where they can be removed with a needle.

myocarditis   An acute inflammatory condition of the myocardium (the heart muscle) caused by viral, bacterial, or fungal infection. It may also be produced as a result of RHEUMATIC FEVER. After a bout of myocarditis, there is usually some residual heart enlargement. People with a virus infection that affects the lungs may have a mild myocarditis that may be detected with an electrocardiogram (an ECG).

The most common cause of myocarditis in Central and South America is the parasitic infection called CHAGAS DISEASE. Many years after the initial infection, these patients can have extensive damage to the heart muscle ending in death.

Symptoms   The symptoms depend on the type of infection that causes the inflammation, the degree of damage, and the capacity of the heart muscle to recover. Symptoms may be mild or nonexistent; if they do occur, they may include fatigue, pain, fever, and rapid heartbeat. Rarely, the inflammation can lead to chest pain and heart failure, followed by cardiac arrest and death. Acute inflammation of the outer lining of the heart (pericarditis) often accompanies myocarditis.

Treatment   Most cases clear up without treatment, although corticosteroid drugs are occasionally prescribed to reduce inflammation. Treatment of the cause of the inflammation together with painkillers, oxygen, and rest are helpful. Most physicians believe that exercise is not helpful for people with myocarditis; they recommend that patients not engage in strenuous exercise until their ECG returns to normal.

myxovirus   Any of a group of medium-sized viruses that include those that cause INFLUENZA, MUMPS, and PARAINFLUENZA.

nanophyetiasis The name for a human disease caused by infection with parasitic flatworms (flukes); it is also called "fish flu." Not a great deal is known about this disease.

There have been no reported massive outbreaks of the disease in North America; the only scientific reports are of 20 individuals referred to in one Oregon clinic. However, a report in the popular press suggests the frequency is much higher.

The disease is endemic in Russia, where the infection rate is reported to be more than 90 percent and growing.

Cause The disease is caused by the *Nanophyetus salmincola* or *N. schikhobalowi,* the North American and Russian troglotrematoid trematodes (respectively). It is transmitted by the larval stage of a worm that embeds itself in the flesh of freshwater fish; North American cases were all associated with salmon. Raw, underprocessed, and smoked salmon and steelhead were implicated.

Symptoms The first reported U.S. cases were characterized by diarrhea, usually accompanied by abdominal discomfort and nausea. A few patients reported weight loss and fatigue.

Diagnosis The disease is diagnosed by finding the eggs in feces. However, it is hard to tell the difference between these eggs and those of another parasite, *Diphyllobothrium latum.*

Treatment Treatment with bithionol or niclosamide appears to resolve the problem.

National Center for Infectious Diseases National center dedicated to surveillance, research, prevention, and training in the area of infectious diseases, affiliated with the U.S. Centers for Disease Control and Prevention in Atlanta, Georgia. Created in 1981, NCID is committed to the prevention and control of traditional, new, and reemerging infectious diseases in the United States and around the world. Six divisions and three programs plan and conduct the center's disease prevention and control activities.

The Division of Vector-Borne Infectious Diseases is part of the NCID and was established in Utah in the 1950s as the Disease Ecology Section of the CDC to deal with arboviral ENCEPHALITIS in the western United States. In 1963 the unit moved to Greeley, Colorado, and in 1967 relocated to its present location in Fort Collins, Colorado. Its PLAGUE program was moved from San Francisco to the unit at that time. In 1989 it was given the responsibility of developing a national LYME DISEASE program and was given its present name to reflect its responsibilities for Lyme disease, plague, and other zoonotic bacterial infections.

DVBID serves as an international reference center for vector-borne viral and bacterial diseases. As one of the few remaining centers responsible for these agents, it tries to develop and maintain surveillance, conduct field and lab research and epidemic aid investigations, define disease etiology, provide diagnostic reference and consultation to state or local health departments.

The division emphasizes research to improve diagnosis, prevention, and control of diseases such as Lyme disease, DENGUE FEVER, YELLOW FEVER, arboviral encephalitis, and plague. It includes three branches: the Arbovirus Diseases Branch, the Bacterial Zoonoses Branch, and the Dengue Branch in San Juan, Puerto Rico.

National Institute of Allergy and Infectious Diseases The federal research institute that provides the major support for scientists conducting research aimed at developing better ways to diagnose, treat, and prevent the many infectious, immunologic, and allergic diseases.

NIAID has four divisions: AIDS; Allergy, Immunology and Transplantation; Microbiology and Infectious Diseases; and Extramural Activities. In addition, NIAID scientists conduct intramural research in labs in Bethesda, Rockville, and Frederick, Maryland, and in Hamilton, Montana.

Among other diseases, NIAID investigates these major conditions:

AIDS: NIAID conducts and supports basic research on HIV and AIDS, develops new drugs, conducts clinical trials of experimental drugs, and develops and tests HIV vaccines.

Emerging diseases: NIAID supports research on LYME DISEASE, HANTAVIRUS, drug-resistant TUBERCULOSIS, and other emerging diseases to develop better ways to diagnose, treat and prevent them.

Enteric diseases: NIAID supports research into diarrheal diseases such as CHOLERA and ROTAVIRUS that are major causes of death among infants and children.

Immunologic diseases: NIAID researchers focus on the basic biology of the immune system and related diseases, including autoimmune diseases such as scleroderma and lupus.

Malaria and other tropical disease: NIAID conducts research into a variety of tropical diseases, including MALARIA, FILARIASIS, TRYPANOSOMIASIS, and LEPROSY and supports centers for tropical medicine research in countries where these diseases are endemic.

Sexually transmitted diseases: NIAID studies support research into GONORRHEA, SYPHILIS, CHLAMYDIA, GENITAL HERPES, and human PAPILLOMAVIRUS, focusing on better diagnostic tests, improved treatments, and effective vaccines.

Vaccine development: NIAID has introduced new vaccines for a variety of serious diseases and is currently testing new vaccines at a number of U.S. centers.

Other areas of research include fungal diseases, HOSPITAL-ACQUIRED INFECTIONS, CHRONIC FATIGUE SYNDROME, respiratory diseases, ANTIVIRAL AGENTS, and ANTIMICROBIAL DRUG studies.

necrotizing fascitis See FLESH-EATING BACTERIA.

Neisseria gonorrhoeae A gram-negative bacterium that causes GONORRHEA, also called gonococcus or diplococcus. This circular bacterium was identified in 1879 by the German dermatologist Albert L. S. Neisser. It was not until 1937 that scientists discovered sulfa drugs could kill the microorganism. Unfortunately, today there are penicillin-resistant strains (known as PPNG, for penicillinase-producing *Neisseria gonorrhoea*), coming primarily from the Philippines. Other strains are resistant to tetracycline.

Neisseria meningitidis See MENINGOCOCCUS.

nematodes See ROUNDWORMS.

neurocysticercosis See TAPEWORM.

neurotoxic shellfish poisoning See SHELLFISH POISONING, NEUROTOXIC.

nitric oxide A simple molecule—with one atom of oxygen and one of nitrogen—that may be used by the immune system to fight a wide variety of infections. So varied is this molecule's role in the body that in 1992, *Science* voted it "Molecule of the Year."

It was best known as a toxic gas and an ingredient in air pollution until 1987, when scientists discovered it was produced by cells throughout the body. Since then, it was identified as a player in a vast number of body activities. In addition to its ability to fight infections, it boosts cell communication, regulates blood pressure, causes penile erections, transmits messages between nerve cells, kills certain parasites, and may play a part in learning and memory.

Scientists have known for some time that nitric oxide disables or kills certain protozoans, worms, fungi, and bacteria. Now, new research suggests that nitric oxide is a potent antiviral that attacks both poxviruses and HERPES simplex, type 1 (HSV1), which causes COLD SORES in humans. It appears to be triggered by cytokines such as INTERFERON (proteins secreted by immune system cells).

Nitric oxide appears to have potential as a broad-spectrum antiviral because it affects many different kinds of viruses. Scientists believe if they can design ways to deliver the right amount of nitric oxide to the site of infection without causing side effects, they could produce a new approach to antiviral therapy.

Other recent studies suggest that nitric oxide may help the body defend itself against diseases such as MALARIA and that nitric oxide levels may play a key role in determining whether a child develops the most dangerous complication of the disease—cerebral malaria. Cerebral malaria, which causes convulsions and coma, kills many of its victims. Scientists don't know why only some people develop the complication, but they found that those who do had the lowest levels of nitric oxide.

nocardiosis   An infection by a funguslike bacterium found throughout the world. This infection is not normally found in healthy patients, but it occurs in those with a compromised immune system, beginning in the lungs and spreading to tissues under the skin.

Cause   The disease is caused by infection with *Nocardia asteroides,* an aerobic species of actinomycetes. The organism enters the respiratory tract and spreads throughout the bloodstream.

Symptoms   Fever and cough similar to pneumonia that does not respond to normal short-term antibiotics, with lung damage and brain abscesses. Occasionally, this bacterium causes skin abscesses only (especially in gardeners).

Treatment   Sulfonamide drugs for 12 to 18 months, sometimes in conjunction with other antibiotics, together with surgical drainage of abscesses, cures between 50 percent and 60 percent of cases.

Norwalk agent (virus) infection   Infection by a family of several small viruses that can cause viral GASTROENTERITIS featuring a mild diarrhea. Only the common cold is reported more often than viral gastroenteritis. Although viral gastroenteritis may be caused by a number of viruses, the Norwalk family are responsible for about one third of all cases not involving young infants.

Moreover, Norwalk virus is the most common cause of viral contamination in shellfish. The specific agent is named for the area where the outbreak of the virus first occurs, such as Norwalk, Hawaii, or Marin agent.

During the Gulf War of 1991, more than 10 percent of the troops were infected by the Norwalk virus when they ate local unwashed fruits and vegetables. Other outbreaks commonly occur in nursing homes, schools, camps, or hospitals. Outbreaks are particularly common in tropical countries with inadequately treated water.

Widespread outbreaks reaching epidemic proportions occurred in Australia in 1978 and in New York in 1982 among consumers of raw clams and oysters. From 1983 to 1987, 10 well-documented outbreaks caused by Norwalk virus were reported in the U.S. involving fruits, salads, eggs, clams, and bakery items.

Studies show that more than 60 percent of adults develop antibodies to Norwalk agent infection by the time they reach age 50.

Cause   Norwalk gastroenteritis can be transmitted by ingesting contaminated food or water. In addition, the infection can be transferred from person to person. Water is the most common source of outbreaks and may include water from city supplies, wells, recreational lakes, swimming pools, and water stores in cruise ships.

Shellfish and salad ingredients are foods most often implicated in Norwalk outbreaks. Eating raw or insufficiently steamed clams and oysters poses a high risk for infection with Norwalk virus. Foods other than shellfish may be contaminated by food handlers who have the virus.

Everyone who ingests the virus and who has not recently had an infection with the same strain is susceptible to infection and can develop symptoms. Infection is most common in adults and older children.

Symptoms Within two to three days of infection, symptoms of vomiting, abdominal cramps, mild diarrhea, fatigue, and muscle aches appear. Most people experience only a mild illness and recover within 48 hours.

For about three months following an infection, patients will develop a short-term immunity. After this period of time, however, it's possible to become reinfected. Severe illness or hospitalization is very rare.

Diagnosis Research labs can look for virus in stool specimens; a blood test can uncover antibodies to the virus. Specific diagnosis of the disease can only be made by a few labs that possess reagents from human volunteer studies. Identification of the virus can be made on early stool specimens using immune electron microscopes. However, this disease is usually diagnosed by the characteristics of the illness itself, without tests.

Treatment Because the diarrhea is caused by a virus, there is no cure. When a person becomes infected, the body develops antibodies that destroy the virus. Rest, clear fluids, and acetaminophen for headaches and body aches will help. Patients who don't experience vomiting can continue to eat solids.

Prevention There are no specific preventive measures, since scientists don't know enough about how the virus is transmitted. However, it's wise to follow guidelines for avoiding food-borne illness, and follow precautions for food and beverage safety when traveling to tropical countries.

nosocomial infection An infection acquired in a hospital. See HOSPITAL-ACQUIRED IN-FECTIONS.

notifiable disease See REPORTABLE DISEASE.

O

onchocerciasis A chronic tropical disease that causes infection of the skin and that may lead to eye inflammation and blindness. The disease, which is a type of FILARIASIS, affects 17.6 million people, most of whom live in Africa. However, the disease is also common in Central and South America. American travelers appear to be at low risk for infection; the risk only rises for those who stay in an area for a long time, such as missionaries, field scientists, and Peace Corps workers.

Cause The disease is caused by the parasite *Onchocerca volvulus* transmitted by the bite of the blood-sucking female *Simulium* black fly. The flies live near rapid rivers and streams (hence the disease's alternative name, "river blindness"), and they come out during the day to bite. Eye lesions are more common among people of the African savannah, whereas gross skin lesions are more often seen among rain forest inhabitants.

The black fly deposits infected larvae beneath the skin of humans; the larvae penetrate the human tissue and develop into an adult worm after about a year. The female adult, which can live for 15 years, produces large numbers of microfilariae that migrate throughout the body. Blindness may result as an allergic reaction to dead worms near the eye.

Symptoms About a year after the black fly bite, symptoms appear and may include severe localized or generalized itching of the skin. The victim may scratch so hard that the skin is broken; hard lumps then appear in the skin. Other symptoms may include fever, headache, and tiredness. Eye inflammation can lead to blindness. In the Americas, lesions are seen usually on the scalp; in Africa, they are found mostly around the pelvis and on the trunk. The development of blindness depends on the number of larvae around the eye.

Treatment In some cases, treatment may include surgical removal of the nodules, together with medication. Ivermectin kills the parasite at the stage where it causes symptoms. Merck, Sharp & Dohme provides this drug free to countries where river blindness is common. It is available in the United States from the CDC under an agreement with the Food and Drug Administration. Ivermectin and other drugs for tropical diseases available through the drug service are not approved in the United States but are provided under investigational drug exemptions granted by the FDA. They are provided free to other countries as a public health service. The drugs must be given carefully because of the severe reaction caused by dead worms.

Researchers are studying a possible vaccine for river blindness using antibodies produced by the few individuals who appear to be resistant to river blindness. (Nearly everyone else who is exposed to the parasites becomes infected.)

o'nyong-nyong An arbovirus that causes disease in Africa and Asia similar to DENGUE FEVER. The name, which means "weakening of the joints" in a Uganda dialect, first appeared in that country in 1959 when it infected millions of Africans. See also CHIKUNGUNYA FEVER.

Cause O'nyong-nyong is transmitted by the bite of the *Anopheles* mosquito, which is also responsible for spreading MALARIA.

Symptoms Symptoms include fever, swollen lymph nodes, and severe joint pain.

Treatment Treatment is symptomatic.

Prevention Killing or repelling insects and sleeping under bed nets is the only way to prevent this disease.

opportunistic infections An infection caused by normally harmless organisms that do not usually produce disease in healthy people. These infections usually occur among patients whose resistance has been impaired by such disorders as diabetes, AIDS, or cancer; by a surgical procedure such as a urinary tract catheterization; or by immunosuppressive drugs.

Long-term use of antibiotics or other drugs also may interfere with the normal function of the immune system, creating a chance for normally harmless organisms to become harmful.

Most AIDS patients die not of their disease but of the accompanying opportunistic infections (especially *Pneumocystis pneumonia*). Other infections often contracted by AIDS patients include fungal infections (such as CRYPTOCOCCOSIS and CANDIDIASIS) and some viral infections (such as CYTOMEGALOVIRUS and HERPES). Because of the underlying immune system problems of AIDS patients, opportunistic infections are often unavoidable. However, they can be prevented to some extent with prophylactic antimicrobial drugs.

oral polio vaccine See POLIOMYELITIS.

orbital cellulitis See CELLULITIS.

ornithosis Also known as psittacosis or parrot fever, this is a serious bacterial disease that is caught from infected exotic imported birds. It is not possible to catch the disease from another human. The disease is found throughout the world and occurs all year long. Adults are more likely to be infected than children.

Cases must be reported to the local health department so the source of the infection can be traced. Infected birds that cannot be treated with tetracycline must be killed to prevent spread of the disease. The cage of an infected bird must be cleaned, disinfected, and thoroughly aired, since the droppings contain the bacteria. When purchasing a pet bird, consumers should always ask whether the bird has been checked for parrot fever.

Symptoms Symptoms appear within 4 to 15 days after infection, and include headache, loss of appetite, muscle aches, chills, sore throat, congestion, chest pain, and sometimes pneumonia. As the fever rises, a dry cough develops. Chest X-rays will show pneumonia. The fever may last for up to three weeks, only gradually falling back to normal. Patients with a particularly bad case (and older people usually are sickest) may not feel completely well for a long time.

Cause Parrot fever is caused by the bacteria *CHLAMYDIA PSITTACI*, carried by parakeets, parrots, pigeons, turkeys, ducks, geese, and canaries. Rarely, the snowy egret or seagulls carry the disease. The bacteria is shed in droppings and feathers, which are infectious for months; the more stressed the infected bird, the higher percentage of virus shed. A human can become ill by inhaling dust containing the bacteria or by being bitten by an infected bird. Pet birds kept indoors or in an enclosed area (such as a pet shop) are at higher risk for the disease.

Diagnosis Because parrot fever is similar to other pneumonias, a physician will reach a diagnosis in part if there is a history of proximity to birds, since it's not easy to isolate the bacteria. A blood sample taken during the illness can be compared with another sample taken three weeks later; an increase in antibodies to the bacteria confirms the diagnosis.

Treatment Tetracycline will cure parrot fever. Acetaminophen can bring down fever above 101 degrees F, and bed rest and fluids will help ease symptoms. Codeine or other cough suppressants may be prescribed for an especially bad cough.

Complications Rarely, parrot fever can lead to infections of the brain and heart. About 30 percent of untreated victims will die.

osteomyelitis A local or generalized infection of bone and bone marrow, most commonly affecting the long bones in children and the vertebrae in adults. A chronic form of the disease may persist for years, with periodic flareups, despite treatment.

Cause Osteomyelitis is usually caused by bacteria (usually staphylococci) introduced into the bone directly during surgery or trauma, from a nearby infection or from the bloodstream.

Symptoms Persistent, severe, and increasing bone pain; tenderness; regional muscle spasm; and fever. During the early stages of the disease, pain is severe.

Treatment Bed rest, antibiotics for months. Surgery may be necessary to remove bone and tissue and to stabilize affected bone. Absolute rest of the affected part may be necessary, with careful positioning using pillows and sandbags.

otitis externa Also known as "swimmer's ear," this is an inflammation of the outer ear caused by infection or because of a generalized skin disorder (such as atopic eczema or seborrheic dermatitis). It is most common in people with dry or waxy ears.

Cause A generalized infection of the ear that may be caused by bacteria, viruses, fungi or trauma. It may affect the entire ear canal and sometimes also the external ear, producing a persistent inflammation called otomycosis. STAPHYLOCOCCUS AUREUS, PSEUDOMONAS AERUGINOSA, and *Streptococcus pyogenes* are common bacterial causes. HERPES simplex and HERPES ZOSTER viruses may be involved.

Malignant otitis externa is a rare (and sometimes fatal) form of the disease caused by the bacterium *Pseudomonas aeruginosa*. This type of otitis sometimes spreads into surrounding bones and soft tissue and usually affects elderly diabetics with a lowered resistance to disease.

Treatment Usually the only required treatment is a thorough cleaning and drying of the ear together with local antibiotic, antifungal, or antiinflammatory drugs. Patients should avoid getting the ear wet until the condition is completely healed; ear canals that are badly swollen may need to use a wick to instill drops into the ear. Nonprescription painkillers may ease pain. Consult a doctor if there is blood, pus, or serum flowing from the ear, or if the ear is red and tender to touch.

Prevention Avoid swimming in dirty water and after swimming dry ears with a blow dryer.

otitis media See EAR INFECTION.

otomycosis A fungal ear infection also known as mycotic otitis externa.

Cause Otomycosis is caused by a mycotic infection of the outer ear canal, including either *Aspergillus fumigatus, A. niger, Candida albicans,* or *C. tropicalis.* Secondary bacterial infections are common.

Symptoms Symptoms include inflammation, itching, scaling, and severe discomfort.

Treatment This can become a chronic, recurring infection; it is treated with Burrow's solution or 5 percent aluminum acetate solution to reduce swelling. Debris is removed in the physicians's office. Antifungal drops are often helpful.

P

pandemic A widespread epidemic occurring throughout the population of a country or the world.

papillomavirus, human (HPV) A group of more than 70 viruses that cause WARTS, including genital warts (See WARTS, GENITAL), PLANTAR WARTS, and a host of other types that cause warts on the hands or feet. There is no cure for the HPV virus.

paragonimiasis A disease caused by a lung fluke (parasitic flatworm) that is found throughout the Far East, West Africa, South Asia, Indonesia, New Guinea, Central America, and northern South America. It is not likely that casual travelers would come in contact with this disease because it is not found in areas frequented by tourists.

Cause It is caused by a type of flatworm which infects humans who eat raw crabs or crayfish. The eggs of the infective lung fluke reach water through sputum or feces and hatch in three to six weeks. These first develop in the freshwater snail, then enter crayfish and freshwater crabs, where they develop tissue cysts. Humans become infected when they handle or eat the raw or pickled crabs and crayfish; the immature flukes are then released and penetrate the peritoneal cavity in the stomach area and travel to other tissues (such as the lungs).

Symptoms Some people with mild infection have no symptoms. In others, about six weeks after ingestion, the worms develop in tissue and start to reproduce. The most common symptoms of a lung infestation begins with a low fever and dry cough followed by a productive cough that may be bloody. The infection progresses slowly, eventually causing fatigue, weight loss, shortness of breath,

and weakness. Other symptoms may depend on the area of the body that is involved, such as the abdomen or central nervous system.

Treatment Drugs are available to treat this disease. Surgery may be needed to remove the cysts.

Prevention The best way to avoid this disease is not to eat raw, undercooked, or pickled crabs, crayfish, or other crustaceans.

parainfluenza A common respiratory virus of childhood that causes respiratory infections in infants and young children and more rarely, in adults. Types I and II may cause CROUP; type III is also a cause of croup, BRONCHIOLITIS, and bronchopneumonia in children; types I, III, and IV are associated with sore throats and the COMMON COLD.

There is currently no vaccine or treatment to protect against PIV-3 infection. Researchers are currently studying a vaccine against the parainfluenza virus type 3 (PIV-3). Unlike the flu, PIV-3 undergoes only slight variation from year to year, and therefore would not require annual updates.

The parainfluenza virus are included in the paramyxovirus group (a group of RNA-containing viruses) that includes the RESPIRATORY SYNCYTIAL VIRUS and the agents causing MEASLES and MUMPS.

parasites Any living thing that dwells in or on another living organism. The parasite, which may spend part or all of its time on the host, gets food and shelter from the host and contributes nothing to its welfare. It satisfies its nutritional requirements from the host's blood or tissues, or from the host's diet, which allows the parasite to multiply.

Some parasites carry disease, irritate tissue, and interfere with bodily functions. Others release toxins into the body's tissue. Human parasites include FUNGUS, BACTERIA, VIRUSES, PROTOZOA, and WORMS.

parasiticide An agent that destroys PARASITES (excluding bacteria and fungi).

paratyphoid fever A bacterial infection caused by any SALMONELLA BACTERIA species other than S. typhi, characterized by symptoms resembling a mild case of TYPHOID FEVER. See also SALMONELLOSIS.

paronychia An infection of the skin at the base of the nail usually caused by the yeast CANDIDA ALBICANS, although bacteria are sometimes at fault. The condition is most often found among women with poor circulation or who must wash their hands often.

Treatment Antifungal or antibiotic drugs will cure this problem. The hands must be kept dry; any abscess must be surgically drained.

parrot fever See ORNITHOSIS.

parvovirus B19 The virus that causes FIFTH DISEASE (erythema infectiosum), a mild and common childhood illness. Fifth disease got its name in 1899 because it was the fifth of six common childhood illnesses discovered that caused a rash.

The virus was discovered in 1975 by English scientists, but they didn't know what disease it caused. Six years later researchers were able to link parvovirus with aplastic crisis (a serious complication that affects people with sickle-cell disease when exposed to the virus). In 1983 scientists finally discovered that it caused fifth disease. The virus is present in blood and mouth or nose secretions.

Pasteurella A genus of bacilli, including species that cause disease in both humans and animals. *Pasteurella* infections may be transmitted to humans via animal bites. The plague bacillus *Pasteurella pestis* is now called

YERSINIA (PASTEURELLA) PESTIS; P. tularensis (which causes TULAREMIA) has been reclassified as FRANCISELLA TULARENSIS.

Pasteurella multocida A species of gram-negative bacteria that usually infects animals but can be transmitted to humans through a bite or scratch. It causes wound and skin infections and occasionally blood poisoning. The bacteria live in the mouths and throats of 90 percent of cats and up to 60 percent of dogs. See also PASTEURELLOSIS.

Pasteurella pestis The PLAGUE bacillus that is now known as YERSINIA (PASTEURELLA) PESTIS.

Pasteurella tularensis A type of bacillus that causes TULAREMIA and has been reclassified as FRANCISELLA TULARENSIS.

pasteurellosis A bacterial disease transmitted by cats or dogs, who harbor the bacteria PASTEURELLA MULTOCIDA in the mouths and throats. About 90 percent of cats, and about half of all dogs, are colonized.

Cause The disease is usually transmitted by the bite or scratch of an infected cat; dog bites are much less likely to cause an infection. About half of the people who are bitten by cats develop the infection. It's also possible (although very unlikely) to pick up this infection simply by breathing in the bacteria, if the victim lives in close proximity with a pet.

Wild animals also carry this bacteria.

Symptoms One to two days after being bitten or scratched, symptoms of pain, heat, redness, or swelling will appear. The area of the bite may begin to drain (either clear or puslike), and there may be fever or chills. The glands nearest the wound may swell.

If the infection was transmitted by breathing in bacteria, symptoms may include cough, fever, chills, and ear or chest pain.

Diagnosis A lab can easily identify the bacteria found in drainage from the wound by culturing the organism.

Treatment   Augmentin (amoxicillin-clavulante) will cure the infection; those who are allergic to penicillin can take tetracycline. Wounds that swell and fill with pus must be drained.

Prevention   All bites and scratches should be washed immediately with soap and water. A serious infection can be prevented by prompt antibiotic treatment, so seek medical treatment if the bite wound is significant.

There are no animal vaccines to protect against pasturella, although TETANUS antibody shots are often given if the victim hasn't had a recent tetanus shot.

pasteurization   The process of applying heat for a certain amount of time (usually to milk or cheese) in order to kill bacteria. By law, milk pasteurization requires a temperature of 145 degrees F to 150 degrees F. for not less than 30 minutes, followed by a temperature of 161 degrees F for 15 seconds, followed by immediate cooling.

The process was developed by French chemist Louis Pasteur (1822–95), who founded the germ theory of infection and masterminded the development of several types of vaccines.

pea pickers' disease   See LEPTOSPIROSIS.

pediculosis   An inflammation of the hairy parts of the body or clothing with LICE—head lice, body lice, or pubic lice. Head lice are usually found on the scalp; crab lice in the pubic area; and body lice, along seams of clothing.

Cause   The crawling stages of lice feed on human blood. Anyone can become louse-infested under suitable conditions; lice are easily transmitted from person to person during direct contact. Head lice infestations are often found in schools or institutions, where children have shared hats or combs. Crabs can be found among sexually active individuals. Body lice can be found among people living in crowded, dirty conditions where clothing is not often changed or washed. The lice can be spread as long as lice or eggs remain alive on the body or clothing.

Symptoms   It may take up to two or three weeks between infestation and intense itching. The first indication of lice infestation is usually itching or scratching in an area of the body where the lice feed. Head lice often cause itching around the back of the head or around the ears. Itching in the genital area may be caused by pubic lice, and can be so severe that it leads to a secondary bacterial infection.

Treatment   Medicated shampoos or cream rinses containing pyrethrins are used to kill lice, and are available without prescription. While products containing lindane are still available through prescription, lindane is no longer the recommended drug of choice because of concerns about side effects. Retreatment after 7 to 10 days is recommended to assure no eggs have survived. Nit combs are available to help remove nits from the hair.

Prevention   Physical contact with infected individuals and their belongings (especially clothing, headgear, and bedding) should be avoided. Bedding and clothing should be washed in hot water (140 degrees F for 20 minutes) or dry-cleaned to kill the lice and eggs.

Pediculus humanus capitis   A species of head LICE. Unlike bacteria and viruses (which are microbes), the head louse is a wingless insect that lives only on the human scalp, where it feeds by sucking blood.

Pediculus humanus corporis   A species of body LICE.

Pediculus humanus pubis   The medical term for crab LICE (crabs).

pelvic abscess   A pelvic infection that contains pus.

pelvic inflammatory disease (PID) Infection of the female reproductive organs (ovaries, uterus, or fallopian tubes), one of the most common causes of pelvic pain and infertility in women. It affects more than 1 million women every year and can lead to fatal complications. Experts worry that if current trends continue unabated, half of all women born since 1955 will have had PID by the year 2000. One case of PID does not confer immunity; it's possible to have many reinfections.

Cause While it may not have an obvious cause, it often occurs from an untreated sexually transmitted disease such as GONORRHEA or CHLAMYDIA. It may also occur after childbirth, abortion, or miscarriage. Young, sexually active women and those who use the intrauterine device are at higher risk for infection.

The bacteria travel from the cervix to the fallopian tubes and ovaries; leading to permanent scarring of the tubes. The more times a woman contracts PID, the higher the chance she will become sterile because of scarring. Younger women are more at risk for the disease because their reproductive organs are not as good at fighting off infection.

Symptoms Most women have no symptoms in the early stages. As the disease progresses, symptoms may include burning during urination, pelvic pain, heavy menstrual flow with severe cramps, bleeding between periods, pain during sex, unusual vaginal discharge, fever, low backache, nausea, and vomiting. The cervix is tender if palpated during physical exam. Youngest women tend to have the most severe symptoms.

Diagnosis A sample from the cervix can be cultured, and blood counts will help reveal the infection. If the diagnosis is still unclear, a physician can examine the fallopian tubes with a laparoscope in the hospital to assess the condition of the tubes.

Treatment Many women are admitted to the hospital for intravenous antibiotic treatment. Mildly ill patients can be treated at home with oral antibiotics. A pelvic abscess or excessive scar tissue may require surgery.

A woman taking antibiotics for PID should not have sex until the treatment is finished; the woman's partner should also be treated.

Prevention PID can be prevented by avoiding exposure to sexually transmitted diseases. Any unusual discharge or pelvic pain should be checked out by a physician.

Because PID is a very serious disease that can permanently damage the reproductive organs, it is important for patients who engage in unprotected sex or who have many partners to have regular checkups.

penicillin The first antibiotic to come into general use, penicillin was developed from a type of mold first discovered by Scottish scientist Alexander Fleming. His discovery led to the development of a wide range of antibiotics, one of the most powerful weapons in the war against bacterial infection.

The biggest difference between bacterial and normal cells is the thick cell wall that protects the bacterial cell membrane. Normal human cells don't have this cell wall, and so any substance that interferes only with cell wall formation couldn't damage a human host. Penicillins and related antibiotics work by interfering with the synthesis of the bacterial cell wall. This is why they are among the safest of drugs—they can't harm healthy cells.

Fleming first reported his findings in the British medical journal *Lancet* in 1941, together with Ernst Chain, Howard Florey, and other Oxford University scientists. Four years later, Fleming shared the Nobel Prize in medicine with Chain and Florey.

It is difficult today to fully comprehend the profound danger of bacterial infection before the late 1930s. Even in young and strong patients, PNEUMONIA was a common cause of death. Each year, many women died from "childbed fever"—strep infection of the uterus (puerperal septicemia), and infections caused 40 percent of all children's deaths in the United States.

The story of penicillin's discovery began in 1928, when Fleming noticed mold had contaminated a dish in which he had been growing staphylococci bacteria. Oddly enough, the bacteria had almost completely disappeared in areas where the mold was growing, destroyed by some substance the mold had produced. Because the particular mold was called *Penicillium notatum,* Fleming named the substance penicillin.

It was not until 1938 that Ernst Chain, a refugee from Nazi Germany, came across Fleming's work; he and Howard Florey obtained a grant from the Rockefeller Foundation for further research. By 1940 the two had recorded incredible results from their experiments. In 1941, *Lancet* reported their amazing findings, in which penicillin had been prescribed for "hopeless" cases. A year later, a Russian-American microbiologist coined the term *antibiotic* for this new type of drug.

It was very difficult to produce enough penicillin, especially since Britain's chemical industry was dedicated to meeting wartime needs. As a result, Oxford scientists grew penicillin-producing cultures in bedpans and cookie tins, and doctors recovered penicillin from the urine of treated patients. Not until the end of World War II was there enough penicillin available for general use outside the military. It was still so hard to find that in liberated Europe in 1945, there was a substantial black market for penicillin.

Penicillin had a significant impact on war casualties, dramatically improving the survival rate of soldiers with infected wounds. At the time, the only antimicrobial drugs available were quinine, quinacrine, the arsenicals, and the SULFONAMIDES. Of these, only the sulfa drugs fought bacterial infections, and they had only limited use because of their toxicity.

Once scientists understood the structure of the original penicillin molecule, they began to modify it, leading to semisynthetic penicillins. Today, there are at least 20 different kinds of penicillin (see box) used to treat many different kinds of infections, such as ear, nose, and throat infections; respiratory and urinary tract infections; prostate infections; and certain sexually transmitted diseases. None of the penicillins (or any other antibiotic) will fight colds, flu, or other viral infections.

Some of the penicillins (such as ampicillin and amoxicillin) have a broader spectrum of action (that is, they affect more bacteria, including some that have never been susceptible to the original penicillin). Others (such as methicillin) strongly resist "penicillinase," an enzyme that destroys penicillin and is produced by many bacteria.

By 1960, seven classes of antibiotics had been identified. The cephalosporins were the second major family of antibiotics, discovered in the late 1950s.

Today, 25,000 metric tons of penicillin are produced each year, most of which are used to help produce other antibiotics.

Today, scientists are faced with a growing problem of bacterial resistance to many of the penicillins. Bacteria are broadly classified into two types, gram-negative and gram-positive, depending on how they respond to a particular staining technique. The gram-negative bacteria (such as ESCHERICHIA COLI, *Proteus,* and *Pseudomonas*) are far less susceptible to the penicillin family than are the gram-positive bacteria, such as STREPTOCOCCI. Later antibiotics (including newer forms of penicillin) are much more effective against the gram-negative organisms.

Still, the bacterial ability to adapt to antibiotics seem almost limitless. As antibiotic use became common, the incidence of bacterial resistance increased to the point where some scientists consider it an overwhelming problem. Sometimes, the extensive use of an antibiotic eliminates sensitive bacterial strains and favors the development of strains that possess natural resistance. This occurred with

---

PENICILLINS

amdinocillin
amoxicillin
amoxicillin and clavulanate
ampicillin
ampicillin and sulbactam
azlocillin
bacampicillin
carbenicillin
cloxacillin
cyclacillin
dicloxacillin
methicillin
mezlocillin
nafcillin
oxacillin
penicillin G
penicillin V
piperacillin
ticarcillin
ticarcillin and clavulanate

---

the proliferation of penicillin-resistant staphylococci. This resistance can be transferred from resistant bacteria to nonresistance forms because genetic material tends to be shared and traded among bacterial.

In addition, using inadequate doses of antibiotics encourages resistance because instead of killing them, it allows bacteria to adapt. Using antibiotics inappropriately has also played a significant role. Physicians who prescribe certain types of broad spectrum antibiotics instead of reserving them for resistant infections curtail the drugs' useful life.

pertussis   See WHOOPING COUGH.

pets and infectious disease   Pet owners can point to a plethora of benefits from their furry cats and dogs, including reduced stress, higher survival rates, increased self-confidence, and improved self-esteem among children. But pets can also carry very real health risks.

In addition to love, cats, dogs, birds, reptiles, and other small animals can transmit diseases to humans.

The understanding that pets can carry disease is not a new one. Ancient Greeks knew exactly where rabies comes from—the bite of a rabid dog. And the bubonic PLAGUE that wiped out half of the population of 15th-century Europe as understood to move from rodents to animals by way of fleas.

The list of animal-transmitted conditions is constantly lengthening. Fortunately, most of these diseases are rare and almost all can be treated. They include:

Cat-scratch disease   This infection is caused by a cat bite or scratch. The bite wound is slow to heal and may cause other mild symptoms. The disease is rarely serious, but antibiotics can help treat it if necessary.

Lyme disease   This disease is not in itself caused by animals but by a tick that can be carried in the home on cat or dog and then bites a human. Lyme disease has many symptoms including rashes and arthritis. Antibiotic treatment is imperative to prevent the disease from progressing. There is now a vaccine for dogs who live in high-risk areas, but its effectiveness is as yet uncertain.

Psittacosis   "Parrot fever" is a bacterial disease infecting 130 species of domestic and wild birds, most commonly ducks, turkeys, chickens, parrots, and pigeons. Humans get the disease from parrots or parakeets by contact with feces and feather dust, experiencing cough, fever, chills, and vomiting. Bird symptoms may include poor eating habits or droopy feathers. Wearing a surgical or dust mask and rubber gloves while cleaning a bird's cage will help protect against this disease. A blood test can confirm the diagnosis and antibiotics will treat the disease in both bird and human.

Rabies Currently epidemic among certain wild animals in the northeast, rabies can be transmitted to humans by a bite from a rabid animal. In the Northeast, canine rabies is controlled and the main source of infection is from bats, although unvaccinated cats and other wildlife are also sources. Vaccination of pet dogs and cats is imperative to stop the spread of this deadly disease. In humans bitten by an infected animal, the disease can be prevented if treatment with rabies shots is begun immediately.

Rocky Mountain spotted fever This tick-borne disease is found throughout the United States; early antibiotic treatment can head off serious complications, including a sometimes-fatal inflammation of lungs, liver, and heart.

Ringworm Cats (especially long-haired kittens), dogs, horses, and cows can all pass on this fungal skin disease that has nothing to do with worms. Pets are the usual carriers. The fungus infects cat hair, which passes it on to humans during petting. It causes an inflamed lesion on the skin or in the scalp. Antifungal drugs and iodine-based soap cure the problem in humans.

Roundworm This parasite is carried most often by nursing dogs and their puppies, and less often by cats. Virtually all puppies have roundworm, and because children play in the dirt they are most likely to pick up the parasite. The disease is transmitted through contact with the dog's feces or contaminated soil. So common is the presence of the dog roundworm that worm-free pups can only be produced by raising several generations in isolation, or giving high doses of worm medication to the pregnant mother. Both pups and humans can be treated with worm medication (ANTI-HELMINTIC DRUGS).

Salmonellosis Infections with the *Salmonella* bacteria can cause GASTROENTERITIS. The bacteria are carried by birds and dogs, although turtles present the largest risk. The sale of pet-sized turtles (less than 4 inches) was banned in 1975. Since a wild turtle is just as likely to have *Salmonella*, it should not be considered as a pet either.

Strep throat Unknown to many people, the streptococcal bacteria that cause strep throat can be carried in a dog's throat and can cause repeated infections in its human family. In cases of repeated infection in a family, the dog's throat should be checked as a possible source of infection.

Toxoplasmosis This disease is transmitted to humans most often by a parasite in cat feces or contaminated dirt. All cat breeds can become infected with the parasite. Cats become infected by killing and eating small rodents. Most people contract the disease not from cats, however, but from raw meat. The meat becomes infected because sheep and cattle graze in pastures contaminated with toxoplasmosis. The disease, which causes few symptoms, except in AIDS patients,

---

HOW TO BUY A HEALTHY PET

Before buying a pet, consumers should make sure the animal is healthy.

- Watch out for dull coat, drooping feathers, lethargic behavior, weeping eyes or nose.
- Check out the animal's surroundings. Are the cages and pens clean and free of feces?
- If the pet is in a pet store, are the other animals clean and healthy?
- Ask a vet or animal welfare group if the store or breeder is reputable.
- Get a vet checkup as soon as you bring a pet home.

HOW TO PROTECT PETS AND FAMILY

- Keep cages/pens scrupulously clean and free from droppings.
- Remove solid waste from cat litter box daily.
- Keep pets clean and free from ticks, fleas, and mites.
- Don't feed pets raw meat.
- Don't allow children to handle unfamiliar pets.
- Don't allow children to handle a sick animal.
- Teach children to wash hands after handling an animal.
- Don't adopt wild animals as pets if they are injured; call an animal rehabilitator or humane society.
- Avoid walking dogs in tick-infested areas in summer.
- Never use pet waste as fertilizer; this material has little value and can spread disease.
- Keep sandboxes covered when not in use.
- Check pets daily for ticks; remove any immediately.

when it can be lethal, can be treated with antibacterial drugs. Expectant mothers can suffer miscarriage, premature birth, or birth defects if they are infected during the first three months of pregnancy.

Pfiesteria piscicida   A member of a 450-million-year-old family of one-celled marine organisms that live in warm brackish waters of tidal estuaries and cause huge fish kills similar to RED TIDE. The microscopic organism sometimes behaves like a plant and sometimes like an animal.

Pfiesteria has many life stages; in some forms it produces a toxin that penetrates through membranes, according to its discoverer, botany professor JoAnn Burkholder, Ph.D., of North Carolina State University.

According to Dr. Burkholder, the organism is apparently capable of infecting humans as well—including Dr. Burkholder and one of her lab assistants, in addition to about 100 North Carolina fishermen who apparently breathed in the toxin while working in infested waters. The symptoms they report include disorientation, memory loss, and skin infections. While North Carolina state officials insist they have no solid evidence that *Pfiesteria* can be harmful, Dr. Burkholder recently received a state research grant of $250,000 to identify the toxin that *Pfiesteria* produces, and to find ways to control the microbe's growth.

According to the government, health risks appear to be associated with contact with water when the toxin is present. There have been no reports of health problems from eating tainted fish. However, people should not eat fish with lesions or that appear unhealthy.

Symptoms seem to be most severe in those with long-term extensive exposure to water and fish with lesions.

pharyngitis   Acute inflammation of the pharynx (part of the throat between the tonsils and the larynx). The chief symptom is a sore throat.

Cause   The illness is most often caused by a viral infection, although it also may be due to a bacterial infection such as STREPTOCOCCI, MYCOPLASMA, or chlamydial infection. It is a common symptom of a COLD or INFLUENZA, of MONONUCLEOSIS or SCARLET FEVER. DIPHTHERIA is a rare cause of pharyngitis.

Symptoms   In addition to the sore throat, there may be pain when swallowing together with a slight fever, earache, and tender, swollen lymph nodes in the neck. In very severe cases the fever may be quite high and the soft palate and throat may swell so that breathing becomes difficult. Extensive swelling and fluid buildup in the larynx can be life threatening.

Treatment   Warm salt water gargles and treatment depending on cause. Bacterial infections can be treated with antibiotics.

Complications   Especially severe or prolonged sore throats should be reported to a physician, who may take a THROAT CULTURE and prescribe antibiotics.

Phthirus Genus of lice that includes the species *Phthirus pubis,* the pubic louse (or crab).

pian See YAWS.

PID See PELVIC INFLAMMATORY DISEASE.

pink eye See CONJUNCTIVITIS.

pinta A skin infection found in some remote tropical South and Central American villages, caused by the organism *Treponema carateum,* a close relative of the bacterium (*Treponema pallidum*) that causes SYPHILIS. Also called azula, carate or mal del pinto.
  Cause The bacterium enters the body through a break in the skin; prolonged exposure and close contact seem to be required for transmission.
  Symptoms The infection begins with a large spot surrounded by smaller spots on the face, neck, buttocks, hands, or feet; up to a year later these spots are followed by red skin patches that turn blue, brown, then white. Lymph nodes are also swollen, followed in one month to a year by a generalized red to slate blue rash. Eventually these lesions lose their color.
  Treatment Penicillin G or tetracycline will cure the disease, but patients may be permanently disfigured.

pinworm infestation The most common parasitic infection in the United States; infection with pinworm is known medically as ENTEROBIASIS. The human pinworm (*ENTEROBIUS VERMICULARIS*) lives only in the intestine. While it's not technically a worm, it does look like one. The species may sometimes be called "threadworm" or "seat worm."
  Cause The female pinworm is white, about a third of an inch long. Pinworms lay eggs in the skin around the anus. When a child scratches the area, the eggs are transferred directly by the fingers to the mouth to cause reinfestation. The eggs may also be carried on toys or blankets to other children. Once swallowed, the eggs hatch in the intestine, where they grow and reach maturity in about six weeks. Animal pinworm does not infect humans.
  Symptoms Pinworms cause tickling or itching in the anal region at night. Despite common folklore, neither teeth grinding, bed wetting, stomach aches, weight loss, poor appetite, nor appendicitis are caused by pinworms. Pinworms actually cause very little harm, but they do itch quite a lot.
  Diagnosis A physician can pick up some of the eggs from the patient's anal area via sticky tape; they can then be identified under a microscope.
  Treatment Ointment or carbolated petroleum jelly can relieve the itch, as can a sitz bath followed by cleaning with witch hazel around the anal area. A deworming drug (pyrantel pamoate) will kill the infestation; mebendazole is the alternative for children over age two. In order to kill the newly hatched adults, it's best to repeat the treatment in two weeks. All members of the household should be treated, whether or not they have symptoms. Bed linens of the affected patients should be changed daily without shaking the eggs into the air.
  Complications In rare cases, pinworms migrate into the vagina or bladder, leading to cystitis or infection of the fallopian tubes. Severe infestations can interfere with sleep or cause secondary bacterial infections because of constant scratching.
  Prevention In order to prevent reinfection, make sure all family members have been treated and bathe frequently. Everyone should wear pajamas to limit the number of eggs on the bed sheets, and all bed linens and clothing should be washed in hot water to kill the eggs. All sleeping areas should be vacuumed daily for one week after treatment.

plague The scourge of early history, plague is a serious infectious disease transmitted by the bites of rat fleas. There are three major forms of the disease: bubonic, septicemic, and pneumonic, each of which can occur alone or together as the disease moves throughout the body. Plague types differ as to what part of the body the disease affects. *Bubonic plague* is centered in the lymphatic system, creating swelling lymph nodes, or buboes, from which it gets its name. *Septicemic plague* indicates that the disease has entered the bloodstream. *Pneumonic plague* occurs when the bacteria enters the lungs.

Plague has been responsible for three great pandemics, which caused millions of deaths around the world and significantly affected the course of history. Although the cause of the plague was not identified until the third pandemic in 1894, scientists are virtually certain that the first two pandemics were plague because a number of the survivors wrote about their experiences and described the symptoms, including the appearance of buboes.

The first great pandemic began in A.D. 542 during the reign of Emperor Justinian, and lasted for about 60 years. Plague affected parts of the Mediterranean region most heavily, and an estimated tens of millions of citizens died.

The second pandemic was nicknamed the "black death" during the 14th century because its primary symptom was black patches on the skin caused by bleeding around the buboes (swollen lymph glands). This was the most severe and historically significant of the three; it began in the mid-1300s in central Asia, and some historians believe it lasted for more than 400 years. About one fourth of the entire population of Europe died within a few years after plague was first introduced into the continent in 1347. The Middle and Far East also suffered during this time.

The final pandemic (or Modern Pandemic) began in northern China, reaching Canton and Hong Kong in 1894. From here, plague quickly spread to all of the continents, spreading death among millions. The bacteria also became established during this pandemic in wild rodent flea populations in areas that previously were plague-free, including some parts of North and South America and southern Africa.

Recent outbreaks among humans have occurred in Africa, South America, and Southeast Asia. It is also found among ground squirrels, prairie dogs, and marmots in parts of Arizona, New Mexico, California, Colorado, and Nevada. Between 10 and 50 Americans each year contract plague during the spring and summer months. The last rat-borne epidemic in the United States occurred in Los Angeles in 1924–25; since then, all plague cases in the United States have been sporadic, acquired from wild rodents or their fleas.

Rock squirrels and their fleas are the most frequent sources of human infection in the southwestern states. In the Pacific states, the California ground squirrel and its fleas are the most common source. Many other rodents (prairie dogs, deer mice, wood rats, chipmunks, and other squirrels) suffer plague outbreaks and sometimes can infect humans.

In the United States during the 1980s, there were about 18 cases a year, usually in people under age 20. About one in seven people who got plague died.

Each of the great pandemics eventually came to an end, probably due to a number of factors. Seasonal or weather changes can adversely affect the survival of rodent hosts and fleas, together with control measures aimed at controlling rodents and fleas, sanitation measures, and use of antibiotics to prevent disease.

Major epidemics are most likely to occur when rats live closely with humans in poverty-stricken areas with poor sanitation and also share habitat with wild rodents infected with plague bacteria. Major outbreaks of primary pneumonic plague are most likely to occur under crowded conditions.

Recently, an outbreak of pneumonic plague struck the western Indian city of Surat. In addition, at least 41 cases of bubonic plague had also been reported in the city. There are 1,000 to 2,000 cases of plague around the world each year. At present, there is no plague in Australia or in western Europe. In Asia and Eastern Europe, plague is distributed from the Caucasus Mountains through much of the Middle East, eastward through China, southward to Asia. Plague also occurs in Africa, North America, and South America.

Cause   Fleas found on rodents may carry the bacterium YERSINIA PESTIS (formerly *Bacillus pestis* or *Pasteurella pestis*). More than 100 species of fleas have been reported to be naturally infected with plague; in the western United States, the most important source of plague is the ground squirrel flea. On a global basis, the most important is the oriental rat flea.

The great pandemics of the past occurred when wild rodents spread the disease to rats in cities and then to humans when the rats died. A bite from an infected flea leads to bubonic plague; pneumonic plague is a complication of bubonic plague but is also spread via infected droplets during coughing.

Since 1924, there has been no documented case of human-to-human transmission of plague from droplets in the United States. All but one of the few pneumonic cases have been associated with handling infected cats. Dogs and cats can become infected after capturing or eating infected rodents. Dogs rarely exhibit signs of illness and are not known to transmit the disease to humans. However, plague *has* been transmitted from infected coyotes to humans. Cats often survive severe disease, and can pass their infections to humans via direct contact or the inhalation of infectious droplets from cats with plague pneumonia.

Person-to-person transmission without symptoms is very unlikely, but close contacts with pneumonic plague patients could lead to contraction of the disease through exposure to infected droplets.

Most experts believe that Swiss bacteriologist Alexandre Yersin first identified the bacterium that causes plague in 1894, while studying a plague outbreak in Hong Kong. The bacterium was later renamed in his honor.

Three different types of plague bacteria have been associated with the three pandemics. The first pandemic (Justinian's Plague) was caused by the "antiqua" type, the Black Death was related to the "medievalis" type, and the Modern Pandemic to the "orientalis" strain.

Symptoms   Two to five days after infection, patients experience sudden fever, shivering, seizures, and severe headaches followed by buboes—smooth, oval, reddened, and very painful swellings in the armpits, groin, or neck.

Pneumonic plague causes severe, overwhelming pneumonia, with shortness of breath, high fever, and blood in the phlegm. (Onset of these symptoms begins only one to three days after exposure.) If untreated, half the patients will die; if blood poisoning occurs as an early complication, patients may die before the buboes appear.

The most commonly affected sites are the lymph nodes nearest the site of first infection. As the bacteria multiply in the lymph nodes, they become swollen; as they collect fluid, they become extremely tender. If the bacteria invade the bloodstream, they can spread to other sites, including liver, kidneys, spleen, lungs, and sometimes the meninges and eyes. Occasionally, the bacteria will cause an ulcer at the point of first infection.

Diagnosis   Findings of a painful bubo, together with fever, exhaustion, and a history of possible exposure to rodents, rabbits, or fleas in the western United States, leads to a suspicion of plague. As soon as a diagnosis is suspected, the patient should be isolated, and local and state health departments should be notified. Blood cultures and examination of lymph node specimens can help diagnose the disease.

Treatment Plague can be treated successfully if it is caught early. Untreated pneumonic plague is almost always fatal, and the chances of survival are very low unless specific antibiotic treatment is started within 15 to 18 hours after symptoms appear.

Administration of streptomycin as soon as possible is the preferred treatment; alternatives include gentamicin, chloramphenicol, tetracyline, and trimethoprim/sulfamethoxazole. Chloramphenicol is specifically indicated in treating plague meningitis. Drug treatment reduces the risk of death to less than 5 percent.

Contacts of anyone with pneumonic plague are given antibiotics as a preventive measure at the first sign of disease.

Prevention Untreated pneumonic plague patients can pass on their illness to close contacts throughout the course of the illness. All plague patients should be isolated for 48 hours after antibiotic treatment begins. Pneumonic plague patients should be completely isolated until sputum cultures are negative.

Residents of areas where plague occurs in the wild animals should make sure their home is rodent-proof. Anyone working in a rodent-infested area should use insect repellent on skin and clothing; pets should be treated with insecticidal dust and kept indoors. Handling sick or dead animals (especially rodents, rabbits, and cats) should be avoided.

Plague vaccines have been used since the late 19th century, but their effectiveness has not been proven. Field experience indicates that vaccination lowers the incidence and severity of disease caused by the bites of infected fleas. But the degree of protection against primary pneumonic infection is not known.

In the United States, plague vaccine comes in an injectable form, but it is not required by any country as a condition of entry. Because immunization requires multiple doses over a 6 to 10 month period, plague vaccine is not recommended for immediate protection during outbreaks. Its unpleasant side effects mean that it should not be considered unless the long-term risk of infection is substantial. Ordinary travelers do not need this vaccine.

Even those who receive the vaccine may not be completely protected; this is why it is still important to take precautionary measures against rodents, fleas, and people or animals with plague. For significant risk, antibiotic preventive treatment may boost immunity.

Those who should receive the plague vaccine include the following:

- those in direct contact with wild or domestic rodents or other animals where an epidemic is occurring among animals
- those who reside or work in plague-infested areas where it is hard to avoid rodents and fleas, especially in developing countries
- lab personnel or vets who work regularly with *Yersinia pestis* organisms or potentially plague-infected animals in risk areas
- military personnel deployed in plague-risk areas

However, the safety of the vaccine for those under age 18 or older than 61 has not been established. Anyone with a moderate or severe illness should delay receiving the vaccine. Pregnant women should not be vaccinated unless the need for protection surpasses the risk to the unborn child. Since beef protein, soy, casein, sulfite, phenol, and formaldehyde are all components of the vaccine, anyone with an allergy to any of these substances should inform the physician providing the vaccine. Anyone with a severe bleeding disorder should discuss their options, since the vaccine is given intramuscularly.

Side effects of the vaccine include tenderness at the site; a small percentage experience sore, swollen lymph glands, headache, and malaise. In rare cases, some people have nausea and vomiting or joint pain. There is a rare chance that other serious problems and even death may occur after getting the vaccine. Travelers should allow at least six months before departure for the three-dose primary vaccination schedule.

Plague is one of three diseases still subject to the International Health Regulations, which require that all confirmed cases be reported to the WORLD HEALTH ORGANIZATION within 24 hours. The rules also state that all human cases be investigated to make sure the disease is not spread, and that passengers arriving on an infected (or one suspected of infection) ship or aircraft may be treated with insecticides and held for a period of up to six days after arrival. Health authorities also can require disinfection of baggage and any portion of the ship or aircraft.

According to the regulations, passengers on an international voyage who have been to an area where there is an epidemic or pneumonic plague must be placed in isolation for six days before being allowed to leave.

plane wart   See WARTS.

plantar warts   A hard, rough-surfaced and painful WART found on the sole of the foot that may appear alone or in clusters.

Cause   This type of wart is usually spread when infected people walk on communal shower floors, contaminating them with the common wart virus papillomavirus

Symptoms   Plantar warts are soft with a central core surrounded by a firm ring, much like a callous. Because of the constant pressure from the body, the wart is compressed, flattened, and forced into the sole of the foot. The wart usually has tiny black spots on the surface that are actually bits of coagulated blood.

Treatment   Like many warts, plantar warts may disappear without treatment; others may persist for years or may recur. A foam shoe pad may relieve discomfort. Alternatively, the warts may be removed by burning or cutting with laser treatment, or by salicylic acid plasters.

Plasmodium   A genus of protozoa, four species of which cause MALARIA, transmitted to humans through the bite of an infected *Anopheles* mosquito. The two most important malaria-causing protozoa are *P. vivax*, and *P. falciparum*, which causes falciparum malaria (the most severe form of the disease). *P. malariae* and *P. ovale* are not as common, but are tropically endemic.

Plesiomonas shigelloides   A gram-negative rod-shaped bacterium isolated from freshwater, freshwater fish, and shellfish. It causes one type of gastroenteritis.

Most infections occur during the summer in tropical or subtropical areas in places with polluted freshwater, when a person ingests contaminated water or raw shellfish. Because most infections are so mild people don't seek medical treatment, the occurrence rate in the United States is not known. Infection with this bacterium may be included in the group of diarrheal disease of "unknown origin," which are treated with and respond to broad spectrum antibiotics.

Moreover, most cases that are reported in the United States involve individuals with preexisting health problems or very young patients. A recent cluster of cases occurred in North Carolina in November 1980 after an oyster roast, when 36 out of 150 people who ate roasted oysters experienced symptoms two days later.

Cause   Most human *P. shigelloides* infections seem to be connected with tainted water; the organism is found in unsanitary water used for swimming, drinking, or rinsing foods that are eaten raw. The infectious dose is presumed to be very high (at least more than 1 million organisms).

Symptoms   *P. shigelloides* gastroenteritis is usually a self-limiting disease with fever, chills, abdominal pain, nausea, watery diarrhea, or vomiting. Symptoms usually begin about a day after eating contaminated food or water. In severe cases, diarrhea may be foamy, green-yellow, and tinged with blood.

Diarrhea is usually mild, but in infants and children under age 15 there may be high fever and chills. Blood poisoning and death may occur among those who have impaired immune systems or who are seriously ill with cancer or blood disorders.

Diagnosis   This infection can be identified through bacteriological analysis.

pneumococcal vaccine   A reasonably effective vaccine that has been available for a number of years to prevent pneumococcal PNEUMONIA. Although it is safe and inexpensive, it has been underutilized. Patients in high-risk categories should get this vaccine, including those over age 50, people with no spleen, anyone with chronic lung problems (including asthma), heart disease, kidney disorders, diabetes, alcoholism, and adult residents of institutions. See also PNEUMONIA, PNEUMOCOCCAL; PNEUMOCOCCUS.

pneumococcus   A type of bacteria that causes PNEUMONIA, MENINGITIS, acute EAR INFECTION, or a bloodstream infection (BACTEREMIA). Pneumococcal disease tends to occur in the elderly or in those with serious underlying medical conditions, such as chronic lung, heart, or kidney disease. Others at high risk include alcoholics, diabetics, and people without a spleen or with an impaired immune function.

Cause   Pneumococcus (also called *Streptococcus pneumoniae*) is transmitted by airborne or direct exposure to respiratory droplets from people who are carrying the bacteria. Infections occur most often during the winter and spring, and less often during the summer.

Symptoms   Within one to three days after infection, a variety of symptoms appear, including fever, chills, headache, cough, chest pain, disorientation, shortness of breath, and sometimes a stiff neck.

Diagnosis   Symptoms and specific lab cultures of sputum, blood, or spinal fluid can help to diagnose the disease.

Treatment   Prompt administration of antibiotics (such as PENICILLIN or cephalosporin) is usually effective. However, there are now some strains of pneumococcus that are penicillin resistant; these may require use of stronger medications, such as vancomycin.

Prevention   A reasonably effective, safe vaccine that protects against many forms of pneumococcus has been available for a number of years, but many high-risk patients have not yet been vaccinated. By the year 2000, experts hope an improved vaccine will be available to include in routine childhood immunization programs. See PNEUMOCOCCAL VACCINE.

Pneumocystis carinii   A species in the genus of protozoans *Pneumocystis* that causes *Pneumocystis carinii* pneumonia. (See PNEUMONIA, *PNEUMOCYSTIS CARINII*.)

pneumonia   An infection of the lungs of variable cause, considered to be the most common infectious cause of death in the United States. It is a common complication of INFLUENZA. There are many different types of pneumonia, classified according to what causes the condition; for example, it may be a bacterial, viral, fungal, parasitic, or mycoplasmic. Pneumonias associated with mycoplasmas, fungus, Q FEVER, LEGIONNAIRES' DISEASE, psittacosis, and viruses are included in a category known as atypical pneumonia syndromes.

If a large portion of one or more lobes of the lung is involved, the disease is called a lobar pneumonia. Bronchopneumonia, more common than lobar, implies that the disease process is distributed in different places in the lungs, originating in a localized area within the bronchi and extending to the adjacent surrounding lung area.

There are a number of risk factors that can predispose a patient to develop pneumonia. Any condition that produces mucus or an obstruction (such as cancer or chronic lung disease) can make the patient more susceptible to pneumonia. Also at risk are people with an impaired immune system, smokers, people confined to bed, alcoholics, or the very old.

Patients with cystic fibrosis are prone to respiratory infection with *Pseudomonas* and *Staphylococcus*; *Pneumocystis carinii* pneumonia has been associated with AIDS patients. Anyone with congestive heart failure, diabetes, or chronic lung disease is also more susceptible.

Pneumonia in the elderly may occur spontaneously or as a complication of another disease. These pulmonary infections are often difficult to treat and are more often fatal than similar infections in younger patients. The onset of pneumonia in the elderly may begin with a general deterioration, confusion, rapid heartbeat and breathing. To reduce the serious consequences of pneumonia in this group, vaccination against pneumococcus and influenza viral infections is recommended.

Cause   Pneumonia is usually caused by inhaling a microorganism, although the germ can occasionally pass to the lungs from the bloodstream.

Symptoms   Shaking chills are very common, and coughing becomes frequent and may produce a colored discharge. The fever is high and may reach 105 degrees F. Pain in the chest may occur as the lungs become more inflamed. During the most serious phase of pneumonia, the body loses fluids, which must be replaced in order to prevent shock; pus in the lungs cause severe respiratory distress.

Treatment   Bacterial pneumonia is usually treated with antibiotics (such as PENICILLIN). When given early enough in the course of the disease, antibiotics are very effective.

pneumonia, bacterial   Pneumonia (lung inflammation) caused by bacterial infection. *Streptococcus pneumoniae* is the most common bacterial cause and occurs most often in winter and spring, when upper respiratory tract infections are most frequent. *S. pneumoniae* is commonly referred to as the *pneumococcus*.

Cause   In addition to *S. pneumoniae*, other bacteria that can cause pneumonia include *Staphylococcus aureus, Klebsiella pneumoniae, Pseudomonas aeruginosa, Haemophilius influenzae, Legionella pneumophila*, and *Mycoplasma pneumoniae*.

Symptoms   Classic bacterial pneumonia usually begins with a sudden onset of shaking chills, a rapid rising fever (101 degrees F to 105 degrees F), and a stabbing chest pain made worse by breathing and coughing. The patient is severely ill and breathes with grunting and flared nostrils, leaning forward in an effort to breathe without coughing.

Diagnosis   History (especially of a recent respiratory tract infection), physical exam, chest X-rays, blood culture (because BACTEREMIA occurs often), and sputum exam.

Treatment   The treatment of bacterial pneumonia involves antibiotics; PENICILLIN G is the antibiotic of choice for infection with *S. pneumoniae*. Other effective drugs include erythromycin, clindamycin, the cephalosporins, other penicillins, and trimethoprim-sulfamethoxazole (Bactrim). Bed rest is required until the infection clears. Oxygen may need to be given.

pneumonia, chlamydial   This type of PNEUMONIA is caused by a newly recognized strain of CHLAMYDIA. Chlamydial pneumonia was formerly known as Taiwan Acute Respiratory agent pneumonia (or TWAR agent pneumonia) because it was first diagnosed in Taiwan.

Today, cases have been reported all over the world, including Europe, Canada, the United States, Australia, and Japan.

Chlamydial pneumonia among people aged 5 to 35 is the second leading cause of pneumonia after mycoplasma pneumonia. Between 5 and 10 percent of older people admitted to the hospital with pneumonia have this condition.

Most infections in young adults are mild and recovery is slow but complete; the cough may last two or more weeks. However, between 5 and 10 percent of elderly patients may die.

Patients are infectious as long as they cough, and antibiotics do not reduce the infectious period. Some people may be infectious for weeks; epidemics in military locations have persisted for up to eight months. It appears that healthy carriers may transmit this disease to others.

While one attack conveys a short-term immunity, it is possible to get chlamydial infection more than once.

Cause Chlamydial pneumonia is caused by a tiny organism (*Chlamydia pneumoniae*) similar to both viruses and bacteria that live inside human cells. But because it responds to antibiotics, it is classified as a bacterium. It is related to *Chlamydia psittaci* (transmitted by birds) and *Chlamydia trachomatis* (which causes the sexually transmitted disease CHLAMYDIA).

It is transmitted much the same way as any other bacterial pneumonia; by direct contact with infected individuals or by breathing in the bacteria when an infected person coughs or sneezes nearby. The disease may be passed by handling a coughing infected person's towels or sheets.

Symptoms Symptoms are similar to mycoplasma pneumonia, beginning with fatigue and weakness, sore throat, hoarseness, low fever, and cough. Some sputum may be coughed up. Older patients have fever with severe lung congestion and rapid, difficult breathing.

The incubation period after exposure varies but is usually between one and four weeks.

Diagnosis An antibody test is the best way to diagnose the disease, but many doctors diagnose the disease on the basis of symptoms and on tests that rule out other types of bacterial pneumonias. Chest X-ray may reveal a pneumonia in the lower lobe of one lung. Throat or sputum cultures will reveal the disease, but many labs are unable to culture this.

Treatment Erythromycin or tetracycline for 10 to 21 days will cure the disease. Adults should try to rest and return to normal activities slowly. Children should be given humidified air from a cool-mist vaporizer, clear fluids, chest raised while sleeping, and acetaminophen for fevers over 101 degrees F.

Complications Those elderly people who recover may experience chronic BRONCHITIS or SINUSITIS.

pneumonia, pneumococcal One of several types of PNEUMONIA (serious inflammation of the lungs) caused by bacterial infection; it kills about 40,000 Americans each year.

Adults over age 50 are most at risk; 85 percent of the deaths occur in this group. Others at risk include those with no spleen or with disorders of the spleen; those with impaired immune systems; those with chronic lung disease, heart disease, kidney disorders, diabetes, or alcoholism; adult residents of institutions.

Cause Pneumococcal pneumonia is an infection caused by a type of bacteria called *Streptococcus pneumoniae* (also called PNEUMOCOCCUS). It is spread by airborne or direct exposure to respiratory drops from a person who is infected.

Symptoms Within one to three days after infection, symptoms of fever, chills, headache, cough, chest pain, shortness of breath, and sometimes a stiff neck may appear. Infections occur most often during the winter and early spring, and less often during the summer.

Diagnosis Doctors can diagnose the disease based on the type of symptoms and specific cultures of sputum, blood, or spinal fluid.

Treatment In most cases, this disease is treatable with antibiotics.

Prevention The PNEUMOCOCCAL VACCINE will generally prevent this disease and should be given to those who are at risk.

pneumonia, *Pneumocystis carinii* A type of pneumonia (PCP), also known as AIDS pneumonia, that is the most common AIDS lung infection. Most people who get PCP have a weakened immune system. PCP is an OPPORTUNISTIC INFECTION dangerous only to those patients with immune system impairment, such as patients with AIDS or leukemia. It is a major cause of death among AIDS patients.

Cause PCP is caused by the species *Pneumocystis carinii*, spread in the air from person to person by breathing or coughing. Healthy people will not be affected by these germs, but anyone with an impaired immune system may be vulnerable.

Symptoms Early signs include breathing problems, fever, or a dry, hacking cough. Lips and nailbeds may turn blue if there are severe breathing problems. Symptoms may last from a few weeks to a few months.

Diagnosis A physician can diagnose the disease by examining the sputum (phlegm) or a lung biopsy.

Treatment The infection is fatal if untreated, but it can be cured with high doses of cotrimoxazole or other antibiotics. Mild cases may be treated at home, but more serious infections require hospitalization.

pneumonia, walking The common name for MYCOPLASMA PNEUMONIA.

pneumonic plague See PLAGUE.

poliomyelitis A contagious viral disease that in its severe form can cause permanent paralysis and sometimes death. This extremely dangerous disease causes mild disabilities in about half of all patients; the rest may suffer permanent paralysis. However, due to modern vaccination practices, the disease has all but been wiped out in the United States. Most American doctors have never seen an active case of polio, but in the first half of this century polio was called the last of the great childhood plagues.

Polio was known for hundreds of years, but the disease was not much discussed in ancient medical literature and did not occur in large epidemics until modern times. In fact, it was only in the late 18th century that the disease was first identified as polio. In ancient times, sanitation was so appallingly poor that there was plenty of opportunity for people to contract polio, carried as it is in feces. The viruses infected each new generation of infants, who were protected in part by antibodies passed from their mothers. These early infections were usually mild, and were rarely diagnosed as polio.

But when improved public sanitation and other health measures arrived (such as water purification and milk pasteurization), there was less chance for babies and young children to contract the mild form of the disease and become immune. When the disease struck older children and adults, it was more likely to paralyze. In northern Europe and the United States, small epidemics began to appear in the late 19th and early 20th centuries. But it wasn't until the summer of 1917 when 27,000 U.S. citizens were paralyzed and 6,000 died that the real threat emerged. The northeast was especially hard hit; in New York City and its suburbs, more than 9,000 cases were reported and 2,448 people died. The 1917 epidemic set off a panic as thousands fled the city to mountain resorts. Movie theaters were closed, meetings were canceled. Because no one know what spread the disease, public gatherings were shunned. Doctors stopped performing tonsillectomies until fall, and warned youngsters not to drink from public water fountains, not to take rides in amusement parks, or swim in public beaches.

In some towns, New York City natives who came to visit were turned away by armed citizens who feared the spread of the disease. Yet despite these precautions, an epidemic appeared each summer after that, with the most serious outbreaks in the 1940s and 1950s. It was the 1952 epidemic that was the worst, with nearly 58,000 reported cases and 3,145 deaths.

And then came the vaccine developed by Dr. Jonas Salk. The 1954 field trial, sponsored by the National Foundation for Infantile Paralysis, tested 1.8 million children, proving that Salk's killed virus vaccine was very effective in preventing polio. Dr. Salk became a national hero.

After the licensing of the vaccine in 1955, an intense public health campaign was mounted to inoculate every American child in the country. Similar scenes were repeated in 1961, when the attenuated live virus vaccine developed by Dr. Albert Sabin was licensed. This time, the vaccine was given in a sugar cube soaked in liquid vaccine. In a few short years, polio was virtually eliminated in this country, since both vaccines contain all three polio strains and prevent the disease.

The last U.S. epidemic occurred in 1979, when 10 Amish children whose parents had refused to have them vaccinated on religious grounds came down with the disease. However, polio still occurs in other parts of the world; there are about 250,000 cases a year. The disease occurs in these areas in the summer and early fall, and concentrates in undeveloped areas with poor immunization.

Cause Polio is caused by a virus with three distinct strains (types I, II, and III) that lives in the nose, throat, and especially the intestinal tract of an infected person. Many people are carriers (that is, they are infected but show no symptoms)—but they can still spread the infection to others. The virus is excreted in large amounts in the feces of a car-

rier, and is probably spread through hand-to-hand or hand-to-mouth contact. Once in the body, the virus multiplies in the throat and intestinal tract. In more serious cases, the virus may attack the nervous system (the brain and spinal cord), where it may kill or injure motor nerve cells. This may lead to extensive paralysis, including paralysis of the muscles involved in breathing, or it may be fatal. Immunity to one type of polio does not confer immunity to the other two.

Symptoms The mild forms of polio usually begin abruptly and last just a few days. Symptoms (if they appear at all) include fever, sore throat, nausea, headache, and stomach ache. Sometimes there will be pain and stiffness in the neck, back, and legs.

The more serious form—paralytic polio—is the form that causes most epidemics; it begins with the same symptoms, but severe muscle pain is usually present. If paralysis occurs, it begins within the first week. Paralysis may affect only a small group of muscles, or it may be widespread. The legs are more often affected than the arms, but the virus may partially or completely paralyze a single limb, half the body, or all four extremities.

Those most at risk for serious neurological damage during epidemics due to lowered immunity included patients who had recently been inoculated or operated on (especially those who underwent tonsillectomies and adenoidectomies) and pregnant women.

Treatment There is no specific treatment for polio. The degree of recovery varies from one patient to the next.

Prevention Mass childhood immunizations with the live-virus polio vaccine has virtually eliminated the once-dreaded paralytic disease in this country. It is an essential part of every young child's preventive care. In fact, the vaccination success has been so great that most of the recent cases have been caused from the rare side effects of the oral vaccine. But while there are few wild polio cases in the United States, there are thousands in the rest of the world. There is therefore a risk of polio being reestablished in the United States if children are not immunized.

A killed-virus vaccine was introduced in the 1950s and reduced the incidence of polio. But the live-virus vaccine a few years later dramatically eliminated polio. It is taken orally, instead of by injection, and provides lifelong protection. Vaccine use can protect people who don't take the vaccine through a phenomenon called "herd immunity"— immunized people shed the weakened virus in their feces, which can be picked up by non-immunized people, thereby protecting them as well.

However, the live vaccine carries an extremely small risk of giving polio to the person being vaccinated, especially if that person has an impaired immune system (5 to 15 cases in the United States each year). The current immunization policy calls for the first two polio vaccines during infancy to be the killed virus (Salk). After that, doctors may rely completely on the Sabin vaccine, which uses a living but weakened virus. The new guidelines were developed following complaints of parents of children who have contracted polio from the live vaccine; they contended that even 5 to 15 cases of polio is too many considering there have been no cases of "wild" polio in the United States for many years. This means that there is no need to establish a "herd immunity," since unimmunized people wouldn't catch polio anymore.

Many experts believe the government may eventually recommend both vaccines—a killed-virus shot followed by the live vaccine. This would provide ultimate protection against vaccine-related disease with a minimum of risk.

Side effects   Very rarely (about 1 in every 7.8 million doses) oral polio vaccine causes paralytic polio in the person who is immunized. The risk is higher after receiving the first dose of OPV and in those with unusually low resistance to infection; it may also be higher in adults being immunized.

CORRECT COOKING METHODS FOR SAFE PORK PRODUCTS

- Cook all pork until internal temperatures reach 171 degrees F or until the meat changes from pink to gray.
- Don't feed raw garbage to swine; don't allow swine access to human feces.
- Freezing pork kills pork tapeworm and roundworm; keep at 5 degrees F for 30 days to kill roundworm cysts; for four days to kill tapeworm cysts.
- Don't eat raw or undercooked pork.

On rare occasions (1 in every 5.5 million doses), paralytic polio may develop in a close contact of a person recently immunized with oral vaccine. This risk is also somewhat higher to contacts of persons receiving their first dose.

Inactivated polio vaccine is not known to produce any side effects other than minor local pain and redness.

Pontiac fever   See LEGIONNAIRES' DISEASE.

pork and infectious disease   Undercooked pork can cause a variety of infectious diseases, including LISTERIOSIS, TRICHINOSIS, and YERSINIOSIS, pork TAPEWORM (taeniasis).

pork tapeworm   See TAPEWORM.

poultry and infectious disease   Undercooked poultry can cause a variety of infectious diseases, including SALMONELLOSIS and YERSINIOSIS. Poultry should be cooked to an internal temperature of at least 180 degrees F or until juices run clear. Poultry should not be thawed at room temperature, and frozen prestuffed turkeys should not be thawed at all, but cooked frozen. After handling raw poultry, wash hands, surfaces, and cutting boards well. Leftover poultry should be divided into small containers and refrigerated for no more than three or four days. See also FOOD POISONING; KITCHEN INFECTIONS.

pregnancy and infectious disease There are many infectious diseases that, when contracted by a pregnant woman, can cause serious harm to her unborn child. They include the following:

Chicken pox While many pregnant women are immune to chicken pox, those who contract the disease during the first three or four months of pregnancy have a 5 percent risk of damaging the fetus, producing small, poorly formed or scarred arms and legs, brain abnormalities, and premature birth. The earlier in the pregnancy a mother gets chicken pox, the higher the risk of fetal damage. However, chicken pox after 14 weeks of pregnancy is very unlikely to affect the unborn baby. Any pregnant woman who has never had chicken pox and who is exposed to the virus during the first trimester should discuss preventive treatment with her doctor.

Chlamydia Some studies—but not all—have linked this infection to a higher risk for premature birth, low birth weight, or premature ruptured membranes.

Cytomegalovirus In most women this does not produce many symptoms, but an infection during pregnancy sometimes can be devastating to an unborn child. Almost all babies infected before birth are born perfectly normal; only about 10 percent are born sick, and of these, 20 to 30 percent may die. Those ill babies who survive may have convulsions, lethargy, a rash, breathing problems, mental retardation, small brain, water on the brain, eye inflammation, hearing loss, poor coordination, learning disabilities, and liver disease. Some long-term studies suggest that a few apparently normal babies who were infected with CMV at birth develop problems later on in life.

Fifth disease Up to 2.5 percent of pregnant women who contract fifth disease during pregnancy have spontaneous abortions or stillbirths. Most babies born to women infected during pregnancy are normal and healthy. If a woman is pregnant and a blood test confirms active infection, the doctor may advise a serial ultrasound to check on the baby's health, since the virus can cross the placenta and infect the fetus.

Genital herpes An initial episode of genital herpes in a pregnant woman is much more dangerous to an unborn child than are recurrent episodes in a previously infected woman. Women with recurrent infections but no active lesions at delivery can have safe vaginal deliveries. Women with active lesions near delivery but before labor need a culture every three to five days. If the cultures are negative, a vaginal delivery is possible. Women with lesions at the time they go into labor will require a Cesarian section to prevent the baby from being infected as it moves through the birth canal.

Genital warts Vaginal delivery may be difficult if the genital warts grow very large during pregnancy, which they often do; the doctor may choose to perform a C-section in this case. Occasionally, a mother with genital warts can pass the infection to the baby during delivery, which can lead to recurrent respiratory papillomatosis (RRP), in which warts grow into the baby's throat and interfere with breathing.

German measles One of the most serious infections a pregnant woman can encounter while pregnant is German measles, a disease so profoundly damaging to a fetus that widespread vaccination is practiced as a way to avoid this problem. If a pregnant woman is infected with German measles during the first 12 weeks of pregnancy, as many as 85 percent of women will miscarry. At 14 to 16 weeks the risk drops to between 10 and 24 percent, and after 20 weeks the risk is close to zero. Infants surviving infection in the womb may be born with defects, including deafness, eye problems (including blindness), heart defects, mental retardation, growth retardation, and bleeding disorders.

Gonorrhea Untreated gonorrhea during pregnancy can cause a uterine infection, premature birth, a smaller-than-normal baby, or an infection in the amniotic fluid. Babies born to infected mothers get gonorrhea conjunctivitis during delivery; an untreated baby will become blind. This is why drops are placed in every newborn's eyes at birth to prevent both gonorrhea and chlamydia conjunctivitis.

Group B strep This form of strep is a normal part of the healthy intestinal tract, but in up to 40 percent of pregnant women the bacteria migrate to the genital tract, where they live without causing any symptoms. In about half of these cases, the mother will give birth to a child carrying group B strep, but only one out of a hundred babies will have symptoms. The baby can be infected either in the uterus or during delivery. Occasionally, an infant will be infected in the hospital nursery as a result of cross-contamination. If the baby becomes sick with group B strep within 48 hours of birth, symptoms may be severe and can include difficulty in breathing, paleness, lethargy, fever, poor feeding, and low body temperature. After delivery, women who develop infections in the uterus, or wound infections after a Caesarian, are often infected with group B strep.

Hepatitis B Infected mothers transmit this infection to their infants during the last three months of pregnancy, during delivery, or while breast feeding. There is less risk of infection if a mother is infected early in pregnancy. All pregnant women should be tested for hep B.

AIDS If a mother is infected with HIV or AIDS, medication during pregnancy can offer significant protection to an unborn baby. Babies born to infected mothers must be carefully followed and checked for infection at birth.

Japanese encephalitis Women who are infected during the first two trimesters may have miscarriages.

Listeriosis Infection with *Listeria* is another very serious infection during pregnancy that is particularly damaging to a fetus or newborn. Babies can be infected via the placenta before birth or during delivery through the birth canal. A pregnant woman with a flulike illness must be tested for this disease if there is a hint that she might have been exposed to *Listeria*. If a baby is infected while in the womb, the infant may be born prematurely, have a low weight, and be very ill with breathing problems, blue skin, and low body temperature at birth. There may be a rash or a sticky eye infection. If the baby survives, the child will be quite ill and may have MENINGITIS or a bloodstream infection. Half of these babies will die, even if promptly treated. Babies who are infected during delivery are born full term with normal birth weight, but may develop meningitis; about 40 percent may die. Some survivors will have permanent brain damage or mental retardation. If listeriosis is suspected during pregnancy, antibiotics given to the mother can prevent disease in the fetus.

Lyme disease It is possible for the spirochete to cross the placenta and harm the fetus, although most babies born to women infected during pregnancy are normal. A pregnant woman infected with Lyme disease does have a slightly higher risk of miscarriage or stillbirth or of having a baby born with heart defects or other problems.

Malaria Pregnant women who become infected with malaria may suffer from miscarriage, premature delivery, or stillbirth.

Shingles Sometimes a young, healthy pregnant woman will develop shingles, since pregnancy does alter the immune system. Because the virus is not in the bloodstream, however, there is no danger to the fetus from this infection. Babies born to mothers who had chickenpox during pregnancy, and babies who get the disease before age two, often have a mild, short-lasting shingles infection as young children.

Syphilis A pregnant woman can pass the infection to her unborn baby at any stage of the disease if she is not treated before 32 weeks of pregnancy, even if she has no symptoms. The bacteria cross the placenta and enter the baby's bloodstream. A baby who is born to a syphilitic mother has congenital syphilis, which can lead to serious illness, birth defects, and death.

Toxoplasmosis This disease is another of the mild infections that can be very serious if contracted by a pregnant woman. If a pregnant woman thinks she has been exposed or has symptoms, blood tests can reveal antibodies; some women with the infection choose to end their pregnancy. There is no way to determine if a fetus has been harmed by the infection, however. Infection is most severe if it occurs during the first three months of pregnancy; complications include miscarriage, premature birth, and poor growth in the womb. Infants who are born apparently normal can develop mental retardation by age 20 and have eye problems.

Trichomoniasis Pregnant women with an untreated infection may experience premature labor or give birth to a low-weight infant.

preseptal cellulitis   See CELLULITIS.

prion   An unusual infectious agent that appears to be neither virus nor bacteria, with no genetic material; a prion consists entirely of protein. Prions cause diseases such as Creutzfeldt-Jakob disease in the human brain and similar disorders in sheep, cows, and animals. It has also been implicated in MAD COW DISEASE (bovine spongiform encephalopathy).

The prion was first identified in 1982 by Stanley Prusiner of the University of California/San Francisco medical school, who suggested that these prion proteins are structurally similar to proteins that are found naturally in the brains of humans and other animals. But prions differ from these other normal proteins in their three-dimensional shape. Prusiner endured ridicule at first, but his theory has gradually won a strong following. Other scientists still insist that prions must be an unknown form of virus.

Prions seem to be able to cause disease by coming into contact with these normal proteins, stimulating them to change their shape to mimic the prion protein. This shape change appears to set off a chain reaction, with normal proteins metamorphosing into the prions, causing a devastating, ultimately fatal, disease.

No treatment has yet been discovered to halt this process. Prions are not destroyed by the usual methods employed to kill infectious agents. They are resistant to everything from boiling temperatures well over 400 degrees F to ionizing radiation.

The prion-related diseases are extremely difficult to diagnose: there is no blood test that reveals the condition, and an infected animal does not mount any immune response to the infection.

Continuing research may help determine whether prions consisting of other proteins might play a part in other degenerative conditions, including Alzheimer's disease,

Parkinson's disease, and amyotrophic lateral sclerosis.

prostatitis Acute or chronic inflammation of the prostate gland caused by either bacterial, fungal, or mycoplasma infection, among other causes. It usually affects men between the ages of 30 and 50.

Cause Prostatitis is often caused by an infection that has spread from the urethra. The infection may or may not be sexually transmitted. A urinary catheter increases the risk of prostatitis.

Symptoms Burning, frequency and urgency of urination, and sometimes a discharge from the penis or blood in the urine. An acute bacterial infection may produce a sudden fever and chills, with rectal, abdominal, or low back pain. However, some patients may not experience any symptoms.

Diagnosis A careful history, culture of prostate fluid or tissue and sometimes an examination of tissue under a microscope. The physician examines the prostate by inserting a gloved finger into the rectum and assessing tenderness of the gland by palpation.

Treatment Administration of antibiotics, sitz baths, bed rest, and fluids. The condition may be slow to clear up and may recur.

protegrin A type of peptide (first discovered in pig white blood cells) that may offer new broad-spectrum microbial treatments for many infectious diseases, including those now resistant to traditional antibiotics.

The peptides seem to be able to kill a wide range of disease-causing organisms quickly, including both gram-positive and gram-negative bacteria. Scientists have evidence that the peptides were able to treat systemic infections by *PSEUDOMONAS AERUGINOSA,* drug-resistant *STAPHYLOCOCCUS AUREUS*, and VANCOMYCIN-RESISTANT ENTEROCOCCUS. In studies, the peptides were also effective against the fungal *CANDIDA ALBICANS* and *HELICOBACTER PYLORI,* the bacteria that causes ulcers. Unlike many antibiotics, which only halt the growth of microorganisms, protegrins quickly kill both bacteria and fungi. They do it while apparently avoiding the normal mechanisms by which bacteria quickly develop resistance to conventional antibiotics. They are not available for clinical use.

protozoa Any of about 30,000 known simple one-celled forms of animal life. Protozoa, which means "first animals," were discovered by the Dutch scientist Antonie van Leeuwenhoek who found them swimming in a rain barrel.

Protozoa include paramecium, a one-celled animal shaped like a shoe, and AMOEBA, another one-celled animal with a constantly changing shape.

Although they consist of only a single cell, they are complete organisms and carry out all necessary life functions, including feeding, moving, excreting wastes, and reproducing. These types of life-forms reproduce very rapidly by cell division. When the cell divides, the nucleus of the cell splits in half; the nucleus of this cell holds the chemical information that the cell needs to function. There may be thousands of new microbes produced in just one day, but most die quickly as well.

Most protozoa are animallike, obtaining their nutrients from the environment. However, a few contain the pigment chlorophyll and, plantlike, can use the sun's energy to manufacture nutrients in the form of carbohydrates.

Because of this overlap, the protozoa have been variously regarded as animals, plants, or as a separate group. Some scientists classify the protozoa as a separate kingdom apart from animals or plants called the Protista, which also includes the single-celled algae.

Protozoa come in many different shapes, but they are usually broadly grouped into three major types related to the way they move: *flagellate, ciliate,* and *amoeboid.* The flagellates move by using a few long, whiplike appendages. Cilia move by short, hairlike appendages. Amoebae move by means of a flowing, shape-changing action.

They may be parasitic and live off hosts, or they may live on their own. They can be found from polar sea ice to tropical rain forests, from the depths of the oceans to the tops of mountains.

Some photosynthetic protozoa (such as species of red-colored dinoflagellates) cause toxic water blooms called RED TIDE.

The parasitic protozoa cause serious disease among humans and animals, especially in tropical climates. This type of protozoa include the malarial trypanosome, a type of organism that invades human red blood cells, causing fatal fever and chills. LEISHMANIA and trypanosome flagellates are found in the tropics, invading body tissue and causing disfigurement and sometimes death. The amoeboid intestinal parasite *Entamoeba histolytica* causes a severe DYSENTERY. Some parasitic species (such as *Pneumocystis carinii*) are more closely related to FUNGI than protozoa, and are especially harmful to humans with an impaired immune function.

pseudomembranous enterocolitis A sporadic, often fatal type of diarrheal disease that has been linked to hospital-acquired infection with CLOSTRIDIUM DIFFICILE in patients taking antibiotics for another infection. The infection is named for the presence of yellow plaques (or pseudomembranes) scattered over the walls of the colon.

Cause The disease is usually associated with antibiotic therapy (especially ampicillin, amoxicillin, and cephalosporins) and develops as a result of overgrowth and toxin production by *C. difficile* within the colon, as the normal bacteria is disturbed (usually when the patient takes antibiotics).

Symptoms There is a wide variety of diarrheal symptoms from mild to severe that begin between 4 to 10 days after the patient starts taking antibiotics; they may start as early as the first day of treatment or as late as three weeks after treatment has been discontinued. Diarrhea is always present in this disease and is generally severe, with dehydration, fever, vomiting and cramps, and abdominal distention.

Diagnosis The diagnosis is best made by finding *C. difficile* toxin in the stool.

Treatment Once the diagnosis is made, immediate therapy includes fluids, electrolyte replacement, and discontinuation of the antibiotic. Many patients respond dramatically once the antibiotic is stopped, within two to three days. The drug of first choice against this disease is oral vancomycin.

Relapses occur in 14 percent of patients between 4 and 21 days after completing the first course of vancomycin; sometimes, repeated bouts of treatment with vancomycin have been needed. Metronidazole is an alternative to vancomycin.

Pseudomonas aeruginosa *(P. pyocyanea)* A species of gram-negative bacteria that has been isolated from wounds, blood, sputum, burns, and infections of the urinary tract. These bacteria are noted for their resistance to disinfectants and antibiotics. The bacilli cause a range of human diseases, from purulent MENINGITIS to HOSPITAL-ACQUIRED INFECTIONS, and can cause life-threatening lung infections in patients with cystic fibrosis. See also URINARY TRACT INFECTION.

psittacosis See ORNITHOSIS.

psychiatric disease and infections Because the central nervous system is susceptible to infection, there are a few mental disorders that have been related to certain infectious agents. These include AIDS dementia, schizophrenia, manic depression, and obsessive-compulsive disorder.

AIDS dementia The HIV virus can cause a wide variety of cognitive and motor problems. The prevalence of dementia among

AIDS patients is between 4 and 7 percent; about one third of adults and half of children with AIDS will eventually develop some sort of mental or thinking deficits. HIV infection has also been associated with mood disorders such as manic depression.

Schizophrenia For the past 70 years there have been reports of a link between some cases of schizophrenia-like psychoses and influenza (especially to fetal exposure during the second trimester of pregnancy and subsequent development of schizophrenia in adulthood). In several studies, the risk of schizophrenia was about 88 percent higher among the offspring of women exposed to the flu viruses during the second trimester as compared to those who weren't exposed. If exposure to the flu virus does increase the risk for schizophrenia, it is estimated that it's not a major risk factor (perhaps accounting for just about 1 percent of all cases). Some researchers suspect that exposure to the virus during the critical period of fetal central nervous system development could lead to a disruption of brain organization.

Obsessive-compulsive disorder Infection by group A beta-hemolytic strep has been linked to specific neuropsychiatric symptoms, probably due to the production of antibodies that react against neurons. Sudden onset or worsening of obsessive-compulsive disorder or tics has been reported after recent group A beta-hemolytic strep infections in children.

Mood disorders BORNA DISEASE VIRUS was first recognized during the 19th century as a cause of severe neurologic disease in animals. Recently, antibodies against BDV has been found in the blood of hospitalized psychiatric patients suffering with major depression, obsessive-compulsive disorder, panic disorder, or organic mood disorder. Researchers suspect that the depressive state may somehow activate a latent infection, but the precise mechanism between the virus and specific mood disorders needs to be determined.

pubic lice See LICE.

pyelonephritis Inflammation of the kidney usually caused by a bacterial infection. This condition may occur as a sudden attack or it may be chronic, in which repeated attacks cause permanent scarring. The acute version of the disease is more common in women and is more likely to occur during pregnancy. (See also KIDNEY DISORDERS, INFECTIOUS.)

Cause Acute pyelonephritis is usually caused by an infection of the bladder that spreads up into the kidney. The chronic version usually begins in childhood, usually as a result of urine flowing back from the bladder into one of the ureters. Persistent backflow of urine causes repeated kidney infections that lead to inflammation and scarring. Over a period of years, this can cause kidney damage.

Symptoms High fever, chills, and back pain.

Treatment Antibiotic drugs, which may need to be given intravenously in serious cases. SEPTICEMIA (blood poisoning) is a possible complication.

Q fever A little-known respiratory illness of animals, also known as Australian Q fever or Query fever, that can be transmitted to humans. The organisms are most plentiful in the uterus and udder of pregnant cattle and sheep.

Q fever is found all over the world and is especially common where cattle are raised and goats and sheep are herded; this includes the western United States and Canada, Africa, England, and the Mediterranean countries. It usually affects veterinarians, dairy workers, and farmers, and those who work in meat-packing plants and animal research.

Cause The nature of the disease and how it was transmitted was unknown for many years. Today, scientists know that a bacterium called *Coxiella burnetii (Rickettsia burnetii)* causes the disease, which is spread through contact with infected domestic animals, by inhaling the rickettsiae from the hides, drinking contaminated milk, or being bitten by an infected tick. The organism survives for a long time in the environment and is hard to kill with disinfectants.

Animals are usually infected by ticks that carry the bacteria; most animals have no symptoms, although they shed the organisms in urine and feces. It's even possible for the disease to spread from the laundry of infected persons contaminated with animal feces; only small numbers of the organisms can cause human disease, and the organism is able to travel through the air for at least a half mile. Even casual visitors to animal research labs have become infected.

However, the bacteria are not passed directly from one person to the next, which means patients are not infectious to others. After one infection, a person becomes immune to Q fever for life.

Symptoms Many people have very mild symptoms, but some are very sick. Onset of symptoms is abrupt, with high fever that may last three weeks or more; fever is often misdiagnosed as INFLUENZA or PNEUMONIA. Other symptoms include chills, muscle pain, severe headache, weakness, fatigue and sweats, with chest pain, dry cough, and a mild pneumonia. The fever may go as high as 104 degrees F. Unless the bacteria reach the heart or liver, the patient will recover completely even without antibiotics.

Diagnosis Anyone with flulike symptoms who is likely to have had contact with infected animals should seek medical advice, stating clearly that contact with the Q fever organism has possibly occurred. A blood test reveals antibodies to the bacteria, which can indicate either a past or current infection.

Treatment Antibiotics such as tetracycline are usually effective in 36 to 48 hours. Chronic infection can be difficult to cure, and may require long-term antibiotics. Other treatment involves bed rest, fluids, and painkillers for fever and aches.

Patients who have diseased heart valves before becoming infected with Q fever may develop severe inflammation and damage to these valves. The liver is also commonly affected.

Complications Chronic HEPATITIS and infection in heart valves or lining of the heart are serious but rare complications. There is a high death rate among people who develop the infection in the heart lining or valves.

Prevention Those who work with domestic animals can be vaccinated against Q fever. Strict hygienic practices must be followed when contaminated hides, wool, straw, or pregnant animals are handled. This involves prevention of inhalation of contaminated dust or fluid droplets, adequate disinfection and disposal of material, and prompt treatment of cuts and abrasions. Placental and other birth material should be burned or buried. Contaminated litter should be burned. All animal milk should be pasteurized or boiled.

A vaccine has been developed in Australia to immunize high-risk groups against Q fever; preliminary trials with the vaccine are promising, but the vaccine is not yet available for general use.

query fever   See Q FEVER.

rabies An acute viral disease of the central nervous system that is usually transmitted to humans by a bite from an infected warm-blooded animal. Untreated, the disease is a swift, deadly killer, and there is no cure; the only hope lies in a vaccine given immediately after a bite by a suspected animal.

Rabies—the name comes from a Latin word meaning "to rage"—has been deeply feared for centuries. First described in 1800 B.C., it was known to the ancient Greeks as *lyssa*, meaning "frenzy," although the Greeks didn't think humans could catch the disease. It was the 16th-century Italian physician Girolamo Fracastoro who discovered that rabies was fatal to humans as well as to animals and called it the "incurable wound," but at least some Romans disagreed. It was not until A.D. 1885 that Louis Pasteur created the first rabies vaccine using live rabies virus. Pasteur's early attempts could cause serious (sometimes fatal) reactions—but it was the only hope a person bitten by a rabid animal could have. Only three people who showed clear evidence of rabies have ever been known to survive the illness without treatment, and all of those patients suffered permanent nervous system damage causing physical or psychological problems.

Although most people tend to associate rabies with dogs, in fact rabies today is more likely to be found in cats. Together with dogs and cattle, these animals make up nearly 90 percent of rabies cases in domestic animals, with horses, mules, sheep, goats, swine, and ferrets making up the rest. Among wild animals, the disease occurs most often in skunks and raccoons, but it also appears in bats, foxes, mongeese, groundhogs, and some rodents.

Rabies has been on the rise in the northeastern United States, increasing dramatically between 1990 and 1993. In 1990, there were 4,880 reported rabies animal deaths; that figure jumped to 9,495 three years later. With proper treatment, human deaths from rabies are rare in the United States, although they occasionally occur: one death in 1990, three in 1991, one in 1992, three in 1993, six in 1994, and four in 1995.

Any wild animal acting unusually tame may have rabies. Because rabies may be contagious before any symptoms appear, a healthy-looking animal can transmit the disease.

Cause Rabies is actually a form of viral ENCEPHALITIS transmitted through infected animal saliva that affects the person's brain and spinal cord. The virus is concentrated in the salivary glands, which is why the disease is usually spread by a bite. The virus also invades and damages muscles involved in drinking and swallowing, causing excruciating pain when swallowing liquids. Although suffering from thirst, animal and human rabies victims can be terrified by the sight of water, hence the other name for the disease—hydrophobia.

Although a bite is the most common way to transmit the disease, rabies can also be transmitted when infected saliva comes in contact with a cut or a skin break. Infected bat droppings may also transmit the disease (at least two people are believed to have been exposed to rabies by breathing the air in caves where rabid bats live). Other unusual causes of transmission occurred when patients received corneal transplants from donors with undiagnosed rabies.

Symptoms The incubation period in humans may range from 10 days to more than a year, although 30 to 50 days is average. (Animals usually develop symptoms between

20 and 60 days.) The length of the incubation period seems to depend both on the location of the wound (the farther from the brain, the longer the incubation) and the dose of virus received. Without treatment, severe bites on the head or upper body could lead to symptoms sooner than a mild scratch on the ankle.

There are two forms of the disease. "Furious" rabies primarily affects the brain and causes an infected animal to be aggressive, highly sensitive to touch, and vicious—the "mad dog" image of a rabid animal. "Paralytic" (or "dumb") rabies primarily affects the spinal cord, weakening the animal so that it cannot raise its head or make sounds because its throat muscles are paralyzed. In the beginning stage of paralytic rabies, an animal may seem to be choking. In both forms, death occurs a few days after symptoms appear (usually from respiratory failure).

Symptoms in humans begin fairly mildly and worsen over time, starting with an itching or burning at the bite site, followed by malaise, fever, headache, fatigue, and appetite loss. The victim begins to grow restless, excitable, anxious, and irritable, with insomnia or depression. The victim may begin to hallucinate, salivate, and have periods of intense excitement and painful muscle spasms of the throat induced by swallowing. As time goes on, other signs of nervous system damage (such as paralysis, disorientation, and coma) follow. Four or five days later, the patient may then either slip into a months-long coma ending in death or die suddenly from respiratory or cardiac arrest.

Diagnosis There are no tests that can detect rabies in humans at the time of a bite, and by the time symptoms appear it's too late for treatment. The transmission of rabies by a bite can be hard to detect. One four year old was exposed to rabies from a bat that flew into her room while she slept. The bat was killed and buried, and the child had no sign of a bite. But when she died a month after of rabies, health officials tested the bat carcass and found both bat and child had the same variant of rabies.

Treatment If a person is bitten by a suspected rabid animal, the wound should be *immediately* washed with soap and water; the bite should be allowed to bleed to help wash out the wound. Medical help is needed at once. (If possible, trap and confine the animal, but only if it can be done safely.)

Unlike other immunizations, the rabies vaccine is administered after exposure to the virus. This unusual technique works because unlike other viruses, the rabies vaccine takes a long time to induce disease. Injections of rabies vaccine may prevent the disease from developing in a person bitten by an infected animal.

There are currently two rabies vaccines licensed in the United States. Both work in the same way, triggering the immune system to produce antibodies to neutralize the virus before it causes disease.

The vaccine is a series of five shots, given on day 0, 3, 7, 14, and 28 after exposure. On day 0, rabies immune globulin is also given, because the vaccine takes about 7 to 14 days to provide an active antibody response. Rabies immune globulin provides a passive immunity until active antibodies are produced from the vaccine.

Over the years, scientists have improved both the effectiveness and safety of human rabies vaccines. Earlier vaccines made from duck embryos required a series of 21 shots, many of which were given in the stomach. (Today, most shots are given in the shoulder muscle.)

The modern vaccines are highly effective and produce few side effects. This vaccine is the only way to treat the disease in humans.

Prevention There is a preexposure vaccine series designed for people at high risk for exposure (veterinarians, researchers, forest rangers, animal control officers, cave explorers, animal handlers, or those who spend time in countries where rabies is common). The

RABIES PREVENTION

To keep pets and humans safe from rabies:

- Keep pet shots up to date, and observe leash laws.
- Don't leave dogs chained alone in the yard; if attacked by a rabid animal, they can't escape.
- Feed pets indoors; keep garbage can lids closed tightly.
- Seal basement, porch, and attic openings; cap chimneys with screens.
- Avoid contact with wild or unfamiliar animals (no matter how cute).
- Report to local authorities strays or animals acting strangely.

preexposure series for all human rabies vaccines is given in three shots—on day 0, day 7, and day 21 or day 28. How often booster shots are taken depends on how good a person is at producing antibodies. People who have received the preexposure series need only two booster shots if they are later exposed to rabies. People in high-risk jobs are encouraged to have their blood tested at regular intervals so boosters can be given if antibody levels fall below a baseline rate. The average high-risk worker only needed boosters about once every two years.

Because of the sharp rise in animal rabies (especially among raccoons), a conditional license was granted for an oral rabies vaccine for raccoons. The license allows the vaccine to be dropped to wildlife habitats in vaccine-laced bait. These conditional licenses are issued to meet emergency situations or special circumstances—in this case, a rabies epizootic (outbreak) from Maine to Florida. The oral vaccine is unique because it was created using genetic engineering. Although most animal cases involve raccoons, there has never been a reported human rabies death directly or indirectly connected to a raccoon. The four human deaths in 1995 in the United States were due to bat bites or from animals bitten by rabid bats.

(Rabid bats have been associated with at least 21 human deaths since 1951 in the United States.)

rash in infectious diseases Rashes have many causes, including reactions to drugs, allergic reactions, and insect bites. But many infectious diseases also cause a rash, and these rashes usually have a distinct characteristic that changes as the infection continues. A good history and description of a rash can help a doctor reach a correct diagnosis.

Rash with fever is most likely an infectious disease. Raised, red, and itchy spots that turn into blisters could mean CHICKEN POX. A rash of dull red spots or blotches, together with runny nose, cough, and sore, red eyes could be MEASLES, especially if the rash is on the face or trunk and if the patient has never had the disease. A rash of pink spots with a tender swelling down the back and sides of the neck could be GERMAN MEASLES (rubella), especially if the patient has not been vaccinated or had the disease. A rash of purple spots with headache, vomiting, dislike of light, and a stiff neck could mean MENINGITIS. A widespread red rash that is especially itchy at night, with tiny gray lines or red infected-looking spots between fingers or wrists, could be a parasitic infection (especially SCABIES). One or more red, scaly patches spreading out in a ring could be a fungal infection.

rat-bite fever A fever caused by the bite of a rat. Although humans usually get the disease from a rat bite, it also can be transmitted by squirrels, weasels, or wild mice. People who work with lab mice have been infected without even being bitten—just from living and working around the rodents. Occasionally, unpasteurized contaminated milk has caused an outbreak; this occurred in 1983 in England, when 208 boarding school children got sick from drinking raw milk. The disease is rare in North America; less than 20 cases have been reported in the last 10 years.

Cause   Either of two types of bacteria can cause the disease; the type usually seen in North America is *Streptobacillus moniliformis.* In the Far East, rat-bite fever is usually caused by the bacteria *Spirillum minus.* Rat-bite fever caused by *S. moniliformis* is also called Haverhill fever; infection caused by *S. minus* is also called sodoku.

Symptoms   About 10 days after being bitten, the victim experiences the sudden onset of fever, chills, headache, and muscle pain followed in three days by rash on arms and legs. Within a week, there may be swelling, redness or pain in the joints. About half of those infected with *Streptobacillus moniliformis* will have joint swelling and pain that comes and goes. Untreated patients may develop endocarditis (an infection of the heart lining). Up to 10 percent of these patients die without antibiotic treatment. Patients with *Spirillum minus* do not experience joint pain but instead notice intermittent fever, swollen glands near the bite site, and a purple-red rash. Without treatment, about 10 percent of the victims die.

Diagnosis   The bacteria can be cultured in either blood, drainage from the wound or joint fluid. Blood counts show evidence of a bacterial infection.

Treatment   Penicillin is effective in treating either form of the disease. Painkillers can treat fever and pain.

Prevention   The most important precaution after any animal bite is to wash the area well with soap and running water and seek medical attention. Rat control is also important.

rats and infectious disease   Rodents live close to humans and in many cities, they actually outnumber people and represent a serious public health threat. Various microorganisms and parasites live in the rat, which can cause illness if spread to people. For example, the organisms responsible for PLAGUE and one sort of TYPHUS are transmitted to humans via the bite of rat fleas. LEPTOSPIROSIS is caused by contact with anything that has come into contact with rat's urine, such as tainted water. The rare bacterial infection RAT-BITE FEVER is transmitted directly by rat bite. The only way to control the spread of these rat-borne infectious diseases is to control the urban rat population.

red measles   See MEASLES.

red tide   Red tides are caused by toxic plankton (called dinoflagellates) that multiply rapidly during the warm summer months; the name "red tide" refers to the plankton's pink or red color. These plankton produce a deadly poison called saxitoxin. Shellfish that eat this plankton become contaminated and can cause disease in anyone who eats them. The toxin is so toxic, even one contaminated shellfish can be fatal if eaten. This is why clams, oysters, and mussels are not sold during the summer months.

Red tides are found in coastal waters in the Pacific from California to Alaska and in the Atlantic from New England to the St. Lawrence. Under good conditions (warm climate, warm water), the plankton may reach 60 million organisms per liter of water. These rapid growths (referred to as a "bloom") discolor the sea and poison fish and marine life. Usually, a person becomes poisoned with the plankton when eating shellfish that have been feeding on them.

Red tides have been known since ancient times; it is believed that the name of the Red Sea was coined by ancient Greeks who were referring to red blooms off the Arabian coasts. In fact, it is believed that the first reference to red tide appears in the Bible: "And all the waters that were in the river were turned to blood. And the fish that was in the river died, and the river stank, and the Egyptians could not drink of the water of the rivers." (Exodus 7:20–21).

Mussels, clams, and oysters are the primary shellfish at risk, and mussels are the most susceptible of all. Healthy bivalve shellfish filter large amounts of toxic plankton, which form the primary ocean food during May through August. During these warm times, the dinoflagellates thrive by photosynthesis and can be so invasive that they kill birds and fish.

The first large epidemic of poisoning caused by red-tide-contaminated shellfish occurred in San Francisco in 1927, when 102 people were sickened and six died. Today, largely because of the prohibition against eating certain shellfish during the summer months, such epidemics are rare.

relapsing fever A comprehensive term for any one of several infectious diseases marked by recurrent fevers, also known as African tick fever, famine fever, recurrent fever, spirillus fever, or tick fever. The disease has occurred in several western states, but is more commonly found in South America, Asia, and Africa.

Cause Relapsing fever is caused by the spirochete *Borrelia*, transmitted by both ticks and lice and often seen during wars and famines.

Symptoms The first episode usually begins with a sudden high fever (104 degrees F. to 105 degrees F) with headache, chills, muscle aches, and nausea. A rash may appear over the trunk and arms and legs, and jaundice is common in the later stages. Each attack lasts two or three days and ends in a high fever, profuse sweating, and rising heart and breathing rates. This is followed by an abrupt drop in temperature and a return to normal blood pressure. Typically, patients relapse about 7 to 10 days later and eventually recover completely. In louse-borne disease, there is usually only one period of relapse; tick-borne illness causes several relapses, each milder than the last.

Diagnosis The spirochete is identified in a blood smear obtained during an attack.

Treatment Long-acting penicillin, tetracycline, or chloramphenicol. However, treatment is withheld during the high-fever stage. Other treatment includes bed rest, sponge baths, and aspirin to alleviate symptoms. Bedding and clothing should be disinfected to destroy any lice or ticks.

reovirus Any of three viruses (found in the respiratory and alimentary tracts of both healthy and sick people) that have double-stranded RNA. They have been linked in some cases to upper RESPIRATORY TRACT INFECTIONS and infantile gastroenteritis.

reportable disease Any contagious disease that must be reported by the physician to the public health authorities, who in turn report some of them to the Centers for Disease Control and Prevention.

This notification of certain potentially harmful diseases is important because it helps public health officers take the necessary steps to control the spread of infection. The reporting also provides valuable statistics on the incidence and prevalence of a disease. This information can then be used to help determine health policies (such as immunization programs or sanitary improvements).

Examples of reportable diseases include AIDS, MALARIA, INFLUENZA, POLIOMYELITIS, RELAPSING FEVER, TYPHUS, YELLOW FEVER, SYPHILIS, GONORRHEA, CHOLERA, and bubonic PLAGUE.

respiratory syncytial virus (RSV) infection A respiratory illness caused by a member of a type of virus known as a MYXOVIRUS (an RNA-containing virus that commonly causes upper respiratory infections and the common COLD). RSV most often attacks infants and very young children; it is responsible for more than 90,000 hospitalizations and more than 4,000 deaths each year in the United States. Most cases occur in children under age four, with the peak of severe illness under six months of age, especially in infants with preexisting heart or lung conditions. RSV also can cause a serious illness in the elderly and in those with impaired immune systems.

The disease can occur at any time, although epidemics usually take place in fall and winter.

The first infection is the worst, but it does not confer immunity; RSV can also cause serious colds in children who have repeat infections.

Cause   The RSV is spread via contact with droplets from the nose and throat of infected patients when they cough and sneeze. RSV can spread through direct respiratory secretions on sheets, towels, and other items. In the winter, this infection is a big problem for hospitalized children who can become seriously ill with PNEUMONIA if they catch RSV.

Air pollution and smoking irritate the lining of the throat and can make it easier to catch RSV; people who live in areas of heavy industrial pollution or live with smokers have more serious and longer RSV infections.

Studies have found that many children under age one who attend day care centers have been infected.

Symptoms   Symptoms can range from a mild cold to severe pneumonia and include coughing, wheezing, runny nose, and severe fatigue. Fever is unusual in young babies. Pneumonia is most likely among high-risk patients; occasionally, the infection can be fatal to infants. Symptoms occur four to six days after exposure, and may persist for a few days to weeks.

In most cases, babies are not seriously ill; it affects infants under age three months the most severely, since they have a hard time breathing. All babies except those with other medical problems should recover within a week.

Children are infectious from 24 hours before symptoms until two weeks after the cold starts. Adults are infectious for a much shorter time, until about five days before the cold starts.

Complications   RSV can cause BRONCHI-OLITIS in infants under age one, pneumonia in babies under age two, or CROUP in children from six months to three years of age. Premature babies who have poorly developed lungs may be quite ill and may survive with permanent lung damage. But it is the babies with heart problems who are most at risk; some of these infants can die from an RSV infection. *Danger signs:* an infant who is not getting enough air into the lungs will have flaring nostrils and dents above and below the breastbone or in between the ribs as she breathes.

Diagnosis   RSV is usually diagnosed on the basis of symptoms; lab tests may be used in cases of severe illness and in special outbreak investigations. If a child has a bad cold, it's not likely that the pediatrician will test for RSV in an office visit. Children admitted to a hospital with pneumonia or bronchiolitis will be tested for the disease during RSV season.

Treatment   There is no cure for this virus. Rest, high humidity, and clear fluids can help. The antiviral drug ribavirin will help a child recover if started in the first few days after symptoms appear. Treatment is reserved for the most serious cases because of potential side effects; an expensive medication, it is given in the hospital as a mist treatment. Most hospitalized children with RSV do not need ribavirin.

Because RSV often improves on its own, treatment of mild symptoms isn't necessary for most people. Antibiotics are not effective, although in certain patients antibiotics may be used to treat underlying secondary bacterial infections.

The FDA approved in 1996 the first drug to protect infants and toddlers from the worst effects of RSV. Respi Gam is an immunoglobulin, made from the blood of healthy people with large amounts of antibodies to RSV. The treatment does not prevent children from getting the virus, as a vaccine would, but it can help protect high-risk children under age two from the most serious complications. It is given intravenously in five monthly doses beginning each November.

Prevention   No vaccine for RSV currently exists, although some researchers are testing various versions of live attenuated RSV vaccines. Since a baby is most vulnerable during the first three months of life (especially those born during the winter), it is possible to take some steps to protect against RSV: don't smoke around the baby, avoid crowds, and keep the baby away from children with obvious colds.

respiratory tract infections Any infection of the upper or lower respiratory tract. Upper respiratory tract infections include the common COLD, laryngitis, PHARYNGITIS, RHINITIS, SINUSITIS, or TONSILLITIS. Lower respiratory tract infections include BRONCHITIS, BRONCHIOLITIS, PNEUMONIA, or tracheitis, lung abscess, emphysema, TUBERCULOSIS, and so on.

retrovirus An RNA virus family that includes HUMAN IMMUNODEFICIENCY VIRUS (HIV), the virus that causes AIDS.

rheumatic fever An inflammatory disease that may appear as a delayed reaction to inadequately treated group A beta-hemolytic streptococcal infection of the upper respiratory tract. Although most symptoms disappear within weeks to months, half the time patients have deformed heart valves. The disorder, which usually appears in young school-age children, also may affect the brain, joints, skin, or other tissues. Once diagnosed, rheumatic fever will tend to recur whenever the patient gets a strep infection.

Fifty years ago the disease was considered to be a serious threat to the health of young U.S. military recruits—so much so that the country set up a special disease lab at Warren Air Force Base in California to handle the problem. When PENICILLIN became available, researchers at the base proved that rheumatic fever could be prevented by an injection of penicillin to everyone with strep throat. By the 1980s, rheumatic fever was considered to be conquered in the United States and other developed countries.

Unfortunately, the disease has not been eradicated; today it involves a much more severe form that causes heart damage and death in many people, from middle class suburban families to those in poor, overcrowded conditions. Since 1985, there have been outbreaks in 24 states, especially in Utah, Ohio, and Pennsylvania.

Researchers believe the resurgence can be traced to a reemergence of certain strains of the bacterium group A *beta-hemolytic Streptococcus* (group A strep). Of the 80 different strains of group A strep, only a few can cause rheumatic fever. This is the same strain of virulent bacteria that killed Muppet creator Jim Henson in 1990.

Cause Rheumatic fever is a delayed complication of group A strep infection, usually either strep throat or SCARLET FEVER. About 1 to 3 percent of untreated people come down with rheumatic fever from 10 days to 6 weeks after getting over these related illnesses. Scientists aren't sure why some people develop rheumatic fever, but it may be a combination of the type of bacteria and the genetics of the infected person. It occurs because the patient's body creates antibodies to the organism and those antibodies mistakenly attack the host's own tissues. Rheumatic fever usually strikes children from 5 to 18 years of age.

Symptoms The onset of the disease is usually sudden, usually about one to five weeks after recovery from scarlet fever or a sore throat. Early symptoms include fever, joint pain, nose bleeds, stomach pain, and vomiting. Other symptoms include palpitations, chest pain, and (in severe cases) heart failure. Sydenham's chorea is usually the only late sign of rheumatic fever and is characterized by an increased awkwardness and a tendency to drop objects. As the chorea progresses, irregular body movements or twitching become severe, sometimes including the tongue and facial muscles.

Diagnosis Rheumatic fever is hard to diagnose because it resembles so many other illnesses; lab studies, throat culture, and EKG. Doctors may use a variety of criteria, including evidence of previous group A strep infection. A diagnosis of rheumatic fever requires one (and preferably two) of these symptoms:

- joint pain (ankles, knees, elbows, or wrists become painful, red, and swollen)
- chorea (clumsy movements that resemble cerebral palsy that last from three to eight months)
- carditis (inflammation of the heart muscle)
- skin nodules or "rheumatoid nodules" (painless swellings under the skin over joints)
- rash (flat, painless rash lasting less than a day with fever and fatigue)
- fever of at least 100.4 degrees F

Treatment   Severe restriction of regular activity and painkillers. Penicillin is often given to eliminate any remaining strep from the old infection, and steroids or salicylates may be used, depending on the severity of joint pain.

While bed rest used to be a part of the treatment, it is no longer considered to be helpful.

Complications   Rheumatic fever can cause carditis in about 50 percent of patients, with heart valve damage that can lead to congestive heart failure. It is one of the most common causes of the need for heart valve replacement.

rhinitis, viral   Inflammation of the mucous membrane lining the nose, caused by the common cold virus. This infection can lead to SINUSITIS. It usually causes nasal obstruction, nasal discharge, sneezing, and facial pain.

rhinoscleroma   An uncommon bacterial infection caused by *Klebsiella rhinoscleromatis* that is chronic and common in rural areas throughout the world with poor hygiene.

Symptoms   The disease begins with increased nasal secretion and crusting, fol-

lowed by an enlargement of the nose, upper lip, palate, or neighboring areas. If the infection spreads to the respiratory tract, breathing may become difficult. The condition may be fatal due to breathing problems or continuing infection.

Treatment   This disease is difficult to treat; systemic antibiotics such as gentamicin and tobramycin have been effective. Alternatively, oral administration of ciprofloxacin may help, although this drug has not been widely studied as a therapy for this condition.

rhinovirus   Any of the more than 200 distinct small viruses that cause about 40 percent of all acute respiratory illnesses. Complete recovery is usual. See also COLDS, COMMON.

Symptoms   Infection is characterized by dry, scratchy throat, nasal congestion, malaise, and headache. There is little fever; nasal discharge lasts two or three days. Children may develop a cough. From onset to end, with or without treatment, the infection lasts two to four weeks.

Treatment   Symptom-relieving medications such as painkillers, antihistamines, and nasal decongestants. Zinc and vitamin C in large doses have been shown to be somewhat effective at shortening the duration of the illness caused by certain strains of rhinovirus.

Rickettsia akari   A type of parasite of insects and insectlike animals such as fleas, lice, ticks, and mites that cause the disease rickettsial pox.

Rickettsia conorri   A type of parasite of insects and insectlike animals such as fleas, lice, ticks, and mites that cause TYPHUS.

rickettsial fever   See ROCKY MOUNTAIN SPOTTED FEVER.

rickettsial infections   Diseases caused by the bite or feces of insects carrying parasitic microorganisms called rickettsia. These diseases include ROCKY MOUNTAIN SPOTTED FEVER, Q FEVER, and various forms of TYPHUS. Rickettsia resemble small bacteria, but they are able to multiply only by invading the cells of another life-form. In this respect, they are more like VIRUSES. The rickettsiae were once classified between bacteria and viruses because they seem to possess the characteristics of both.

Rickettsiae are primarily found in the intestines and saliva of insects and insectlike animals (such as fleas, lice, ticks, and mites). However, these insects can transmit rickettsiae to larger animals (including humans) through their saliva and feces.

They were named for 19th-century American pathologist Howard Taylor Ricketts, who studied them in 1906 when he was at the University of Chicago as part of his studies of Rocky Mountain spotted fever. Ricketts died in Mexico in 1910 from typhus, which he was investigating at the time, and the genus *Rickettsia* was named in his honor.

Rickettsiae that produce disease are usually transmitted by the bite of an infected louse, tick, mite, or flea. The diseases they cause are widespread and are found wherever in the world that humans, rodents, and arthropods live together. The rickettsial human infections are divided into four main groups: the typhus fever group (including classical typhus and rat-borne typhus); spotted fever group (Rocky Mountain spotted fever, South Africa tick fever, boutonneuse fever, and Sao Paulo typhus of Brazil); tsutsugamushi group (Tsutsugamushi disease of Japan, Malayan scrub typhus, and Sumatran mite typhus); and miscellaneous group (trench fever, Q fever, rickettsial pox).

Most rickettsial infections are characterized by a fever and a rash, although the fatality rate differs from one variety of illness to the next. It ranges from less than 1 percent for the milder diseases to 70 percent for some outbreaks of typhus and Rocky Mountain spotted fever.

rickettsial pox   An urban disease transmitted by the bite of a mite from a house mouse. The responsible microorganism is *Rickettsia akari,* which belongs to the spotted fever group.

Rickettsia prowazekii   A type of parasite of insects and insectlike animals such as fleas, lice, ticks, and mites that cause TYPHUS.

Rickettsia rickettsii   A type of intracellular parasitic microorganism that looks like small bacteria but can reproduce only by invading cells of another life-form. These parasites live primarily off insects and insectlike animals such as lice, fleas, ticks, and mites; in turn, these insects can transmit the rickettsia to rodents, dogs, or humans through saliva or feces. Human diseases caused by these organisms include ROCKY MOUNTAIN SPOTTED FEVER and various forms of TYPHUS.

Rickettsia tsutsugamushi   A type of parasite of insects and insectlike animals such as fleas, lice, ticks, and mites that cause TYPHUS or Tsutsugamushi disease.

Rift Valley fever   A disease uncommon in the United States but found much more often in the southern Sahara Desert, caused by an arbovirus that causes fever in humans and stillbirths in cattle.

Cause   The virus is transmitted by the AEDES and other types of mosquito. It was first discovered in the 1930s as a cause of stillbirth in European cattle in Kenya and a cause of fever in veterinarians who studied the problem and were exposed to blood or viscera. After the Aswan Dam was completed in the 1970s, vast new wetlands were created that boosted the local mosquito population. As a result, an epidemic of Rift Valley fever swept through the area, killing 598 of the 18,000 victims of the disease and wiping out entire livestock herds. Over the next 10 years, other epidemics related to dam construction occurred in Mauritania, Madagascar, and

Senegal, followed by a second outbreak in Aswan in 1993. In this latest epidemic, patients were blinded after experiencing fever, headache, and muscle pain.

Symptoms   Symptoms are similar to DENGUE FEVER, with high fever, severe headache, and visual problems. Fatal bleeding can occur in rare cases.

Treatment   Treatment is symptomatic.

Prevention   A vaccination can prevent the disease.

ring rubella   See FIFTH DISEASE.

ringworm (tinea)   A skin infection caused by a fungus that can affect the scalp, skin, fingers, toenails, or feet. The disease has nothing to do with worms or rings. Scalp ringworm is the most common fungal skin infection in children. While anyone can get ringworm, children are more susceptible to certain varieties.

Patients are infectious for as long as the lesions appear on the body; if untreated, the condition may last for years.

Cause   Ringworm is spread by direct skin-to-skin contact with infected people or pets, or with indirect contact with items such as barber clippers, shower stalls, or floors. Children can get it from playing with ring-worm-infected dogs or cats or from sharing combs, brushes, headphones, towels, pillows, hats, and sofas.

Symptoms   The infection usually begins as a small pimple that gets larger and larger, leaving scaly patches of temporary baldness; infected hair is brittle and breaks off easily. Sometimes there is a yellow cuplike crusty area. The infection usually is seen 10 to 14 days after contact.

Ringworm of the scalp (*Tinea capitis*) involves scaly, temporary bald patches with dandruff-like white scales. The hair may be dull, and the infection may affect only one part of the scalp or may spread over the entire head. A severe case may include fever and swollen glands below the hairline.

Ringworm of the nails causes thick, discolored, and brittle or chalky and friable nails.

Ringworm of the body (*Tinea corporis*) is flat and ring-shaped; the edge is red and may be dry and scaly, or moist and crusted. The center area clears and appears normal. Symptoms occur 4 to 10 days after contact. The rings can appear on face, legs, arms, or trunk.

Ringworm of the foot appears as a scaling or cracking of the skin, especially between the toes.

Since so many species of fungus can cause ringworm, infection with one species won't make a person immune to future infections from other species.

Diagnosis   Microscopic inspection of infected hair or skin scrapings will reveal certain characteristics of the fungus. The doctor may use an ultraviolet light called a Wood's light to diagnose ringworm; when the lamp is shone on an affected area, the fungus may show as a yellowish or brilliant green fluorescence, depending on the type of fungus. (The most common type of scalp fungus will not have this effect.)

Treatment   Antifungal medication (such as griseofulvin) by mouth or applied to the skin. An antifungal ointment applied directly to the scalp will stop the ringworm from spreading to other areas of the head, and to a child's friends. Any secondary bacterial infection will be treated with antibiotics. Boggy raised areas of the scalp (keratons) will require a special cream and a cotton cap to cover the scalp until the areas dry. The infected hair will need to be clipped and a special shampoo used.

Body ringworm is easier to treat; a variety of antifungal creams will work. The patient should wash well with soap and water and remove all scabs and crusts. Antifungal cream should then be rubbed into all lesions.

Prevention   People should not share towels, hats, or clothing of an infected person. Good grooming and hygiene and frequent checks of a child's scalp can prevent the disease.

Once an infection has been diagnosed, all contaminated articles must be cleaned to prevent further infection. Combs, brushes, hats, scarfs, and bedding must be cleaned in hot, soapy water.

risus sardonicus   An unusual grinning expression caused by prolonged contraction of the facial muscles; it is a symptom of TETANUS.

Ritter's disease   The former name for STAPHYLOCOCCAL SCALDED SKIN SYNDROME.

Rocky Mountain spotted fever   An infectious disease characterized by a spotted rash, caused by the organism *Rickettsia rickettsii* (similar to bacteria) transmitted from rabbits and other small mammals to humans, primarily by tick bites.

In the eastern United States, children are most often infected, whereas in the West disease is highest among adult males. It is found most often on the Atlantic coast, but it gets its name from its original occurrence in the Rocky Mountain states. The incidence of the disease has been rising steadily since 1980; there are more than 1,000 cases reported each year.

Cause   RMSF is spread by the bite of an infected American dog tick, lone-star tick, or wood tick or by contamination of the skin with tick blood or feces. Person-to-person spread of RMSF does not occur. Any tick may harbor the disease.

Symptoms   Sudden onset of mild to moderate fever, which can last for two or three weeks. Loss of appetite and slight headache may develop slowly about a week after a tick bite. Sometimes, however, symptoms appear suddenly—high fever, prostration, aching, tender muscles, severe headache, nausea, and vomiting. Two to six days after symptoms appear, small pink spots appear on wrists and ankles, spreading over the entire body and darkening, enlarging, and bleeding. The illness subsides after about two weeks. Un-treated cases with very high fever may end in death from PNEUMONIA or heart failure.

One attack probably provides permanent immunity.

Diagnosis   Diagnosis may be difficult because the disease resembles several other infections; lab tests on blood and tissues may confirm the disease.

Treatment   Antibiotic drugs doxycycline or tetracycline usually cure the disease. If patients can't tolerate these drugs, chloramphenicol may be used.

Prevention   People in tick-infested areas should use insect repellent and examine themselves daily for ticks. Local tick populations may be controlled with applications of pesticides to vegetation along trails, and mowing grass in yards often to eliminate areas where small rodents can live.

roseola   (exanthem   subitum)   A common infectious disease of early childhood that primarily affects youngsters aged six months to two years. Only about a third of children with the infection have any symptoms at all. All children recover completely.

Cause   The source of this infection was not known until 1986, when scientists discovered the cause was human herpes virus-6; still, its etiology is not fully understood. Because scientists recently found HHV-6 in the saliva of healthy children, they have concluded that the virus may be spread through contact with saliva of family members or other children who carry the virus but do not have symptoms.

Research suggests that after an active infection, HHV-6 can become latent and hide in the body, later reappearing to cause other illnesses. Some scientists suggest it may be linked to the development of CHRONIC FATIGUE SYNDROME.

Symptoms   Most cases of roseola occur in spring and summer and are characterized by the abrupt onset of irritability and a fever, which may climb as high as 105 degrees F. By the fourth or fifth day, the fever breaks, suddenly returning to normal. At about the same time, a rash appears on the body, often spreading quickly to the face, neck, and limbs, fading within two days. Other symptoms may include sore throat, enlarged lymph nodes, and occasionally a febrile seizure.

Diagnosis   Roseola is usually diagnosed by noting symptoms and ruling out other causes of high fever. Tests have been developed to look for both the virus and its antibodies, but these are available in research labs only.

Treatment   There are no serious complications, and there is no specific treatment other than acetaminophen for the fever; rest and fluids.

Complications   Rarely a child will have seizures due to the high fever, or develop ENCEPHALITIS.

rotavirus   Rotavirus is the common name for a family of viruses that shave several features. The group A rotaviruses are the most common cause of severe diarrhea in children. This virus strikes 130 million people every year, causing diarrhea so severe that 870,000 children die each year worldwide. While few U.S. children die, the disease still sends 50,000 of them to the hospital every year. If an infant or toddler develops diarrhea in the winter, there is a good chance that a rotavirus is the culprit. By age four, most people have been infected and developed antibodies. While the disease is not particularly deadly in the United States among children with healthy immune systems, rotavirus in the developing world is more serious because many infants are malnourished. In the United States, the chance a child will be hospitalized with rotavirus is 1 in 40. One in every 800 hospitalized will die. The rotavirus season begins in late fall and ends in the spring. See also DIARRHEA AND INFECTIOUS DISEASE; ANTIDIARRHEAL DRUGS.

Cause   Rotavirus invades the cells of the small bowel so that it can't absorb liquids, resulting in diarrhea. While the rotavirus also

infects animals, scientists don't believe it is passed from pets to humans; the virus is thought to be spread by the fecal-oral route. The virus must be swallowed in order for it to infect the digestive tract. Children infected once can be infected again.

Symptoms   Symptoms develop quickly; most babies begin with vomiting and a low fever followed by watery diarrhea from three to eight days. The child is infectious until the diarrhea stops. As many as 20 vomiting and 20 diarrhea episodes a day are not uncommon.

Diagnosis   Physicians can diagnose rotavirus from symptoms alone, noting the age of the child and time of year. A new test of stool samples can detect rotavirus in 15 minutes.

Treatment   There is no cure for rotavirus infection. Nonprescription antidiarrhea medicine should not be given to infants and young children. Infants with severe dehydration and vomiting require IV-fluid replacement.

Prevention   A new type of vaccine, formulated by the National Institute of Allergy and Infectious Diseases, was tested in 2,000 children and proved to prevent more than 80 percent of the most severe diarrheal diseases.

The proposed vaccine seems safe; the only side effects are a low-grade fever three or four days after the vaccine. The proposed oral vaccine would be given in a three-dose series, intended to be given at two, four, and six months, with other vaccines.

The vaccine has been recommended for approval by an advisory panel of the Food and Drug Administration. The vaccine, to be called Rota Shield, may become available by fall 1998.

roundworms   Also known as nematodes, this class of elongated, cylindrical worms include at least a dozen or so types that are parasites on humans. In temperate climates such as the United States, the only common type of roundworm disease is PINWORM INFESTATION, which primarily affects children. Ascariasis, whipworms, and TRICHINOSIS are also fairly common. TOXOCARIASIS sometimes occurs, caused by the worm *TOXOCARA CANIS* (in dogs) and the *T. cati* (in cats). (Most North American infections are due to *T. canis*.)

In tropical countries, roundworm diseases are much more common and include HOOK-WORM DISEASE, STRONGYLOIDIASIS, Guinea worm disease, and different types of FILARIASIS.

Symptoms In many cases, the adult worms live in the human intestines without causing symptoms unless there are many worms present. Sometimes symptoms occur as worm larvae pass through various parts of the body. The number of worms present is called the "worm burden."

Treatment Most infestations are treated relatively easily with ANTIHELMINTIC DRUGS.

rubella   See GERMAN MEASLES.

rubeola   Another name for MEASLES.

Russian flu   See INFLUENZA.

S

Salk vaccine See POLIOMYELITIS

Salmonella bacteria The bacteria that cause a type of food poisoning known as SALMONELLOSIS. Included in this type are _Salmonella enteritidis, S. cubana, S. aertrycke,_ and _S. choleraesuis._ These bacteria are known for multiplying rapidly at room temperature and are often found in raw meat, poultry, eggs, fish, raw milk, and foods made from them and in pet turtles. Proper handling and cooking of contaminated food will kill the _Salmonella_ bacteria.

The most dangerous members of the _Salmonella_ family are _S. typhi,_ which causes TYPHOID FEVER. _Salmonella_ is also a common cause of OSTEOMYELITIS (bone infection), especially of the spine.

salmonellosis One of the major types of FOOD POISONING, it is caused by bacteria that multiply rapidly at room temperatures. While salmonellosis is fatal in only 1 percent of cases, it is very dangerous in pregnant women, young children, the elderly, and those with cancer or AIDS.

Salmonellosis is very common in this country; bone meal, fertilizer, and pet foods may all be implicated in the spread of the disease. In particular, recent outbreaks have been linked to chickens and eggs; it is estimated that 60 percent of chicken carcasses in processing plants harbor the bacteria.

The largest outbreak ever recorded occurred in 1994 and involved more than 200,000 Americans. In this case, commercially pasteurized ice cream premix was contaminated by bacteria during transport to a Minnesota ice-cream plant in tanker trailers that had previously carried nonpasteurized liquid eggs. The outbreak ended after sales of the ice cream were stopped. See also DIAR-RHEA AND INFECTIOUS DISEASE; ANTIDIARRHEAL DRUGS; TRAVELER'S DIARRHEA.

Cause Salmonellosis is caused by infection with the _Salmonella_ bacteria; even extremely low doses (too low to be detected by current standards) can cause food poisoning.

The incidence of salmonellosis appears to be spreading in epidemic proportions. Bacteria are now commonly found in eggs and poultry across the country; it is estimated that 60 percent of chicken carcasses in U.S. processing plants harbor the bacteria. _Salmonella_ is also present in raw meats, fish, raw milk, bone meal, fertilizer, and pet foods as well as in pet turtles and marijuana, and it can also be transferred to food from the excrement of infected animals or people. One type of the bacteria, _S. enteritidis,_ has been found in the eggs of chickens with the disease. The more bacteria injested, the faster illness will occur.

Symptoms While tiny amounts of _Salmonella_ can be ingested in otherwise healthy people without problem, a minimal number may cause salmonellosis symptoms from 12 to 48 hours after eating tainted food, smoking tainted marijuana, or handling infected turtles. Symptoms vary, depending on the amount of bacteria that were eaten, but include headache, nausea, vomiting, fever, stomach cramps, and diarrhea. Symptoms usually last two to seven days. Severe cases can lead to shock and can be fatal in infants and the elderly.

Treatment As with most types of food poisoning, there is no specific treatment. Patients should eat a bland diet and drink plenty of fluids to combat dehydration. Antibiotic treatment (chloramphenicol, ampicillin, or tetracycline) should be administered only in cases of severe infection or if there is indication of bacteria in the blood.

Prevention Fortunately for consumers, proper handling and cooking of contaminated food will kill the *Salmonella* bacteria. Proper refrigeration and cooking methods for meat and eggs must be observed at all times. Eggs should be refrigerated and not used raw (such as in Caesar salad or egg nog). Raw chicken should never touch any other food or utensils during preparation, and cooks should wash their hands after touching raw chicken.

In the fall of 1992, the U.S. Department of Agriculture's Food Safety and Inspection Service approved two new methods to combat the rising level of *Salmonella* in chicken; the use of trisodium phosphate in a rinse to destroy bacteria and the use of irradiation to control potential contamination on poultry.

Food-grade trisodium phosphate is a federally approved ingredient that, according to tests, has no discernible effect on the taste, texture, or color of chicken. The compound destroys *Salmonella* by stripping a thin, exterior fat coating on the chickens. No residue is absorbed in the skin or meat of the birds. Another new treatment sprays helpful bacteria on baby chicks. The "good" bacteria crowd out the *Salmonella*.

No labeling is required for trisodium phosphate-treated chickens, but irradiated chicken must prominently carry the international symbol for the process with the words "treated with irradiation" on labels. However, irradiating food is not a guarantee that it won't be contaminated. While irradiation might kill most of the bacteria, it can also make it easier for those that are left to survive.

San Joaquin fever Another name for COCCIDIOIDOMYCOSIS.

Sarcoptes scabiei The mite responsible for the skin infestation of SCABIES.

scabies A highly infectious, fairly common skin infestation caused by the mite *SARCOPTES SCABIEI*, which burrows into the skin and lays its eggs. Scabies infect people from all socioeconomic levels, with no regard to age, sex, race, or standards of personal hygiene. Clusters of outbreaks are sometimes seen in institutions such as child care centers or nursing homes.

Cause Scabies mites are passed by direct skin-to-skin contact; indirect transfer from underwear or sheets can occur only if these have been contaminated by infected people right beforehand. Hatched mites can pass from one individual to another person simply by direct contact, although the mites are usually passed during contact such as sexual intercourse. A person can continue to spread scabies until the mites and eggs have been destroyed.

Symptoms The most common symptom is intense itching (especially at night). Tiny gray, itchy swellings appear on the skin, between the fingers, on wrists and genitals, waist, thighs, nipples, breasts, lower buttocks, and in armpits. Reddish lumps may later appear on limbs and trunk.

Symptoms may appear from two to six weeks in people who haven't been previously exposed to scabies. Those who have had cases in the past may show symptoms within one to four days after a reexposure.

Treatment Insecticide lotion such as prescription lindane, permethrin, or crotamiton should be applied to all skin below the patient's head, which kills the mites (although itching may continue for up to two weeks later). All members of a family should be treated at the same time.

Itching may persist, but this is not necessarily a failure of treatment or a reinfestation. Those with symptoms should be treated with a second course of lotion 7 to 10 days later, followed by a cleansing bath eight hours after application, and a change to clean clothing.

Prevention Scabies can be prevented by avoiding physical contact with an infested person or his or her belongings.

scalded skin syndrome   See STAPHYLOCOCCAL SCALDED SKIN SYNDROME.

scarlatina   Another name for SCARLET FEVER.

scarlet fever   An infectious bacterial childhood disease characterized by a skin rash, sore throat, and fever. It is less common and dangerous than it was years ago. No longer a reportable disease, experts don't know for sure how many cases occur today in the United States, although it is believed that the disease has been on the increase for the past several years.

With the spread of streptococcus infections around the world has come more cases of scarlet fever, which is caused by infection with group A streptococcus, according to the World Health Organization. Scarlet fever strains of group A strep produce toxins that are released in the skin, causing a bright red rash.

In the past, the disease was associated with poor living conditions. In 1737, a scarlet fever epidemic in Boston killed 900 people; another epidemic in New York City in the late 1800s killed 35 percent of children who contracted the disease; that same year, 19 percent of Chicago children who got the disease perished.

Inexplicably, by the 1920s the death rate of the disease dropped to 5 percent for reasons that are still not completely understood. It is believed that the scarlet fever bacteria underwent a natural mutation that made it less of a killer. The introduction of penicillin reduced the death rate even more.

Today, most cases are found among residents of middle-class suburbs, not in the inner cities. Because it is possible to get strep and scarlet fever more than once, and because the incidence of all strep infections is rising, prompt medical attention when strep is suspected is important. A patient with a sore throat and skin rash should seek medical care. Anyone can develop scarlet fever, but most cases are found among children aged four to eight.

Cause   Scarlet fever bacteria are spread in droplets during coughing or breathing or by sharing food and drink. When bacterial particles are released into the air, they can be picked up by others close by. The hallmark rash is caused by a toxin released by the bacteria.

Symptoms   After an incubation period of two to four days, the first sign of illness is usually a fever of 103 to 104 degrees F, accompanied by a severe sore throat. The face is flushed and the tongue develops a white coating with red spots, rather like a white strawberry. The child may seem tired and flushed; 12 to 18 hours after the fever, a rash appears as a mass of rapidly spreading tiny red spots on the neck and upper trunk. The scarlet fever rash is unique in that it feels rough, like fine sandpaper, and is quite distinctive.

Other common symptoms include headache, chills and vomiting, and tiny white lines around the mouth, as well as fine red striations in the creases of elbows and groin. After a few days, the tongue coating peels off, followed by a drop in fever and a fading rash. Skin on the hands and feet often peel.

Complications   As with other types of sore throat caused by the streptococci bacteria, untreated infection carries the risk of immunologic disorders, such as RHEUMATIC FEVER or glomerulonephritis (inflammation of the kidneys).

Treatment   A 10-day course of antibiotics (usually PENICILLIN or erythromycin), with rest, liquids, and acetaminophen. Children are contagious for a day or two after they begin treatment, but after that they can return to school.

schistosomiasis   An infection that occurs worldwide, caused by flukes (parasites) that live and multiply in freshwater snails. There are two types of human schistosomiasis—cutaneous schistosomiasis (SWIMMER'S ITCH) and visceral schistosomiasis, a serious systemic disorder that occasionally causes minor skin symptoms. The disease is caused by one of three types of flukes (called schistosomes) acquired from bathing in infested lakes and rivers.

Visceral schistosomiasis is a parasitic disease (also called bilharziasis) that causes an itchy rash where flukes have penetrated the skin. The disease is found in most tropical countries and affects more than 200 million people around the world.

Cause When the parasite-infected snails release large numbers of very small larvae in the water, the larvae can penetrate unbroken skin of a human host, where they develop within their host into adults; their eggs provoke inflammatory reactions. The worms enter the blood and make their way into the liver and intestines. Travelers are at risk when swimming in an area where the infection is present.

Symptoms Symptoms begin within two to three weeks of exposure. While it also causes problems in other organs, the skin symptoms of this condition include dermatitis, hives, and skin lesions due to the deposits of eggs in the skin. The relatively minor skin symptoms of this form of schistosomiasis are quite different than the marked skin inflammation in SWIMMER'S ITCH (the second form of schistosomiasis).

About one to two months after the penetration of the skin, hives again appear. Skin lesions caused by the egg deposits may appear in the genital and perineal areas.

Treatment The new drug praziquantel has revolutionized the treatment of this form of schistosomiasis since the 1980s, since one dose can kill the flukes and prevent further damage. There is no vaccine to prevent the disease, and visitors to the tropics should assume that all lakes and rivers are unsafe for swimming. Alternative drugs are oxamniquine and metriphonate.

Prevention Since there is no way to tell infested from noninfested water, travelers should avoid freshwater swimming in rural areas of suspected countries. Accidental exposure to water in suspected areas should be followed by immediate, vigorous towel drying or quick application of alcohol to the exposed areas of skin.

There are no preventive drugs yet available, but scientists have developed a new vaccine that protects against damage caused by the worm. In an animal study, it dramatically reduced the scar tissue. The vaccine didn't stop reinfection, but did halt the damage that the organism caused.

scrofula The former term for TUBERCULOSIS of the bones and lymphatic glands (especially in children). The old English name was king's evil, so-called because it was believed that the king's touch could cure the disease.

septicemia (bacterial sepsis) The medical name for blood poisoning, a potentially lethal blood infection characterized by the rapid multiplication of bacteria and the presence of their toxins that kill 175,000 Americans each year. Unlike BACTEREMIA, in which bacteria are present in the blood but don't always cause illness, septicemia is a severe, life-threatening emergency.

Cause Septicemia can occur when certain forms of bacteria enter the bloodstream. These bacteria give off endotoxins—poisonous substances that remain even after the bacteria disintegrate and that can lead to a dramatic drop in blood pressure (SEPTIC SHOCK), with rapid heartbeat and breathing.

Symptoms Symptoms include the sudden onset of fever, chills, rapid breathing, headache, nausea or diarrhea, and clouding of consciousness. Skin rashes and jaundice may occur, and the hands may be especially warm. If large amounts of toxins are produced by the bacteria, the patient may pass into a state of septic shock.

Diagnosis Septicemia is diagnosed by a culture of the blood.

Treatment Antibiotics must be administered, together with IV fluids. The site of infection should be identified and may need to be removed surgically. If the infection is identified and treated promptly, there should be a full recovery.

septic shock   A type of shock in which there is tissue damage and a dramatic drop in blood pressure as a result of SEPTICEMIA (bacteria causing blood poisoning) and TOXEMIA (the multiplication of bacteria and their toxins in the blood). This type of shock usually follows signs of severe infection (often in the stomach or intestines or in the urinary tract).

Septic shock is especially common in those who have an immune system problem, in people taking drugs for cancer, or in people taking prolonged antibiotic treatment.

Cause The toxins (poisons) released from bacteria into the bloodstream are the primary source of the problem because they can damage cells and tissues throughout the body. This leads to clotting of blood in the smallest blood vessels, seriously interfering with the normal blood circulation. Damage occurs especially to tissues in the kidneys, heart, and lungs. The toxins may lead to leaking of fluid from blood vessels, interfering with their ability to constrict, which triggers a drop in blood pressure.

Symptoms Symptoms vary with the extent and type of major tissue damage. In general, the symptoms are the same as those of septicemia, with the additional signs of cold hands and feet; blue coloration; a weak, rapid pulse; and significant drop in blood pressure. Fever, rapid breathing, confusion, or coma are common. There may also be vomiting or diarrhea.

Treatment Septic shock must be treated immediately, with rapid fluid replacement and antibiotics. Surgery may be needed to remove the infection from the body. Measures should be taken to increase the blood pressure. Despite aggressive treatment, septic shock is a grave condition that carries a 50 percent mortality rate.

sexually transmitted disease (STD)   A contagious disease usually transmitted during sexual intercourse or genital contact. In the United States, the most commonly reported infections during 1995 were sexually transmitted, and the incidence has risen over the past 20 years despite improved methods of diagnosis and treatment.

Also known as venereal disease, these conditions are often acquired by people who have many sex partners. Some of the major STDs are also transmitted by blood and can therefore be acquired by drug addicts who share needles.

Until about 25 years ago, the venereal diseases were limited to GONORRHEA, SYPHILIS, CHANCROID, GRANULOMA INGUINALE, and LYMPHOGRANULOMA VENEREUM. To these have been added SCABIES, HERPES, genital WARTS, pubic LICE, PEDICULOSIS, TRICHOMONIASIS, genital CANDIDIASIS, MOLLUSCUM CONTAGIOSUM, HEPATITIS B, nonspecific URETHRITIS, CHLAMYDIA, CYTOMEGALOVIRUS, and AIDS.

During World War II, the incidence of STDs rose in the United States, but these declined with the introduction of PENICILLIN and subsequent cure of syphilis and gonorrhea. However, in the 1960s and 1970s the infections began to increase with the introduction of oral contraception. The pill meant that more women were having more sex partners and fewer couples used barrier methods of birth control, which provide some protection against STDs. At the same time, in the early 1980s doctors began to diagnose nonspecific urethritis in about 25 percent of patients who visited STD clinics; most of these people were found to have chlamydial infection. By 1995, chlamydia was the most common of all the reported infectious diseases (477,638 cases). gonorrhea and AIDS were second and third, according to the Centers for Disease Control and Prevention. Chlamydia was more often reported among women, while gonorrhea and AIDS were reported more often by men.

Throughout the 1970s and early 1980s, most STD patients could expect to be cured with antibiotics. But about the same time, doctors began to realize that new infections such as the chronic disease HERPES and the occasionally fatal illness hepatitis B could not be cured by drugs. With the spread of AIDS in 1982, doctors realized that STDs were again a serious risk to life, and now consider promiscuous sex to be a high-risk venture.

STDs can be diagnosed at special clinics or from specialists in genitourinary medicine and infectious disease. The doctor decides which disease (or diseases) are present and which drugs to prescribe. Once drugs have eased the symptoms, tests are given to make sure the patient is no longer infectious. Treatment is also given to all recent sex partners to prevent transmitting infection. The confidential tracing and treatment of contacts is an essential part of managing STDs.

shellfish poisoning Eating shellfish has been linked to a number of diseases, including those caused by bacteria, a variety of viruses, and toxins.

Shellfish are highly susceptible to bacterial and viral contamination, since they live close to the shore where pollution tends to be worse. While shellfish by themselves are not poisonous, they can become contaminated from their environment, passing infection on up the food chain when eaten by humans. Oysters, clams, and mussels are particularly prone to becoming contaminated because of their metabolic system, which pumps water across their gills to isolate plankton; this makes them vulnerable to bacteria, viruses, and contaminants in the water. (Lobsters and other crustacean shellfish only rarely become contaminated.)

Shellfish contamination caused by bacteria and viruses can be prevented by cooking seafood thoroughly, storing shellfish properly, and protecting them from contamination after cooking. However, traditional methods of cooking seafood (such as steaming clams only until they open) may be insufficient to kill all bacteria and viruses inside them.

Most cases of shellfish poisoning have occurred when people ate raw or undercooked shellfish; in fact, raw shellfish have been linked to nearly 1,000 cases of HEPATITIS a year. For this reason, doctors recommend that no one eat raw shellfish.

Good data on the occurrence and severity of shellfish poisoning are largely unavailable, which reflects the inability to measure the true incidence of this disease; cases are often misdiagnosed and infrequently reported.

The shellfish industry and government regulatory agencies try to control the problem of shellfish contamination at the source, by seeing that shellfish are harvested from unpolluted beds not tainted by sewage. Unfortunately, these efforts can't guarantee that shellfish from unapproved beds don't reach the market.

Viral contamination The most common viral contamination in shellfish is caused by the Norwalk virus which leads to food poisoning when raw or improperly cooked food has been in contact with water contaminated by human excrement. (See NORWALK AGENT INFECTION.)

It's also possible to contract HEPATITIS A from eating raw shellfish harvested from sewage-contaminated waters. Even though federal regulations and posting of contaminated waters offer some protection, there is still a risk of contracting viruses when eating raw shellfish.

Symptoms begin from two to six weeks after eating and include fever, weakness, anorexia, jaundice; severe cases may damage liver and can be fatal.

Toxins Shellfish also can become tainted by eating toxic plankton (called dinoflagellates) that multiply rapidly during the warm summer months; because the plankton have a pink or red color, this phenomenon has come to be called RED TIDE. Red tides are found in coastal waters in the Pacific from California to Alaska and in the Atlantic from New England to the St. Lawrence. Under good conditions (warm climate, warm water), the plankton may reach 60 million organisms per liter of water. These rapid growths (referred to as a "bloom") discolor the sea and poison fish and marine life. Usually, a person becomes poisoned with the plankton when eating shellfish that have been feeding on them.

The plankton produce a deadly poison called saxitoxin that is so toxic that even one contaminated shellfish can be fatal if eaten. This is why clams, oysters, and mussels are not sold during months without an *R* in them (the summer months).

Mussels, clams, and oysters are the primary shellfish at risk, and mussels are the most susceptible of all. Healthy bivalve shellfish filter large amounts of toxic plankton, which form the primary ocean food during May through August. During these warm times, the dinoflagellates thrive by photosynthesis and can be so invasive that they kill birds and fish.

The first large epidemic of poisoning caused by red tide–contaminated shellfish occurred in San Francisco in 1927, when 102 people were sickened and 6 died. Today, largely because of the prohibition against eating certain shellfish during the summer months, such epidemics are rare.

Shellfish poisoning caused by toxic forms of dinoflagellates include paralytic shellfish poisoning, neurologic shellfish poisoning, diarrheic shellfish poisoning, and amnesic shellfish poisoning. Each has different etiology, symptoms, and prognosis for recovery, but of the three, paralytic shellfish poisoning is by far the most serious.

Shellfish containing toxin look and taste normal, and usual cooking methods do not affect the toxin. State shellfish screening programs test shellfish for the presence of these toxins and monitor the safety of shellfish harvest beds.

shellfish poisoning, amnesic   This type of shellfish poison first came to the attention of public health officials in 1987, when 156 cases of acute intoxication occurred after people ate cultured blue mussels harvested off Prince Edward island in eastern Canada. Of those who got sick, 22 were hospitalized and 3 elderly patients eventually died.

Cause   Amnesic shellfish poisoning is the result of an unusual neurotoxic amino acid (domoic acid) that contaminates shellfish. The domoic acid is produced by a phytoplankton called *Nitzschia pungens* f. multiseries. (Phytoplankton are microscopic, photosynthetic, free-floating organisms in the ocean; *N. pungens* is a type of phytoplankton with a particular kind of cell wall.) Many different kinds of phytoplankton exist and only a few of them are toxic.

Symptoms   While everyone is susceptible to shellfish poisoning, elderly people appear to be predisposed to the severe neurological effects of amnesic shellfish poisoning. Within 24 hours of eating contaminated shellfish, the symptoms begin: vomiting and diarrhea, abdominal pain, and a host of neurological problems, including confusion, memory loss, disorientation, seizure, and coma.

Diagnosis   Diagnosis is based on observing symptoms and recent dietary history.

Treatment   There is no antidote for this type of shellfish poison. The only treatment is to ease the symptoms.

shellfish poisoning, diarrheic   This type of shellfish poisoning is rarely fatal and has not been confirmed in U.S. seafood, although the organisms that produce it are present in U.S. waters. It occurs in Europe in a sporadic, widespread fashion, and an outbreak was recently confirmed in Canada.

Cause   It is caused by eating shellfish contaminated by toxin-producing plankton. It is associated in particular with eating mussels, oysters, and scallops.

Symptoms Symptoms appear between a few minutes to three hours after ingestion, and include gastrointestinal problems accompanied by muscular weakness, chills, headache, and fever. Recovery is rapid and death is rare.

Diagnosis Diagnosis is based on observing symptoms and recent dietary history.

Treatment There is no antidote for this type of shellfish poison, but most people recover on their own.

shellfish poisoning, neurotoxic A type of shellfish poison that occurs when humans eat shellfish that have ingested toxin-producing plankton.

While all shellfish are potentially toxic, NSP is generally associated with shellfish harvested along the Florida coast and the Gulf of Mexico. Outbreaks are sporadic and continuous and have been reported along the Gulf coast of Florida and more recently in North Carolina and Texas.

Cause NSP is the result of exposure to a group of toxins called brevetoxins.

Symptoms Both gastrointestinal and neurological symptoms appear in this type of shellfish poisoning within a few minutes to a few hours after eating the shellfish. Symptoms include tingling and numbness of lips, tongue, and throat; muscular aches; dizziness; reversal of the sensation of hot and cold; diarrhea; and vomiting.

Recovery is complete with few aftereffects; no fatalities have been reported.

Diagnosis Diagnosis is based on observing symptoms and recent dietary history.

Treatment There is no treatment other than easing symptoms.

shellfish poisoning, paralytic (PSP) The most serious type of shellfish poisoning, PSP is a toxic neurologic condition caused by eating clams, oysters, or mussels that have ingested toxin-producing plankton. The type of toxin is called saxitoxin, among the most potent toxins known and one that is not destroyed by cooking. The saxitoxin comes from algae eaten by filter-feeding shellfish such as clams and mussels; this toxin can be present even when there is no visible discoloration (or RED TIDE) in the ocean water. The shellfish store the toxin from the algae in their tissues and pass the toxin on to anyone who eats them. In recent years, the toxin has been found in snails and in crab viscera as well.

Most victims of this type of poisoning in the United States are individuals who have gathered shellfish for their own use. PSP has generally been considered to be dangerous only in shellfish harvested from cold water, but the incidence of red tides in warmer waters may be increasing. Outbreaks have recently been reported from Central and South America, Asia, and the Pacific.

Cause The 20 toxins responsible for paralytic shellfish poisonings are all derivatives of saxitoxin.

Symptoms Saxitoxin interferes with functions involving the brain, movement, and senses. Soon after eating (sometimes in less than an hour), symptoms appear. At first, there is a tingling or numbness in lips and tongue, often followed by tingling and numbness in the fingertips and toes, nausea, lightheadedness, followed by vomiting and diarrhea. This may progress to loss of muscle coordination. This is followed by a gradual paralysis, trembling, headache, and weakness. Death as a result of respiratory paralysis can occur within 12 hours of eating PSP-containing shellfish. Eating as little as 0.5 to 1.0 mg. of contaminated shellfish can be fatal, and a person's survival depends on how much has been consumed. If a person survives the first 12 hours, chances of survival are good. However, between 8 and 23 percent of PSP poisonings are fatal. The severity of the illness is less if the water used in cooking is not consumed.

Diagnosis   There is no lab test that can determine the presence of PSP in an individual. Diagnosis is made on the basis of recent food consumption, symptoms, and detection of toxin in uneaten shellfish.

Treatment   There is no known antidote for shellfish poisoning caused by saxitoxin-producing plankton. Administration of prostigmine may be effective, together with artificial respiration and oxygen as needed. It is important that vomiting be induced at the onset of symptoms to help remove remaining toxin-containing shellfish and that medical attention be obtained. Drinking alcohol increases absorption of the toxin.

Prevention   To prevent outbreaks of PSP, samples of susceptible mollusks are tested for toxin by state health departments during certain times of the year. Affected growing areas are quarantined, and sale of shellfish is stopped. Warning signs posted in shellfish-growing areas, on beaches, and in the news warn the public of the danger.

Because of this constant monitoring, shellfish poisoning in the United States is rare; from 1973 to 1987 only 19 outbreaks were reported, with an average of eight cases per outbreak.

Shigella group   A group of four different species of bacteria that lead to the diarrheal disease known as SHIGELLOSIS.

shigellosis   A bacterial diarrheal disease caused by the bacterium *Shigella,* which includes four different species. The disease is common among the developing countries, where lack of sewage treatment leads to contaminated food and water.

Two thirds of cases are found in children between 6 months and 10 years of age, although it is rare in infants under age 6 months. The highest rates of infection occur in child care centers, large camps, and institutions.

A person is infectious from the time the diarrhea appears until the bacteria are no longer in the stool, which could take a month. Antibiotics shorten the infectious period to a week.

Cause   Shiga toxin is named after Kiyoshi Shiga, who in 1898 first described the bacterial origin of DYSENTERY caused by *Shigella dysenteriae.*

The *Shigella* bacteria are found in milk and dairy products, poultry, and mixed salads, but they can develop in any moist food that is not thoroughly cooked. The bacteria multiply rapidly at or above room temperature. *S. sonnei* is the mildest of the four, and is responsible for most cases around the world. *S. dysenteriae* (also known as bacillary dysentery) is fairly common in rural Africa and India, where it causes illness and many deaths.

A person gets sick after ingesting bacteria; it only takes a few organisms to cause illness. The bacteria may be found in contaminated bodies of water or in food that is left out in the open where flies can contaminate it. Dogs who eat infected human feces can spread the infection to humans (especially children), and the disease can also be spread sexually with anal-oral contact.

Symptoms   Symptoms, which usually appear eight hours to eight days after ingestion, begin with nausea and vomiting, watery or bloody explosive diarrhea and stomach cramps, weakness, vision problems, headache, and difficulty swallowing. Those with weakened immune systems may have more serious diarrhea and may take longer to recover. Young children have more serious symptoms, and those children already malnourished or weak will be much sicker.

Diagnosis   Culture of the stool will reveal *Shigella.*

Treatment   Most people with shigellosis recover on their own. Some may require fluids to prevent dehydration. To shorten severe cases, antibiotics will help stop the diarrhea, although *Shigella* has become resistant to some drugs. Trimethoprim-sulfamethoxazole, ciprofloxacin, or orofloxacin are usually effective; some strains are susceptible to tetracycline. Those who are infected in a developing country may respond better to nalidixic acid, since the bacteria in those locations are widely resistant.

Antidiarrheal medications should not be taken. Dilute drinks high in sugar and bland foods high in carbohydrates are tolerated best by the patient.

Prevention Confirmed *Shigella* cases must be reported to the health department, which will begin an investigation and control measures in order to prevent large-scale outbreaks. Although several vaccines have been tested, none have yet been licensed for use in preventing the disease. The single most important way to prevent the spread of disease is to carefully wash hands after using the toilet, since *Shigella* is passed in feces.

shingles A painful, red blistering viral infection of the nerves that supply certain areas of the skin, caused by reactivation of the VARICELLA-ZOSTER VIRUS (VZV), the same culprit that causes childhood CHICKENPOX.

Shingles is a common illness that strikes one in five Americans. The name comes from the Latin word *cingulum,* meaning "belt" or "girdle." By age 85, people have a 50-50 chance of developing shingles if they haven't already had them.

Cause After an episode of chickenpox, the virus lie dormant in sensory nerves along the spine for many years. When the immune system efficiency is weakened, the virus reemerges and migrates along the sensory nerve, breaking out at its receptor ends in the skin. Each year, shingles affects several hundred patients per 100,000 in the United States, usually over age 50.

Scientists suspect that a decline in the activity of white blood cells may allow the virus to reemerge. This idea is bolstered by the fact that shingles also appears in children with leukemia, cancer patients undergoing chemotherapy, and organ transplant patients. The

virus often affects a nerve that has had previous trauma.

Symptoms The first sign is excessive sensitivity in an area of skin, followed by pain; after about five days the rash appears, turning into tense blisters that turn yellow within three more days. The blisters then dry out and crust over, gradually dropping off (leaving small pitted scars behind). Because the nerves have been damaged after the virus attack, after the blisters heal the nerves constantly produce strong pain impulses that may last for months or years.

The older the patient and more severe the rash, the more likely the pain will persist. Shingles often affects a strip of skin over the ribs on one side; sometimes it affects the lower part of the body or the upper half of the face on one side. It can occur in any area of the body.

Treatment There is little that can be done either for the rash or the pain afterward, but prompt use of antiviral drugs such as acyclovir, famcyclovir, or valacyclovir can shorten the rash stage and lessen the chance of pain later. Therefore, patients should seek medical help at the first signs of shingles. Acyclovir slows reproduction of the virus and shortens the course of the infection, although it doesn't prevent the nerve pain following a shingles attack. Some experts maintain that steroid drugs such as prednisone can prevent this pain. Valacyclovir is a chemical cousin of the widely used acyclovir; it received FDA approval in June 1995.

For severe pain from shingles, experts occasionally recommend injecting a nerve block in the appropriate place to block the sympathetic nerves supplying the area of pain. This block typically relieves pain for hours in up to 80 percent of patients.

An over-the-counter product called Zostrix or Valtrex (active ingredient: capsaicin, a red pepper derivative used to make chili powder) may help relieve the post-herpetic shingles pain, once all the blisters have disappeared.

Experts believe that capsaicin blocks the production of a chemical necessary for pain impulse transmission between nerve cells. *Do not apply Zostrix to active shingles blisters.* As a counterirritant, Zostrix is designed to be used on unbroken, healed skin with a pain sensation, not for open oozing infections.

Adenosine monophosphate is the newest potential treatment now being studied by researchers.

Complications   Almost half of the 600,000 patients who get shingles each year suffer from agonizing pain that may last from days to years. If the pain lasts long after the rash, it is known as postherpetic neuralgia. It can also lead to bizarre sensations that can linger for years, including phantom feelings.

Sufferers complain that a light touch can feel like torture and a drop of water feels like a third-degree burn. Even the softest clothing can be unbearable to these patients.

Postherpetic neuralgia is treated with a variety of medications from amitriptyline to opioids.

Sin Nombre virus   The newest strain of HANTAVIRUS (virus carried by rodents) that caused an outbreak of hantavirus pulmonary syndrome in the Four Corners area of the United States. The virus, originally named after the Muerta Canyon on the Navajo Reservation of New Mexico, has killed more than 100 patients across the United States (mostly in Arizona, New Mexico, and Colorado). Hantavirus is the third most deadly virus ever found in the United States, after HIV and RABIES.

This American variety appears to be 10 times more deadly than a related hantavirus from Asia, called the Hantaan virus. Scientists suspect the Sin Nombre virus is not at all a new organism but rather one that has been living for eons in deer mice of the southwest, emerging occasionally to infect humans. Navajo legends appear to have mentioned this disease.

Because the virus has been identified as a cause of disease in patients in New York and Virginia, scientists believe that eventually the organism will be found throughout the United States.

sinusitis   An inflammation of one or more of the sinuses, often as a complication of an upper respiratory infection or dental infection. (It may also be caused by allergies, air travel, or underwater swimming.) Sinusitis is extremely common and afflicts some people with every bout of the common cold. In many people, once a tendency toward sinusitis develops, the condition recurs with each viral infection.

Cause   Sinusitis is often caused by infection spreading from the nose along the narrow passages that drain mucus from the sinuses into the nose. As the nasal mucous membranes swell, the openings from the sinuses to the nose may be blocked. This leads to a buildup of sinus secretions, often teeming with bacteria. The disorder is usually caused by a bacterial infection that develops as a complication of a viral infection (such as the common cold). (See COLD, COMMON.) It is also possible that an infection may occur from an abscess in an upper tooth or from infected water forced into the sinuses while swimming.

Symptoms   Pressure, throbbing headache, fever, and local tenderness, together with a feeling of fullness or tension. It may also cause a stuffy nose and loss of the ability to smell.

Complication   Often, sinusitis leads to the formation of pus in the affected sinuses, causing pain and a nasal discharge. Other more rare complications include orbital CELLULITIS, OSTEOMYELITIS, and MENINGITIS.

Diagnosis   X rays may be taken to determine the location and extent of the disorder, and a culture may be grown from a swab of the sinus to identify the bacteria.

Treatment   Steam inhalations, nasal decongestants, painkillers, and antibiotics.

Surgery to improve drainage may be performed for chronic problems.

sixth disease   See ROSEOLA.

skin infections   Because the skin represents the outer barrier to the world, it is responsible for defending the interior of the body against a wide range of attackers, including bacteria, viruses, insect venom, and fungi. Skin infections can range from a local superficial problem (such as IMPETIGO) to a widespread and possibly fatal infection.

Examples of bacterial skin infections include impetigo, ECTHYMA, FOLLICULITIS, BOILS, CARBUNCLES, ERYSIPELAS, SCARLET FEVER, CELLULITIS, etc. Viral infections with skin symptoms include HERPES SIMPLEX, CHICKEN-POX, and SHINGLES, WARTS, MEASLES, GERMAN MEASLES, FIFTH DISEASE, AIDS, etc.

sleeping sickness   The common name for African TRYPANOSOMIASIS, a serious infectious disease of tropical Africa caused by parasites transmitted by the bite of infected TSETSE FLIES. About 20,000 cases are reported worldwide each year.

Cause   East Africa's version of sleeping sickness is caused by the parasite *Trypanosoma brucei rhodesiense* and is spread mainly to wild animals, only rarely affecting humans. West Africa's chronic *gambiense* variety (caused by the *T. brucei gambiense*) may not cause the "sleeping" part of the illness until years after exposure. This variety is spread primarily from person to person. Within humans, the parasites multiply and spread to the bloodstream, lymph nodes, heart, and brain.

Symptoms   With both versions of sleeping sickness, a painful nodule develops at the site of the fly bite. In the West African version, the disease progresses slowly with bouts of fever and lymph gland enlargement. After a period of months or years, the parasites invade the tiny blood vessels supplying the central nervous system. This causes the legendary

drowsiness, lethargy, and sleepiness. The patient may become completely inactive, with drooping eyelids and a vacant expression (hence, the term *sleeping sickness*). If untreated at this point, the patient may die. The East African form is more virulent; a severe fever develops within a few weeks of infection and effects on the heart may be fatal before the disease gets to the brain.

Diagnosis   Microscopic examination of the blood, lymph fluid, or cerebrospinal fluid reveals the presence of the parasites.

Treatment   The drug Suramin (available from the Centers for Disease Control) can treat both versions of African sleeping sickness. Melarsoprol (a derivative of arsenic) is available from the CDC to treat final stages of both versions. If the patient is known to have the *gambiense* variety, the drug eflornithine (approved by the FDA) is more effective and safer.

Melarsoprol can cause serious or fatal nervous system problems in some patients, according to the FDA. Eflornithine is useful for both early and late stages of *gambiense* sleeping sickness; it is not effective for the *rhodesiense* variety. It works by interfering with the parasite's growth. In most cases, a complete cure is possible, although there may be brain damage if the infection has already spread to the brain.

Prevention   Eradication of tsetse flies can help prevent spread of this disease. Visitors to rural parts of Africa should take measures to protect against tsetse fly bites.

smallpox   A highly infectious serious viral disease (causing skin rash and flulike symptoms) that has been totally eradicated since 1980. A common scourge of the 19th century, smallpox was characterized by a rash that spread over the body, turning into pus-filled blisters that crusted and sometimes left deeply pitted scars. Complications included blindness, pneumonia, and kidney damage. There is no effective treatment for the disease, which kills up to 40 percent of patients.

Smallpox was eradicated through a cooperative international vaccination program. The disease affects only humans, and its victims are easily recognized and only infectious for a short time. As a result of the successful eradication program, smallpox vaccination certificates are no longer required for international travel. Most countries have stopped vaccination because the vaccine itself is now more dangerous than the disease, since the vaccine can cause ENCEPHALITIS and there is now no chance of contracting smallpox.

The virus responsible for smallpox is still maintained at laboratories in Moscow and at the Centers for Disease Control in Atlanta. Some experts suggested that the virus be destroyed, but that idea was met by such criticism among the scientific community that any decision to do so has been postponed.

snail fever   See SCHISTOSOMIASIS.

sore throat   A scratchy, painful throat often accompanying a cold or other infection and caused by a variety of organisms.

Complications   Although a sore throat in itself is not serious, it may indicate a bacterial infection, such as a strep throat: swollen/tender lymph nodes in the neck, fever for more than two days, and pain with swallowing.

Spanish flu   See INFLUENZA.

WARNING SIGNS—EPIGLOTTITIS

It may be more than just a sore throat. If any of the following signs are present, they may signal the onset of EPIGLOTTITIS, which is a medical emergency in children.

- sudden severe pain in throat
- refusal to swallow
- uncontrolled drooling
- difficulty breathing
- especially harsh sounds when breathing in

---

spinal meningitis   See MENINGITIS, MENINGOCOCCAL.

spinal tap   The common name for a lumbar puncture, a procedure in which cerebrospinal fluid is removed by using a hollow needle inserted into the lower back, usually between the third and fourth lumbar vertebrae. In infectious diseases, the main use of the spinal tap is to examine the fluid to diagnose infections of the brain and spinal cord, such as MENINGITIS.

The fluid is checked for appearance, white blood cells, sugar, and protein. Examined on a slide in the lab, the fluid is also sent for a special test to help determine what sort of germ is causing symptoms. After the tap is done, the needle is removed, the puncture site is covered with a sterile tape, and the patient must lie flat for at least an hour to prevent a headache. The procedure itself, however, usually takes less than 20 minutes.

While some people fear the thought of a spinal tap, in fact the procedure is only mildly uncomfortable.

Spirillum minus   A species of bacteria in the *Spirillum* genus that causes RAT-BITE FEVER.

spirochetes   Slender, coiled bacterial organisms that lack a rigid cell wall and move by flexing their coils. Spirochetes used to be considered protozoa, but they are now classified as bacteria of the Spirochaetales. They include the species *Borrelia, Leptospira,* and *Treponema.*

sporotrichosis   A chronic fungal infection of the skin that often follows trauma, characterized by painful abscesses and ulcers. The fungus affects both men and women who come in contact with the fungus through soil, vegetation, plants, or decaying vegetables.

Cause   Sporotrichosis is caused by the fungus *Sporothrix schenckii.* Outbreaks are common among those who handle sphagnum moss, baled hay, or thorny plants. A number of recent cases have occurred among nursery workers (especially those who handle sphagnum moss topiaries). The fungus enters the skin through a small cut or puncture from thorns, barbs, pine needles, or wires; it can't be spread from one person to another.

Symptoms There are several forms of the disorder; most patients develop an acute skin condition beginning with a small, painless bump that looks something like an insect bite. It may be red, purple, or pink and usually appears on the finger, hand, or arm at the site where the fungus first entered the skin. The first bump may be followed by one or more bumps, which may resemble boils. The infection can spread to other parts of the body.

While it is possible for the infection to spread to joints, lungs, and central nervous system, this is very rare. Such systemic infections can be fatal. Usually, this occurs only with those who have a disorder of the immune system.

Symptoms may appear any time from 1 to 12 weeks after exposure; usually, however, the bumps appear within three weeks from the time the fungus enters the skin.

Diagnosis Sporotrichosis is confirmed by culturing the fungus from a swab of the pus or biopsy of a freshly opened skin bump that has been cultured in a lab.

Treatment Droplets of potassium iodide for six weeks is the usual method of treatment. The drug itraconazole (Sporanox) may be prescribed, but experience with this drug is still limited. Amphotericin B and flucytosine also have been used to treat the disease.

Prevention Wearing gloves and long sleeves when handling wires, rose bushes, hay bales, pine seedlings, or other materials may help, since it protects against minor skin breaks. It's a good idea to avoid skin contact with sphagnum moss, since moss has been implicated as a source of the fungus in a number of outbreaks.

St. Anthony's fire The common name for ERYSIPELAS, a potentially fatal streptococcal infection of the skin characterized by red oozing swellings on the face with blistering of the skin and headache. Severe cases require hospitalization and intravenous antibiotics.

staphylococcal infections A group of infections caused by staphylococci bacteria that is characterized by the formation of abscesses in the skin or other organs. Staphylococci, which grow in grapelike clusters, are a common cause of skin infections—but they can also cause serious internal disorders.

Staphylococcal bacteria are normally found on the skin of most people, but if the bacteria get trapped within the skin by blocked sweat or sebaceous glands, they can cause a wide variety of skin infections including pustules, BOILS, STYES, or CARBUNCLES. The bacteria can cause a severe blistering rash in newborn babies called STAPHYLOCOCCAL SCALDED SKIN SYNDROME.

This type of bacteria also is found in the throats and nose in most people; when mucus is not cleared from the lungs (such as after a viral infection), organisms can build up in the lungs and cause PNEUMONIA.

Staphylococcal infections are among the most common infections in surgical patients, according to the Centers for Disease Control and Prevention. More troubling still, the percentage of hospital-acquired staph infections that are resistant to antibiotics has risen from under 5 percent in 1982 to more than 25 percent in 1992.

BACTEREMIA (bacteria in the blood) caused by a staph infection is common and may lead to endocarditis (a type of heart disease), MENINGITIS, or bone infection (OSTEOMYELITIS). Untreated, multiplying bacteria in the blood (SEPTICEMIA) can lead to fatal cases of SEPTIC SHOCK. Staphylococcal pneumonia may follow a viral disease (such as INFLUENZA). Acute GASTROENTERITIS (food poisoning) may be caused by a toxin produced by certain species of staphylococci in contaminated food.

Among menstruating women (especially those who use highly absorbent tampons), toxin-producing staph may multiply in the mucous membranes lining the vagina, causing TOXIC SHOCK SYNDROME. A separate type of staph infection can cause URINARY TRACT INFECTIONS.

Treatment for these types of bacterial infections usually includes bed rest, painkillers, and an antimicrobial drug that is resistant to penicillinase (an enzyme secreted by many species of *Staphylococcus*). Surgical drainage of deep abscesses may be necessary. See also HOSPITAL-ACQUIRED INFECTIONS; VANCOMYCIN-RESISTANT ENTEROCOCI (VRE).

staphylococcal scalded skin syndrome (SSSS) A blistering skin rash in newborns that is caused by toxins on the skin released by staphylococcal bacteria. The disorder primarily affects infants between one to three months of age and occasionally older children and adults.

First recognized as a distinct condition in the mid-1800s, this disease has been incorrectly called by many different names, including Ritter's disease, toxic epidermal necrolysis, and pemphigus neonatorum.

The fatality rate is less than 4 percent. Epidemics have occurred in contaminated nurseries, and the bacteria may be transmitted by a carrier who has no symptoms. The condition has also been reported among adults, most of whom had poorly functioning immune systems.

Cause Recently, scientists discovered the cause of this condition to be a toxin-producing strain of *Staphylococcus aureus*. Infants with poor immunity or kidney problems are more vulnerable to this infection.

Symptoms The skin rash strongly resembles a burn, with blistering and peeling of the skin giving a scalded appearance. Indeed, some parents have been wrongly accused of child abuse in the face of the symptoms of this disease. First symptoms usually include evidence of a primary staph infection, including IMPETIGO, eye infection, EAR INFECTION, or SORE THROAT with fever, malaise, or irritability. The skin of the face becomes tender, and the skin around the mouth becomes reddened, weeping, and crusting in a way that resembles potato chips. The trunk also may become involved.

In some patients the rash stabilizes, whereas in other cases flaccid blisters begin to develop all over the skin within 24 to 48 hours. Large areas of skin slough off, and hair or nails may be lost.

Treatment The condition is treated with prompt administration of antistaphylococcal antibiotics. Patients often appear very ill with dehydration; they are at risk of secondary infection. The skin should be covered with wet dressings and antibiotic ointments such as bacitracin. Patients usually heal without scarring within a week.

It is important to maintain correct body temperature; infants must be kept warm, but any sudden rise in body temperature could indicate blood infection and the immediate need for more aggressive treatment. The skin should be loosely clothed and covered so as to reduce friction. Cotton should be inserted between affected fingers and toes to prevent scarring. Warm baths and soaks help healing and gentle removal of peeling skin will help. Scars from this condition rarely occur.

Staphylococcus aureus A species of *Staphylococcus* that is responsible for a number of infections such as the BOIL, CARBUNCLE, ABSCESS, CELLULITIS, sepsis, and OSTEOMYELITIS.

STD See SEXUALLY TRANSMITTED DISEASE.

sterilization The complete elimination or destruction of all forms of microbial life. In hospitals, equipment is sterilized with steam, dry heat, gas, or liquid chemicals. Sterilization is rarely needed at home. For most in-home needs (such as bottles and nipples for babies), heating by boiling (DISINFECTION) is sufficient.

steroids See CORTICOSTEROID DRUGS.

St. Louis encephalitis See ENCEPHALITIS, ST. LOUIS.

strep throat (streptococcal pharyngitis) A bacterial throat infection caused by *group A beta-hemolytic Streptococcus*, a circular bacterium also known as *Streptococcus pyogenes*. Only group-A strep causes the infection known as strep throat; most kinds of sore throats are *not* strep.

Strep throat occurs all over the world, usually affecting school-age children in winter and spring in the temperate zones of North America. Some people seem to have a tendency toward multiple strep throat infections, while others rarely come down with the disease. It is rare in youngsters under age three.

Because there are many types of group-A strep bacteria, one bout of strep throat does not confer long-term immunity; patients can therefore come down with repeated episodes. Adults may be immune to some types of group-A strep and therefore have fewer infections.

Cause While some people carry group A strep in their throats and nasal passages, they remain healthy; however, they can spread the infection to others, as can those who are actively ill. However, you cannot catch strep throat from touching the clothing of an infected person. A sneeze or a cough can project the organisms up to two feet, so it spreads easily in schools and group living situations.

Some epidemics have been traced to infected health care workers in operating rooms and to infected food handlers; other outbreaks have occurred by eating contaminated food.

Patients are most infectious in the beginning of the illness; untreated, a patient is infectious for 10 days to 3 weeks. Carriers are infectious for two to three weeks, although the bacteria may be carried in nose and throat for weeks to several months. Those who receive PENICILLIN are no longer infectious after 24 hours. This means that a child with strep can go back to school or child care one to two days after receiving penicillin, if they feel well and have no fever.

Symptoms Up to half of all children with strep throat have no symptoms but are considered healthy carriers. In those who do have symptoms, they will appear within one to three days after infection. Young children often have high fevers and red, swollen throats, but their throats are actually less painful than those of adults with the same infection. A few children (1 in 10) become quite ill, with extremely high fevers, nausea, and vomiting. Such a severe reaction is rare, however. Most people have a sore throat, fever, and pain in swallowing.

A strep throat is different from a run-of-the-mill sore throat that comes along with a cold or the flu. With strep throat, there is no runny nose or cough, and symptoms appear abruptly with a fever as high as 104 degrees F, headache, stomach ache, and a red, swollen throat. By the second day, the throat and tonsils may be covered with white or yellow patches that spread together to cover the entire throat. However, it is possible to have a strep throat *without* these telltale white patches, or even without a fever.

Most people also have swollen lymph glands in the front of the neck, just below the point where the ear and jawbone meet. These glands may remain swollen for up to a month after recovery from the infection.

Diagnosis Because almost all of the symptoms of strep throat also can occur with viral infections, lab tests are needed to confirm the diagnosis. Anyone who suspects strep throat should see a doctor for a throat culture or rapid test. A throat culture is the best, most accurate test. Rapid strep tests are also widely used, and can give results within three minutes.

Treatment A positive strep test requires antibiotic treatment to prevent complications. Antibiotics (penicillin) given seven to nine days after the illness starts will prevent RHEUMATIC FEVER. Benzathine penicillin G is usually injected, since this type of penicillin stays in the body for 10 days. Oral penicillin V must be taken four times a day for 10 days; some studies suggest that oral penicillin may lead to more relapses. Those who are allergic to penicillin may take erythromycin. Oral cephalexin and other new drugs are also effective but more expensive.

These bacteria are often resistant to tetracycline or sulfonamide.

High fevers may be treated with acetaminophen. Easy-to-swallow foods or cold food (ice cream, frozen juice bars, warm soup, mashed bananas, puddings, gelatins, noodles, soft drinks) are good choices.

Gargling with warm salt water and warm tea with honey and lemon are effective pain reducers. It is not important if the patient doesn't want to eat, but fluids are critical.

Complications The risk of severe complications is the primary concern with strep throat, and the reason why it is so important to be properly diagnosed and treated. One of the most serious complications is rheumatic fever, a disease that affects up to 3 percent of those with untreated strep infection. Rheumatic fever can lead to rheumatic heart disease.

Kidney inflammation (acute glomerulonephritis) is another possible complication of strep throat, which can appear from 10 days to 6 weeks after the throat infection. The bacteria do not directly infect the kidneys; instead, the body's immune system response can damage the kidney's filtering mechanism. Warning signs of impending kidney problems include swelling of hands, face, and feet; dark or bloody urine; headaches; vision problems; and decreased urinary output. Children usu-

---

WARNING SIGNS OF COMPLICATIONS IN STREP THROAT

The doctor should be notified immediately if any of the following symptoms occur:

- breathing problems
- dark, murky urine
- drooling in older child
- extreme problems in swallowing
- fever that goes away and then returns
- headache
- high fever, above 105 degrees F
- joint pain
- less urine than normal
- no improvement in two days
- rash
- seal-bark cough
- vision changes

---

ally recover albeit slowly, but adults may suffer permanent kidney damage.

EAR INFECTIONS are another possible complication of untreated strep throat.

SCARLET FEVER (scarlatina) is an uncommon strep infection that may follow untreated strep throat within two days, producing a fever and a fine red rash over the upper body. With antibiotics, recovery is complete within two weeks, although skin may peel on fingers and toes afterward. A severe form of scarlet fever can cause serious illness, including high fever, convulsions, and death.

Prevention Stay away from anyone with strep throat who has not received antibiotics. Children with strep should not be sent to school until they have taken antibiotics for 24 hours or if there is still a fever and sore throat.

Streptobacillus moniliformis A species of necklace-shaped bacteria that cause RAT-BITE FEVER in humans.

streptococcal infections A group of infections caused by bacteria of the Streptococcus family, among the most common bacteria in humans. These infections are responsible for a wide range of health problems, including such skin conditions as ERYSIPELAS, SCARLET FEVER, or wound infections.

The name *streptococcus* was first used in 1874, meaning "twisted chain of berries," and refers to the fact that the bacteria grow in long linked chains like strung beads.

Some types of strep bacteria exist harmlessly in the throat; if the bacteria gets in the bloodstream, they are usually destroyed—unless the patient has a heart condition, which may lead to bacterial endocarditis Other types of strep bacteria can lead to sore throats, TONSILLITIS, EAR INFECTIONS, STREP THROAT, or PNEUMONIA. This same bacteria may lead to the serious complications of RHEUMATIC FEVER. Another type of harmless strep is found in the intestines, but if the bacteria gain access to the urinary system, they can cause a URINARY TRACT INFECTION.

Common throughout the world in school-aged youngsters, incidence of infections have decreased since the beginning of this century. The danger of resistance to antibiotics were of little concern with these infections until the 1970s, when penicillin-resistant strains of strep bacteria began to crop up. As strep-A infections became less worrisome, strep-B infections became more virulent; then in the 1980s, strep A became more dangerous again; a much stronger *S. pneumoniae* is part of this resurging tide of infection. By 1993, Kentucky pediatricians reported that 28 percent of *S. pneumoniae* cultures from children with acute ear infections were drug resistant.

streptococcal pharyngitis   See STREP THROAT.

Streptococcus   A genus of gram-positive bacteria classified by letters from A to T. The various species occur in pairs, short chains, and chains. Many of the species can cause disease in humans. See also STREPTOCOCCAL INFECTIONS; STREP THROAT.

streptococcus, group A (GAS)   Group-A strep are bacteria that are responsible for most cases of strep illness. Many people carry the bacteria in the throat or skin and have no symptoms at all. When symptoms do occur, they cause relatively mild illnesses. Other strep serogroups (B, C, D, and G) may also cause infection. Group-B strep cause most of the strep infections in newborns and mothers who have just delivered.

Syndromes caused by group-A strep include STREP THROAT (SCARLET FEVER and RHEUMATIC FEVER are rare complications, usually preceded by a sore throat); skin infections (ERYSIPELAS/CELLULITIS and IMPETIGO), and PNEUMONIA.

Occasionally, group-A bacteria can cause much more severe—even life-threatening—diseases, such as necrotizing fasciitis (FLESH-EATING BACTERIA), BACTEREMIA, and streptococcal TOXIC SHOCK SYNDROME (STSS).

Invasive GAS disease is a severe, sometimes life-threatening infection in which the bacteria have spread to other parts of the body, such as the blood, muscle, and fat tissue or the lungs. Two of the most severe (but least common) forms are necrotizing fasciitis (infection of muscle and fat tissue) and toxic shock syndrome. About 20 percent of patients with necrotizing fasciitis and 60 percent of those with STSS will die; only 10 to 15 percent of those with other forms of invasive group-A strep die.

About 10,000 to 15,000 cases of invasive GAS occur in the United States each year, causing more than 2,000 deaths. The Centers for Disease Control estimates between 500 and 1,500 cases of necrotizing fasciitis and 2,000 to 3,000 cases of STSS each year in the United States; on the other hand, there are several million cases of strep throat and impetigo each year.

Cause Invasive GAS disease occurs when the bacteria gets past the body's immune defenses. The germs are spread by direct contact with nose and throat discharge, or by touching infected skin lesions. The seriousness of the infection is greatest when the person is ill or has an infected wound. Health conditions that impair the immune system make infection with GAS more likely. In addition, there are some strains of GAS that are more likely to cause serious disease.

Most of the people who come in contact with a virulent strain of GAS still won't develop invasive disease; most will have a simple throat or skin infection. Some may not have any symptoms at all. While it's possible for a healthy person to contract invasive GAS, it is people with chronic conditions such as cancer, diabetes, or kidney dialysis, or who use steroid medications, who are at highest risk.

There have been no reports of casual contacts (such as coworkers or classmates) of infected patients developing invasive GAS disease after contact with a patient. However, occasionally close family contacts *have* developed severe disease. There are no current recommendations regarding whether close family contacts should be tested and treated for disease if a family member becomes ill.

Treatment Group-A strep bacteria can be treated with common antibiotics; PENICILLIN is the drug of choice for both mild and severe disease. Erythromycin drugs are used in those allergic to penicillin. In addition to antibiotics, supportive care is needed. In severe tissue infections, surgery may be needed to remove dead skin. Early treatment can reduce the threat of death, although even the best therapy may not prevent death in every case.

Prevention Hand washing may help stop the spread of all types of group-A strep infections, especially after coughing or sneezing, and before preparing food. Those with a strep throat should stay home from work or school or day care until 24 hours after taking an antibiotic. Wounds should be cleansed and watched for signs of possible infection.

Early signs and symptoms of necrotizing fasciitis include fever, severe pain and swelling, redness at wound site. Early signs of STSS include fever, dizziness, confusion, rash, and abdominal pain.

streptococcus, group B (GBS) Group-B streptococcus (GBS) is a type of bacteria that causes illness in pregnant women, newborns, the elderly, and those with impaired immune systems. It is also the most common cause of life-threatening infections in newborns.

GBS is the most common cause of blood infection (sepsis) and MENINGITIS (infection of the fluid and lining of the brain) in newborns and is a frequent cause of newborn PNEUMONIA. About 8,000 infants in the United States are infected each year, and up to 15 percent of these infants die. Those who survive (especially those who have meningitis) may have problems, including hearing or vision loss or learning disabilities.

In pregnant women, GBS can cause URINARY TRACT INFECTIONS, endometritis, and stillbirth. Other common diseases caused by GBS include blood infections, skin or soft tissue infections, and pneumonia. About 20 percent of men and nonpregnant women with GBS infections will die.

Cause While many people carry GBS in their bodies (in bowel, genitals, urinary tract, throat, or lungs), most don't get sick. Between 15 and 40 percent of all pregnant women have GBS in the rectum or vagina.

Symptoms About 2 percent of infants infected with GBS develop symptoms, most appearing during the first week of life—usually within a few hours after birth. It's also possible for infants to contract GBS several months after birth; meningitis is more common with this type of late-onset disease.

Diagnosis GBS can be diagnosed by growing bacteria from spinal fluid or blood cultures, which can take a few days.

Treatment Antibiotics (penicillin or ampicillin) are the treatment of choice.

Prevention Most GBS among newborns can be prevented by giving certain pregnant women antibiotics intravenously during labor. Any pregnant woman who has had a baby with GBS disease or who has a urinary tract infection caused by GBS should receive antibiotics during labor. Women who have been diagnosed with GBS infection at labor are at higher risk if they have fever during labor, rupture of membranes 18 hours or more before delivery, and labor or rupture of membranes before 37 weeks. Women who have GBS but don't have these risk factors have a relatively low chance of delivering a baby with GBS disease.

Unfortunately, some babies still get GBS in spite of testing and antibiotics. Vaccines to prevent GBS disease are being developed.

Streptococcus pneumoniae Any of 70 different types of pneumococci that can cause PNEUMONIA and other diseases in humans. This type of bacteria is one of the most common and clinically important bacterial germs. More and more strains of this bacteria are appearing to be moderately to highly resistant to PENICILLIN.

The most common infections caused by *S. pneumoniae* include SINUSITIS, BRONCHITIS, and pneumonia, followed by BACTEREMIA and MENINGITIS. Other, more unusual infections include soft tissue infection. Pneumococci may also rarely cause pericarditis or endocarditis.

Streptococcus pyogenes Another name for a type of B hemolytic strep group-A strep).

strongyloidiasis An intestinal infestation of tiny parasitic roundworms that cause itching and raised red patches where the worms enter the skin. The disease, caused by *Strongyloides stercoralis*, is found throughout the tropics, especially in the Far East. The worms are picked up by walking barefoot on soil contaminated with feces; the larvae enter the skin of the feet and migrate to the small intestines, where they develop into adulthood, burrowing into the intestinal walls and producing larvae.

Symptoms After infestation, the worms cause redness, swelling, itching, or hives, that fade within two days. If the larvae penetrate the perianal area, skin lesions begin to radiate from the anus down the thigh or across the buttocks or abdomen as itchy bands. While the individual lesions may fade away within a few days, an infestation may continue in the host for many years and cause recurrent problems.

Complications Rarely, death may occur from blood poisoning or MENINGITIS many years after the worms enter the body. PNEUMONIA may occur because of immune system damage.

Treatment Thiabendazole is the drug of choice.

stye (sty) A small pus-filled ABSCESS (also called a hordeolum) near the eyelashes caused by a bacterial infection.

Cause Stye is often caused by a staphylococcal organism.

Symptoms Pus-filled swollen bump near the eyelashes that can be reddened and painful.

Treatment If the stye is painful, warm compresses may help eliminate the pain; antibiotic ointment designed for the eyes can help prevent a recurrence.

sulfonamides (sulfa drugs) A large group of synthetic drugs used to treat bacterial infections derived from a red dye (sulfanilamide). Drugs in this class prevent the growth of bacteria; they do not *kill* bacteria. Used in combination with other drugs, they are used to treat a wide variety of conditions such as URINARY TRACT INFECTIONS, BRONCHITIS, PNEUMONIA, skin infections, and EAR INFECTIONS. Most (including sulfamethoxazole and sulfaphenazole) are quickly absorbed from the stomach and small intestine and should be taken at regular intervals. Others are long-acting (such as sulfadoxine, used to treat LEPROSY and MALARIA) and only need to be taken once a day.

Side effects Side effects may include anemia or jaundice, especially if taken for longer than 10 days. More severe side effects include blood disorders, skin rashes, and fever. These drugs are not given during the last trimester of pregnancy or to young babies because of the risk of mental retardation. The drugs are prescribed with caution to patients with kidney or liver problems. In general, patients using these drugs should avoid exposure to direct sunlight, which could provoke a rash.

sweating sickness, English A contagious disease that appeared in the 15th century that struck and killed victims quickly and violently. It is believed to have been introduced into England by French soldiers recruited by King Henry VII for his army in 1485. Subsequent outbreaks occurred in 1507, 1516, 1529, and 1551. Unlike most other epidemics of infectious diseases, its appearance was relatively brief, and it permanently disappeared in 1551.

Unlike other infectious epidemics of the 14th and 15th centuries, which tended to strike the poor, the English sweating sickness struck the wealthy with equal vengeance. The most famous victim of "the sweat" was Cardinal Thomas Wolsey of England, who came down with the disease three times in 1517, but survived each time. Also infected were the aldermen and two lord mayors of London, both of whom died within a week during the epidemic of 1485. During this first epidemic, the royal court issued a decree forbidding anyone from appearing at court except on official business.

While it is difficult to tell for sure how many people died from this epidemic, it is believed that the sweats of 1485 and 1507 each killed 10,000 people throughout England. The sweat of 1551 was particularly severe in Devon and Essex.

Although the sweat resembled INFLUENZA, SCARLET FEVER, and the PLAGUE, medical historians have not been able to identify it. Although some experts believed it to be a lesser form of plague, it remains an unsolved medical puzzle.

Striking with fearsome rapidity, the disease lasted only about 24 hours and produced a profuse and drenching sweat from head to foot, together with pains in the back, shoulder, arms, legs, and head, as well as intestinal problems and "passion" in the heart. Reportedly, the disease could kill in as little as two hours.

While primarily a disease of England, it also occurred in Germany, Scandinavia, Poland, Lithuania, Russia, and the Netherlands. Angry German Catholics swore the disease was God's retribution for Martin Luther's Protestant heresies. The disease never spread into Spain or Italy.

swimmer's ear See OTITIS EXTERNA.

swimmer's itch The common name for cutaneous SCHISTOSOMIASIS (or cercarial dermatitis), this is an itchy skin inflammation caused by bites from flatworms. It is characterized by a distinctive patchy, red pinpoint skin rash after swimming in or having contact with freshwater populated by ducks and snails. On the saltwater tributaries of Long Island Sound it is known as "clamdigger's itch"; it is called "duck-feces dermatitis" or "sawah itch" in rice paddy workers of China or Malaysia.

This type of dermatitis is a potential risk whenever people use an aquatic area with animals and mollusks who are infested with the flatworms. In the United States, the worst outbreaks occur in the lake regions of Michigan, Wisconsin, and Minnesota, although it may also occur in saltwater areas.

Cause   The rash is caused by the flatworm parasites of migrating birds and mammals; the animal defecates the worm into the water; snails ingest the worm; when the larval parasites are released from infected snails, they migrate through water, where they can infect swimmers. Children are most often infected due to their swimming habits. If the victim swims or wades in infested water and then allows water to evaporate off the skin instead of regularly drying off with a towel, the parasites can then burrow under the skin. The problem occurs in summer when the water temperature reaches the right level for snails to reproduce and grow rapidly. At the same time, migrating birds infected with the parasite return from their winter habitats, and swimmers enter the water.

Symptoms   After exposure to water affected by the schistosomes, a prickling or itchy feeling begins that can last up to an hour while the flukes enter the skin. Small red macules form, but there may be swelling or wheals among sensitive people. As these lesions begin to disappear, they are replaced after 10 or 15 hours by discrete, very itchy papules surrounded by a red area. Vesicles and pustules form one or two days later; the lesions fade away within a week, leaving small pigmented spots. Different symptoms depend on how sensitive the patient is to the schistosome; each reexposure causes a more severe reaction.

Diagnosis   Diagnosis is difficult; skin biopsies are not helpful. There is no widely available blood test that gives a specific indication that cercariae are the source of the itch. Diseases that have been confused with swimmer's itch include IMPETIGO, CHICKENPOX, poison ivy, or HERPES.

Treatment   Treatment may not be needed if there are only a few itchy spots. Calamine lotion or oral antihistamines may help control the itch until the lesions begin to disappear on their own. If symptoms persist for more than three days, consult a doctor.

Prevention   The best way to alleviate the problem is to destroy the snails by treating the water with copper sulfate and carbonate or with sodium pentachlorophenate. A thick coating of grease or tightly woven clothes can protect against infestation; bathing with a hexachlorophene soap before swimming may help to some degree. Briskly rubbing the skin with a towel after swimming may help remove some organisms.

syphilis   A sexually transmitted infection that causes (among other symptoms) a skin sore and rash. Also present as a congenital (at birth) infection, syphilis was first recorded as a major epidemic in Europe during the 15th century, after Columbus returned from his trip to America. Today, the infection is transmitted almost exclusively by sexual contact. Since the 1970s and early 1980s, the incidence of syphilis in the United States has been on the rise.

Cause   Syphilis is caused by a spirochete *Treponema pallidum* that enters broken skin or mucous membranes during sexual intercourse, by kissing, or by intimate bodily contact with an open syphilitic sore. The rate of infection during a single contact with an infected person is about 30 percent.

Symptoms   During the first (or *primary*) stage, a sore (chancre) appears between three to four weeks after contact; the sore has a hard, wet, painless base that heals in about a month. In males, the sore appears on the shaft of the penis. In women it can be found on the labia, although it is often hidden so well that the diagnosis is missed. In both sexes, the sore may be seen on the lips or tongue.

Six to 12 weeks after infection, the patient enters the *secondary* stage, which features a skin rash that may last for months. The rash has crops of pink or pale red round spots, but in black patients the rash is pigmented and appears darker than normal skin. In addition, the lymph nodes may be enlarged, and there may be backache, headache, bone pain, appetite loss, fever, fatigue, and sometimes meningitis. The hair may fall out and the skin may exhibit gray or pink patches that are highly infectious. The secondary stage may last up to a year.

The *latent* stage may last for a few years or until the end of a person's life. During this time, the infected person appears normal; about 30 percent of these patients will develop tertiary syphilis.

Tertiary syphilis (end stage) usually begins about 10 years after the initial infection, although it may appear after only about 3 years or as late as 25 years later. The person's tissues may begin to deteriorate (a process called gumma formation), involving the bones, palate, nasal septum, tongue, skin, or any organ of the body. The most serious complications in this stage include heart problems, brain damage (neurosyphilis) leading to insanity, and paralysis.

Treatment PENICILLIN is the drug of choice for all forms of the disease; early syphilis can often be cured by a single large injection; later forms of the disease require multiple doses of penicillin over time. More than half of syphilis patients treated with penicillin develop a severe reaction within 6 to 12 hours caused by the body's response to the sudden killing of large numbers of spirochetes.

Prevention Infection can be avoided by maintaining monogamous relationships; condoms offer some protection, but they are not absolutely safe. People with syphilis are infectious during the primary and secondary stages, but not in the latter stages of the latent and tertiary stages.

taeniasis See TAPEWORM.

tapeworm A parasitic intestinal worm that belongs to the class Cestoda. There are three major species of tapeworms, and all are acquired in humans by eating raw, undercooked, or smoked contaminated meat or fish. In most tapeworm infestations, the animal or fish has ingested eggs, which develop into larvae, invading the animal's muscles and organs. A human acquires the infection by eating the infected animal meat.

Beef tapeworm   (Taenia saginata) The beef tapeworm is commonly found in undercooked beef in Mexico, South America, Eastern Europe, the Middle East, and Africa. Symptoms may include stomach pain, diarrhea, and weight loss, although it doesn't usually cause any symptoms. Detached white segments of the worm can emerge spontaneously from the rectum, which is the sign of infestation. Medications are available to treat beef tapeworm.

Pork tapeworm (Taenia Solium)   The pork tapeworm is commonly found in South America, Eastern Europe, Russia, and Asia. Humans can acquire the tapeworm by eating undercooked pork or raw pork sausage. There are not usually any symptoms other than vague abdominal complaints. Diagnosis is made from white translucent segments of the tapeworm in feces.

Pork tapeworm can lead to a serious complication called cystocercosis, a sometimes-fatal disease. In this illness, a person ingests the eggs, and the larvae then penetrate the stomach wall, invading the tissues (especially the skeletal muscle and the brain) where they form cystlike masses. After several years, the cysts begin to degenerate and produce an inflammatory reaction. At this stage the person may experience epileptic seizures or visual or mental disturbances. Treatment includes drug therapy as well as surgical removal of the cysts.

It is important not to EVER eat raw, undercooked, or smoked pork.

Fish tapeworm (diphyllobothriasis) Fish tapeworm occurs after ingesting raw freshwater fish and is found throughout the world. It is particularly common in Scandinavia and the Far East, where consumption of raw fish is high. The infection usually produces a single worm and does not usually cause symptoms other than a vague intestinal discomfort. Pernicious anemia may develop as a result of the worm impairing absorption of vitamin B_{12}. Drug therapy is available.

TB See TUBERCULOSIS.

T cell A type of lymphocyte (white blood cell) involved in the cellular immune response. *Helper T cells* participate in the activation of other T cells; they are targets of the HIV virus, the agent of AIDS. *Suppressor T cells* inhibit the responses of other T cells to antigens. *Cytotoxic T cells* are the cells of the cellular immune system; they recognize and eliminate virus-infected cells.

tetanus An acute, often-fatal infectious disease commonly known as "lockjaw" because the presence of the disease causes the jaw muscles to lock. In the United States, 4 out of every 10 people who get tetanus will die. The disease is not passed from one person to the next because the illness is caused by toxins produced by the bacteria.

Anyone who was not vaccinated as a child or who has not received a booster since then is at risk. The tetanus vaccine has been available since the 1940s, so those born before then may never have been vaccinated.

A previous infection does not confer immunity; it is possible to get tetanus more than once if the victim was not properly immunized with vaccine. Experts suggest repeat vaccination every 10 years.

Cause The disease is caused by a bacterium belonging to the Clostridium family, which thrives in the absence of oxygen and is found almost everywhere in the environment—most commonly in soil, dust, manure, and in the digestive tract of humans and animals. The bacteria form spores, which are thick-walled reproductive cells that are hard to kill and highly resistant to heat and many antiseptics. Tetanus cannot be transmitted from person to person but enters the body via a wound—even as small as a pinprick or tiny scratch. Usually, however, a wound that leads to tetanus is a deep puncture or laceration caused by a nail or a knife; because these wounds are hard to clean, bacteria remains deep within the wound. In the presence of dead tissue, tetanus spores can grow and produce the deadly exotoxin that causes symptoms. While tetanus bacteria are found almost everywhere, natural immunity is rare, which is why immunization is so important.

Most cases are caused by puncture wounds, but it's also possible to contract tetanus from animal scratches and bites, in wounds where the flesh is torn or burned, in crushing wounds, and in frostbite. It may even follow minor wounds such as splinters and can develop after surgery, dental infections, and abortion.

Ear infections can lead to a rare form of tetanus called cephalic tetanus, wherein tetanus bacteria are found in the inner ear. Occasionally, tetanus is also found in those with no known injury, wound, or medical condition.

Symptoms Tetanus affects the central nervous system, producing both stiffness or muscular rigidity and convulsive muscle spasm.

While symptoms usually appear within three days to three weeks after infection, the incubation period can be as long as 50 days. The shorter the incubation period, the greater the risk of death. The first symptoms include headache, irritability, and muscular stiffness in the jaw and neck. As more toxin is produced, the jaw, neck, and limbs become locked in spasms, the abdominal muscles become rigid, and the patient may be racked with painful convulsions. The most common symptom is the telltale stiff jaw, caused by spasm of the muscle that closes the mouth. The affected patient may have other symptoms: difficulty swallowing, restlessness and irritability, fever, headache, and sore throat. As the disease continues, the patient may develop a fixed smile and raised eyebrows because of muscle spasms in the face. Spasms of the diaphragm and the muscles between the ribs may interfere with breathing so that mechanical ventilation may be necessary.

In severe cases, patients become so sensitive to stimulation of any kind (such as a draft or a noise) that their bodies become racked with painful spasms and profuse sweating. These convulsions can be strong enough to break bones.

In addition, overstimulation of the involuntary nervous system may boost blood pressure to dangerous levels or cause irregular heartbeats. Coma may follow repeated convulsions.

Tetanus can be localized so that there are muscle contractions just in the part of the body where the infection began. It can also affect the entire body; about 80 percent of cases are generalized in this latter way.

Treatment Powerful tranquilizers and antispasmodic drugs can control symptoms, which last for several weeks and require intensive hospital care. Tetanus immune globulin can confer passive immunization for a few months. Tetanus victims are also given penicillin IV for two weeks and tetanus toxoid vaccine.

Dead skin from the wound must be removed and any pus drained.

Complications Tetanus complications may include PNEUMONIA, which is found in 50 to 70 percent of fatal cases. Other complications may include bone fractures or simple exhaustion due to the muscle spasms. As the disease worsens, victims cannot open the mouth. Constipation and difficulty passing urine may occur.

In 1947, 91 percent of the 560 people who got tetanus died. In the period from 1989 to 1990, U.S. doctors reported 117 tetanus cases; 25 patients (all over the age of 40) died. Today, the mortality rate in the United States is about 25 percent and 50 percent worldwide.

Prevention Tetanus is totally preventable by routine immunization, which causes the body to respond to an inactivated form of the toxin, producing antitoxin (not antibodies) that neutralizes the toxins. A booster is needed every 10 years. The only side effect of vaccination is a sore arm for a few days.

Primary immunizations are given in combination with diphtheria and pertussis (DPT) at 2, 4, 6, and 15 months of age. A booster is given when a child enters school sometime between age four to six years. Every 10 years after, another booster is needed.

There are few side effects with the vaccine, which is virtually 100 percent effective in preventing tetanus. The DPT shot in children may produce redness or formation of a small hard lump at the site. Some children may have allergic reactions; rarely, serious adverse reactions include rare anaphylaxis (difficulty in breathing or swallowing) and possibly Guillain-Barre syndrome. People who have had a severe reaction should not have any more doses.

Since adults aged 50 or older are responsible for more than 70 percent of tetanus infections, adults must be sure to receive boosters every 10 years.

tetanus immune globulin An injectable solution prepared from the globulin of an immune human that is effective and much safer than tetanus antitoxin. It is administered for short-term immunization against tetanus after possible exposure to tetanus and tetanus treatment.

It should not be substituted for tetanus toxoid (the vaccine that can prevent tetanus). The most serious side effect of immune globulin is an allergic reaction (anaphylaxis). There may also be fever and pain at the injection site.

Thirty Years' War epidemics A wide variety of infectious diseases plagued the soldiers of the Thirty Years' War (1618–48), including TYPHOID FEVER, bubonic PLAGUE, and DYSENTERY. The constant troop movements across Germany led to repeated outbreaks of disease, although a number of local epidemics were unrelated to the war.

Still, many features of the drawn-out conflict boosted the transmission of infectious disease, including the neverending shift of the fronts, the constant troop movements, influx of fresh soldiers from foreign countries, displacement of the German population, and cities swollen with refugees. In this particular war, the extensive contact between soldier and civilian served only to worsen the spread of infectious disease. It has been reported that up to half of the German population died from infections during this war.

throat culture A test to determine the type of organism causing disease in the throat. For this test, a health care worker obtains a specimen from the throat with a long-handled sterile swab. The specimen is placed on a culture plate and read at 24 and 48 hours.

Rapid strep tests are now widely used. These tests react with certain proteins in the bacteria, giving results in just three minutes. They are about 90 percent accurate. Many health care workers do both the rapid test and a backup throat culture to make sure all cases of STREP THROAT are diagnosed.

thrush   A yeast infection of the mouth, found often in infants and young children and in those with an impaired immune system.

Cause   A yeast infection is a fungal infection, but not all fungi are yeasts. In the case of thrush, the yeast that causes the infection is CANDIDA ALBICANS. While there are many different kinds of *Candida* species, albicans causes most human infections and almost all cases of thrush.

An infant may be infected during delivery if its mother has a vaginal yeast infection at birth; infants also may contract thrush from infections on a caregiver's hands or from bottle nipples. Babies born to diabetic mothers are more susceptible to thrush, as are those born with birth defects of the palate or lip. A person is infectious as long as there are lesions in the mouth.

Symptoms   Pain in the mouth area, together with raised patches in the mouth that look like milk curds on cheek and tongue and roof of the mouth.

Diagnosis   Tests aren't needed; the disease can be identified by inspecting the mouth. However, the patches may be swabbed and examined for yeast cells under a microscope; alternatively, the fungus can be cultured.

Treatment   The mouth can be painted with nystatin suspension. Rinsing the mouth often can discourage the spread of thrush.

Prevention   Mothers with the symptoms of yeast infections should be treated in the last three months of pregnancy. No one should put fingers in a new baby's mouth. If the infant is bottle fed, nipples and bottles should be boiled and hands washed before feeding.

Adults with impaired immune systems, including those with AIDS or patients taking corticosteroid drugs, should be careful to brush the mouth and tongue regularly and rinse the mouth often.

ticks and disease   The tiny bloodsucking pests that commonly plague American dogs and cats can also transmit disease to pet owners. These diseases include BABESIOSIS, EHRLICHIOSIS (see EHRLICHIOSIS, HUMAN GRANULOCYTIC), and LYME DISEASE, now epidemic in the northeast. Ticks can also transmit a type of "tick paralysis" in dogs. There are about 200 species of ticks in the United States, found in woods, beach grass, lawns, forests, and cities.

Unlike fleas, ticks are not insects but are arachnids, as are mites, spiders, and scorpions. They have a four-stage life cycle, beginning with eggs, then larvae, nymph, and adult. Adult females of some species lay about 100 eggs at a time; her more prolific cousins can lay between 3,000 and 6,000 eggs. Six-legged larvae hatch from these eggs, and after at least one blood meal, the larvae molt into six-legged nymphs (in some species, this happens more than once). Finally nymphs molt into adult males or females with eight legs.

Depending on its species, a tick may take less than a year or up to several years to travel through its entire four-stage life cycle. Ticks need a blood meal at each stage after hatching; some species can survive years without eating anything.

A vaccine to prevent Lyme disease in dogs was licensed in June 1992 and is recommended for dogs at risk for ticks, not those who live in apartments or who live in regions where Lyme disease is not a problem. In most cases, immunity lasts up to about six months with the vaccine.

In addition, the Environmental Protection Agency has licensed a product, named Damminix, that consists of tubes stuffed with cotton balls treated with the pesticide permethrin. The theory is that the cotton balls mimic the nesting material for deer mice; when placed outdoors in areas inhabited by mice, the cotton kills and repels ticks on the mice. See also EHRLICHIA; EHRLICHIA CHAFFEENSIS; EHRLICHIOSIS, CANINE; EHRLICHIOSIS, EQUINE; EHRLICHIOSIS, HUMAN MONOCYTIC.

tinea Any of a group of common FUNGAL INFECTIONS of the skin, hair, or nails. Most infections are caused by a group of fungi called DERMATOPHYTES and are often called RINGWORM. These common fungus infections are caused by various species of the fungi *Microsporum*, *Trichophyton*, and *Epidermophyton*. Tinea is highly contagious and can be spread by direct contact or via infected material; infections may be picked up from other people or animals, soil, or an object (such as a shower stall). The term *tinea* is often followed by the Latin term for the part of the body affected by the fungus, such as *tinea pedis* (ATHLETE'S FOOT).

Symptoms The symptoms vary according to the part of the body affected by the infection; the most common area is the foot (causing athlete's foot), with cracking, itchy skin between the toes. Tinea cruris (JOCK ITCH) is more common in males and produces a red, itchy area from the genitals outward over the inside of the thighs; tinea corporis (ringworm of the body) is characterized by itchy circular skin patches with a raised edge. Tinea capitis (ringworm of the scalp) causes round, itchy circles of hair loss found most commonly in children in large cities or overcrowded conditions. Tinea unguium (ringworm of the nails, or onychomycosis) is characterized by scaling of soles or palms with thick, white, or yellow nails. Ringworm can also affect the skin under a beard (TINEA BARBAE).

Treatment Antifungal drugs (creams, lotions, or ointments) can successfully treat most types of tinea. For widespread infection (or those affecting hair or nails), the drug is given as a tablet (usually griseofulvin). Treatment should continue after symptoms have faded to ensure the fungi have been destroyed. Mild infections on the surface of the skin may be treated for four to six weeks; toenail infections may require treatment for up to two years.

tinea barbae Ringworm infection of the skin under the beard, caused primarily by *Tinea mentagrophytes* or *T. verrucosum*. See TINEA.

tinea capitis The medical term for RINGWORM of the scalp.

tinea corporis The medical term for RINGWORM of the body.

tinea cruris The medical term for JOCK ITCH.

tinea manuum RINGWORM infection most often caused by *Tinea rubrum*, usually found together with a foot infection. The condition is characterized by thickened outer skin of palms and fingers, especially in the creases of the skin. See also TINEA.

Treatment New topical imidazole antifungals are the treatment of choice, but topical agents alone don't usually cure this problem; an oral antifungal drug (such as griseofulvin, terbinafine, or ketoconazole) is usually required for between two to three months.

tinea nigrapalmaris A superficial RINGWORM infection of the stratum corneum of the palms, although the soles of the feet may also be affected. While the condition is found throughout the world in both men and women of all ages, it is uncommon in North America. Compared to other types of ringworm infections, the incidence of tinea nigrapalmaris is low, even in South America.

While this condition is not fatal, it may mimic malignant melanoma (a type of skin cancer).

Symptoms   The condition is characterized by a single brown-black macule with sharply defined margins (found on the palm or sole) that tend to spread in a circular pattern.

Treatment   Most infections respond to imidazole cream together with removal by scraping with an emery pad. Recurrence is rare. Surgery is not effective, and there are no established oral medications.

tinea pedis   The medical term for ATHLETE'S FOOT.

tinea versicolor   A common fungal skin infection (also known as pityriasis versicolor) characterized by patches of white, brown, or salmon-colored flaky skin on the trunk and neck. It primarily affects young and middle-aged adult men and is not contagious.

Cause   A fungus (living as a yeast on most people's skin) called *Malassezia furfur* causes the condition when it colonizes the dead outer layer of skin.

Symptoms   The infection is characterized by pale tan patches on the upper trunk and upper arms that may itch and do not tan. In dark-skinned people the lesions may be depigmented.

Diagnosis   The patches will show up as fluorescent patches under a special Wood's light and may be easily identified in skin scrapings.

Treatment   Thorough application of antifungal cream or lotion from ears to knees at night will eradicate the fungus, provided not one spot is missed. It is also important to wash underwear and night clothes thoroughly. The treatment will cure the condition, but it may take many months for the skin patches to return to a normal color.

toe web infection   Disorders of the spaces between the toes are usually called ATHLETE'S FOOT, and most are caused by fungal infections. Although the fungus is the primary cause of tissue destruction, subsequent bacterial infiltration can contribute to the problem and interfere with treatment success.

Treatment   Because so many different types of organisms are involved in toe web infections, several different types of treatment must be used in order to be effective. If the lesions are dry and scaly, topical antifungal agents (such as *miconazole*, clotrimazole, or ciclopirox olamine) are effective. For soft, wet lesions, treatment must include removal of excess moisture, daily compresses, broad-spectrum topical antimicrobial agents, long-term use of antifungals, and oral griseofulvin.

tonsillitis   Infection or inflammation of a tonsil caused by a virus or bacteria. Acute tonsillitis is often caused by STREPTOCOCCUS infection. If tonsillitis caused by a strep infection is untreated, it may lead to RHEUMATIC FEVER or kidney disease. Tonsillitis most often occurs in childhood. See also STREP THROAT, PHARYNGITIS.

Cause   The tonsils are believed to help stop infection and protect the upper respiratory tract. However, it is possible for the tonsils themselves to become infected. This happens most often in youngsters under age nine; occasionally, it occurs in teenagers or young adults. Infectious MONONUCLEOSIS often causes tonsillitis.

Symptoms   Severe sore throat, fever, headache, fatigue, swallowing problems, earache, and enlarged, tender lymph nodes in the neck. Acute cases may also be accompanied by SCARLET FEVER. Once in a while, the illness can cause a temporary deafness or an abscess on the tonsil. If symptoms last for longer than 24 hours or if pus is seen on the tonsils, a physician should be consulted.

Treatment Tonsillitis can be treated with systemic antibiotics. While a tonsillectomy is still sometimes performed for recurrent cases, this surgical procedure is done much less often today than it was in earlier decades.

tonsils The tonsils—a mass of oval lymphoid tissue on either side of the back of the mouth—are one of the body's ways of dealing with invading infections. The tonsils make up part of the lymphatic system, an important part of the body's defense system against infection. Along with the adenoids at the base of the tongue, and posterior oropharynx, the tonsils protect against upper respiratory tract infections. They gradually get bigger after birth, reaching full size at about age seven; after that, they shrink substantially.

An infection of the tonsils is called TONSILLITIS, a common infectious disease of childhood. Quinsy (abscess on the tonsil) is a rare complication. While removal of the tonsils because of infection was once a common treatment in childhood, it is rarely done today.

toxic shock syndrome *(TSS)* An uncommon, severe condition characterized by a distinctive skin rash resembling sunburn on the palms and soles. It peels within one or two weeks. TSS is caused by strains of *Staphylococcus aureus* and Group-A/B strep. (See STREPTOCOCCUS, GROUP A and STREPTOCOCCUS, GROUP B.)

The condition, first recognized in the 1970s, is associated with the use of certain brands of highly absorbent tampons (now taken off the market). About 70 percent of cases occur in women who are using tampons when symptoms begin. The FDA estimates that 1 to 17 of every 100,000 menstruating women develop TSS each year.

Scientists first described TSS as a distinct disease in 1978; two years later, reports of the problem increased among young women who had become ill during or just after menstruation. Studies showed that the use of the high-absorbency tampons was associated with the problem, but the exact connection remains unclear.

About 5 percent of TSS cases are fatal. Since 1984, there have been 69 reports of death related to tampon use; all but three resulted from TSS. The risk of death is higher in cases not related to menstruation, according to experts at the Centers for Disease Control.

Cause The condition is caused by a toxin produced by *Staphylococcus aureus*, enterotoxin F. It is most common in menstruating women using high-absorbency tampons but has also been seen in newborns, children, and men. Scientists believe that for TSS to develop, the staph bacteria release one or more toxins into the bloodstream. While the bacteria normally live in the nose, skin, and vagina and cause no problem, they can also lead to serious infection after a deep wound or surgery or during tampon use.

Symptoms Symptoms may not begin until the first few days after a woman's period and tend to appear quickly. In addition to the skin rash, symptoms include sudden high fever, vomiting and diarrhea, headache, muscular aches and pains, dizziness, and disorientation. Blood pressure may drop rapidly, and shock may develop. Death occurs in about three percent of cases, usually due to a prolonged drop in blood pressure or lung problems.

The sunburn-like rash may not develop until the patient is very ill or may go completely unnoticed if it appears on a small area. The skin on palms and soles may flake or peel.

Once a person has had TSS, he or she is more likely to get it again.

Treatment Antibiotic drugs and IV fluids (to prevent shock), plus treatment for any complications as they occur. Recurrence is common; women who have had toxic shock syndrome should not use tampons, cervical caps, diaphragms, or vaginal contraceptive sponges.

Prevention A woman can dramatically reduce the risk of TSS by not using tampons. Because the TSS risk increases with tampon absorbency, it is a good idea to use products with the lowest absorbency possible. To help women compare absorbency from brand to brand, the FDA requires that manufacturers use a standard test to measure absorbency and state the findings on the label. The FDA also requires manufacturers to give information about TSS on the box or in a package insert. This information must include a warning about the association between TSS and high-absorbency tampons.

Toxocara canis One of two types of roundworm, this is the variety found in dogs. *T. canis* is the more infectious of the two, and causes the infestation known as TOXOCARIASIS.

Toxocara cati One of two types of roundworm, this is the variety found in cats. *T. cati* is the less infectious of the two and causes the infestation known as TOXOCARIASIS.

toxocariasis Infection with the larvae of *Toxocara canis* (the common ROUNDWORM of dogs and cats). Children between age one and four who eat dirt are at particular risk for this disease. Older children and adults in households with an infected younger child may show evidence of light infection. The disease is also known as visceral larva migrans.

Cause Ingesting the eggs that are often found in soil leads to the spread of tiny larvae throughout the body. In the United States, dogs are often infected with worms that are passed to them as pups before birth or while nursing. Adult worms pass eggs in the dogs' feces, which then may find their way into soil or sandboxes. These eggs can remain viable

for many weeks—even months. When a child eats soil or sand containing these eggs, the larvae hatch in the child's small intestine, penetrating the intestinal wall and migrating throughout the body. After some time, the larvae in the child will die.

It is also possible to be infected by eating unwashed vegetables grown in contaminated soil. However, humans cannot pass the infection from one to another.

Symptoms Most people have no signs of the infestation, and there is a long incubation period. Children who swallow large numbers of worms may be sick with breathing problems or PNEUMONIA, enlarged liver, fever, anemia, fatigue, skin rash, and eye problems. In rare cases, seizures may develop or the child may lose her eyesight as larvae enter the eye and die there.

Diagnosis An abnormal blood count with a high number of a certain type of white blood cells and antibodies suggest a diagnosis. Tests for specific antibodies to the worm can be obtained from the CDC. The infestation may also be diagnosed by sputum analysis and by a liver biopsy.

Complication If the larvae migrate to the liver, lungs, or abdomen, they can cause an enlarged liver, pneumonia, and stomach pain. They may reach a child's eyes, thus damaging the retina.

Symptoms of complications include breathing problems, rash, and fever.

Treatment There is no specific drug treatment that will cure the infestation. The disease is usually self-limiting even without treatment. In severe cases, the patient should be hospitalized and given the ANTIHELMINTIC DRUG thiabendazole to control the infestation. Anticonvulsant drugs may also be administered. Steroids have helped some people with heart or nervous system problems.

Prevention Worming of pets can help prevent the spread of this disease. All pets at age three weeks should be dewormed, followed by a deworming every two weeks until the pet has had three treatments. They should be checked for worms regularly.

toxoid A bacterial toxin that has been treated with chemicals or with heat to decrease its toxic effect. Inactivation renders the toxin nonpoisonous but preserves its ability to stimulate antibody production by the immune system. Certain toxoids are used to immunize people against specific diseases, such as DIPH-THERIA or TETANUS.

Toxoplasma A genus of crescent-shaped parasites that live within the cells of various tissues and organs of vertebrate animals (especially birds and mammals). They complete their life cycle in the cat. One strain (*T. gondii*) causes TOXOPLASMOSIS.

toxoplasmosis A disease of mammals and birds, especially the cat that causes a mild illness except in the case of those with impaired immune systems or pregnant women. Cats get the disease by eating infected mice.

At least 50 percent of everyone in the United States has been infected with toxoplasmosis by the age of 50; the vast majority of infections produce no symptoms. In New York, researchers discovered that between 20 and 40 percent of pregnant women were immune; research figures in Paris showed that 84 percent of tested pregnant French women were immune.

Cause The parasite (*Toxoplasma gondii*) is transmitted to humans via undercooked meat, contaminated soil, or by direct contact. Most often, a cat is involved. The parasite excretes eggs into the cat's feces, where it then travels to humans and other animals. The eggs of the *T. gondii* migrate to an animals' muscles, where they remain infectious for a long time. Eating undercooked beef, mutton, or lamb from an infected animal can transfer the infection. Humans can also get the disease by drinking unpasteurized goat's milk from infected goats, drinking water contaminated with cat feces, or

by handling cat feces or infected soil. In humans, the parasite enters the blood and in pregnancy can infect the fetus.

Symptoms If clinical signs show up, they are usually mild, with a slight swelling of lymph nodes at various sites in the body together with a low-grade fever, tiredness, sore throat, or slight body rash. The disease is often misdiagnosed as infectious MONONU-CLEOSIS. Symptoms usually appear between 5 and 20 days after exposure. Humans are not infectious to each other.

In patients with an impaired immune system, however, the infection can be quite severe, involving multiple organs in the body.

The infection is most serious during pregnancy. While 90 percent of such infected babies are born without disease, 7 percent have minor abnormalities and 3 percent have severe damage. The highest risk occurs if the mother is infected during the first six months of pregnancy. Infant abnormalities include eye problems, water on the brain (or micro-cephaly), low levels of iron in the blood, jaundice, vomiting, fever, convulsions, or mental retardation. In a newborn, the parasite continues to divide, but symptoms may not appear for several years. Postnatal disease may include fever, headache, facial pain, and lymph node swellings. Severe disease includes heart problems (myocarditis), MENIN-GOENCEPHALITIS, and PNEUMONIA.

Diagnosis Blood tests can reveal the disease; antibodies will remain for life. If a pregnant woman thinks she may have been exposed or her symptoms resemble the disease, blood tests can detect antibodies; some women with an infection during early pregnancy may choose to end the pregnancy. Unfortunately, there is no test that can show whether or not the fetus has been infected by the disease.

Tests taken of newborns can detect those who may have been infected while in the womb; those babies with possible infection can be treated with antibiotics for one year, which can reduce the risk that the baby will have permanent damage. At present, however, this test is not done routinely in all states.

Complications Complications of infection during pregnancy in the first trimester can include miscarriage, premature birth, and poor growth in the womb. Infants who appear normal at birth may develop eye problems or mental retardation by age 20.

People with impaired immune systems (such as in AIDS) are at risk for complications, including pneumonia, heart infection, and death. These patients often suffer with infection in the brain, especially if dormant organisms that have remained in the muscle for years reactivate. (This does not happen to people with healthy immune systems.)

Treatment Severe cases are treated with sulfonamides and pyrimethamine. Healthy nonpregnant adults and children don't need treatment. Pregnant women cannot take pyrimethamine, which can damage the fetus.

Pregnant women with suspected or proven toxoplasmosis need counseling to understand the risks and options. No safe and effective drug exists that can be used during pregnancy.

In Europe, the drug spiramycin is used in these cases, where it has proven to decrease (but not eliminate) the risk of infection to the fetus. This drug is not approved for use in the United States and is available here only as an investigational drug requiring special permission to be dispensed.

Prevention Pregnant women and those with impaired immune systems should avoid eating raw or undercooked meat. Pregnant women should not touch or even clean cat litter. Cat boxes should be cleaned daily before the feces dry; the eggs are most infectious from dry feces for at least three days. Hands should be washed after handling cats (especially before eating). Indoor cats should be kept indoors, away from infected mice. Stray cats should not be allowed in the house; raw meat should not be fed to cats. At-risk individuals should not work in gardens accessible to cats.

trachoma A chronic infectious disease of the eye caused by the bacterium CHLAMYDIA TRA-CHOMATIS that is fairly rare in the United States today, although it is still found in the southwest in hot, dry climates. The disease is the chief cause of blindness in Third World countries. About 500 million people are infected, causing up to 8 million cases of blindness.

Trachoma is one of the earliest-known human diseases, recorded on papyrus in 1500 B.C. It was named in A.D. 60 from the Greek word meaning "rough" (a reference to the pustules on the eyelids). The disease spread from the Holy Land during the Crusades, becoming known as Egyptian or "military" ophthalmia.

Cause It is found most often today among children and women who care for them, especially where there is lack of clean water. The organism is spread by direct contact and possibly by flies.

Symptoms Tearing, inflammation, and eye pain in the presence of light. If untreated, rough thickened scar tissue forms on the upper eyelids, studded with lumps that get bigger until they affect the cornea, eventually causing blindness. Damage to the mucous-secreting cells of the conjunctiva and the tear-producing glands may cause "dry eye." An abnormal growth of blood vessels can reach down into the upper part of the cornea, causing a loss of transparency and loss of vision. More severe damage to the cornea occurs when scarring of the inside upper lid force lashes to rub against the cornea, causing ulcers and secondary bacterial infection.

Treatment In the early stages, doctors try to eradicate the organisms causing trachoma, which are sensitive to antibiotics (tetracycline, erythromycin, and topical sulfonamides) given directly into the eye and also by mouth. Established trachoma with scarring is much more difficult to treat. Surgical treatment of the lid deformities and corneal grafts to restore transparency and vision may be needed.

Prevention Education and providing water for washing hands, towels, and handkerchiefs are important in eliminating the disease.

traveler's diarrhea Up to half of all Americans who visit the tropics pick up traveler's diarrhea (also known as "Montezuma's revenge" or *turista*). Areas of high risk include the developing countries of Africa, the Middle East, and Latin America.

The risk of infection varies depending on where the person eats, from low risk (in private homes) to high risk (food from street vendors). Travelers' diarrhea is more common in young adults than in older people and is usually acquired by ingesting food and water contaminated with feces. See also DIARRHEA AND INFECTIOUS DISEASE; ANTIDIARRHEAL DRUGS.

Cause Most traveler's diarrhea is caused by a special strain of the common intestinal bacteria ESCHERICHIA COLI. Other bacteria responsible for SALMONELLOSIS and SHIGELLOSIS can also cause diarrhea, as can the parasitic conditions of GIARDIASIS and AMEBIASIS.

Symptoms Diarrhea, nausea, bloating, and malaise that usually lasts from between three to seven days. Even untreated traveler's diarrhea will go away by itself in most cases. Diarrhea that lasts more than four days or is accompanied by severe cramps, bloody stools, or dehydration should be reported to a physician, however.

Treatment Drink plenty of fluids to replace water; add oral rehydration packets to fluids to replace lost minerals. Several prescription and over-the-counter drugs will relieve symptoms or kill bacteria. One of the best treatments for early diarrhea is the antibiotic combination trimethoprim/sulfamethoxazole, which is 90 percent effective against the organisms that cause traveler's diarrhea. Antibiotics can usually shorten the illness and ease the symptoms.

The most widely used antidiarrheal medications are over-the-counter drugs, Pepto-Bismol (bismuth subsalicylate) and Immodium (loperamide). Both treat the symptoms instead of killing the bacteria. Pepto-Bismol should not be used by pregnant women, people subject to seizures, or those taking aspirin or other blood thinners, according to the FDA. Immodium can decrease the number of stools, but it can bring complications for those with serious infections. It should not be used by anyone with a high fever or bloody stools.

Prevention Since most diarrhea-causing organisms are found in water, they can be passed on in untreated water or on food handled by people who have not properly washed their hands. In order to prevent this type of diarrhea while traveling, travelers should avoid

- drinking tap water or using it to brush teeth (even in good hotels)
- using ice in sodas or alcoholic drinks
- mixing alcohol with water
- drinking milk or dairy products unless they have been pasteurized

Instead, travelers should

- boil water for tooth brushing for five minutes, or add water purification tablets
- avoid bottled water unless it's carbonated (the carbonation process inhibits bacterial growth)
- drink carbonated beverages, beer, wine, coffee, or tea
- wipe off bottle or can tops before drinking
- avoid eating raw vegetables, fruits, meat, or seafood
- avoid cold buffets left in the sun for several hours
- avoid garden or potato salads or food from street vendors
- eat only hot cooked meals, fruit with peels, and packaged foods

Before leaving for a trip, a physician can provide a prescription to take along for antidiarrheal medicine.

Alternatively, Pepto-Bismol appears to be effective in preventing traveler's diarrhea

(2 oz four times a day, or 2 tablets 4 times a day), but this is not recommended for more than three weeks at a time. Side effects of this preventive treatment include temporary blackening of the tongue and stools, occasional nausea and constipation, and rarely, ringing in the ears. Pepto-Bismol should be avoided by those allergic to aspirin or who have kidney problems or gout. This preventive treatment should be discussed with a doctor before trying it on children, adolescents, and pregnant women.

New research Scientists at West Virginia University have discovered that wine is capable of killing bacteria that cause diarrhea much faster than did Pepto-Bismol, tap water, tequila, or pure alcohol. In the case of *Salmonella*, for example, the wines destroyed about 10 million bacteria in just 20 minutes; it took the Pepto-Bismol two hours to reach the same effect.

trematodes   See FLUKE.

trench mouth   See VINCENT'S DISEASE.

Treponema   A genus of spirochetes, some of which cause diseases in humans including PINTA, SYPHILIS, and YAWS.

Treponema pallidum   An active spirochete that causes SYPHILIS.

Trichinella spiralis   The intestinal roundworm that causes TRICHINOSIS that can be ingested when eating uncooked infected meat (usually pork).

trichinellosis   See TRICHINOSIS.

trichinosis   A food-borne disease caused by the microscopic intestinal ROUNDWORM *Trichinella spiralis*. Anyone who eats undercooked meat of infected animals can develop trichinosis; pork products are most often responsible, although cases have appeared after eating infected bear and walrus.

The parasite may be found in a wide variety of animals, including pigs, dogs, cats, rats, and many wild animals (such as fox, wolf, and polar bear).

Up to 5 percent of Americans have had an infestation, usually without symptoms. It is almost never a problem in countries such as France, where pigs eat root vegetables, not garbage.

Cause   Worm larvae exist as cysts in the muscles of infested animals. Within four to six weeks after eating the undercooked or raw meat of an infested animal, the larvae are released from the cysts and develop into adults in the person's intestines. The adult worms produce fresh larvae, which travel in the blood to tissues and organs including the heart, tongue, eye, and brain and to the muscles, where they form cysts. The disease does not spread by person-to-person contact, but infected animals are infectious for months, and the meat from these infected animals remains contaminated unless properly cooked.

Symptoms   The incubation period varies depending on the number of parasites in the meat and how much was eaten. Infestation with only a few worms causes no symptoms, whereas a heavy infestation may cause diarrhea and vomiting, PNEUMONIA, heart failure, or respiratory failure.

Usually within 10 to 14 days after infection, symptoms of fever, muscle aches, pain, and swelling around the eyes will begin. Thirst, profuse sweating, chills, weakness, and tiredness may develop. If the parasite becomes imbedded in the diaphragm (thin muscle separating lungs from abdominal organs), chest pain may result. When the larvae attach to the lining of the intestines, the intestines become inflamed, causing abdominal pain, diarrhea, and weakness. As the larvae begin to increase in length and form cysts in the muscles, muscle soreness and pain in muscle fibers will begin.

Very rarely, a person becomes seriously ill and dies. Those who survive maintain a partial immunity.

Diagnosis A physician may suspect trichinosis from the symptoms; it is confirmed by blood tests that detect antibodies to the larvae or by a muscle biopsy that reveals the larvae themselves.

Complications Warning signs include breathing problems, swelling, or shortness of breath. Heart failure may be fatal either in the first two weeks after infection or between the fourth and eighth week.

Treatment Painkillers and thiabendazole and corticosteroids may relieve symptoms. Bed rest is recommended to prevent relapse and possible death. After two or three months, the organisms cause no more symptoms. Once the larvae migrate to muscle, mebendazole is the treatment of choice.

Prevention The best way to prevent the disease is to ensure meat—especially pork products or wild game—is properly cooked to at least 150 degrees F for 35 minutes per pound. Freezing infected meat no higher than -13 degrees F for 10 days will destroy the parasite. Pork or pork products should never be eaten raw, and even smoked or salted meat may still harbor organisms. Pork should not be ground in the same grinder as other meats; the grinder should then be cleaned well after grinding pork. Hunters should cook walrus, seal, wild boar, and bear meat well before eating.

Routine inspection of carcasses for *Trichinella* organisms is not performed in the United States because the disease is on the decline. Irradiation of pork carcasses can also eradicate the larvae.

Trichomonas vaginalis A protozoan (single-celled microorganism) that causes infection of the vagina (TRICHOMONIASIS).

trichomoniasis A vaginal protozoan infection that is usually sexually transmitted, although it also may be transmitted from an infected washcloth or towel or to a baby during childbirth. The infection may also occur in men, who have an infected urethra, although this does not usually cause symptoms.

A fairly benign condition, trichomoniasis is believed to infect about 3 million people each year in the United States.

Cause The protozoa *Trichomonas vaginalis* causes trichomoniasis.

Symptoms The protozoa may exist in the vagina for years without causing symptoms, but if they do occur they include painful inflammation and itching of the vagina and vulva, with a profuse, yellow, frothy, foul-smelling discharge. Sex is usually painful.

While men don't usually have symptoms, they may experience urethral discomfort, inflammation of the head of the penis, and signs of urethritis.

Diagnosis Lab examination of vaginal discharge will reveal the disease. Diagnosis is usually difficult in men.

Treatment Metronidazole is the treatment of choice; an infected person's partner should be treated at the same time to prevent reinfection.

Trichophyton A genus of fungus that infects skin, hair, and nails.

trichosporosis A fungal condition in which the hair shafts are coated with hard masses of white (*Trichosporon cutaneum*) or black (*Piedraia hortaei*) fungus. The best treatment is to remove the affected hairs by clipping or shaving.

tropical diseases Most diseases found in temperate areas are also widespread in the tropics, but many other infectious diseases are largely confined to tropical areas. This is primarily because the people there live in poverty, not because of temperature, humidity, or disease-carrying insects prevalent in this part of the world. War refugees migrating to other areas carry infections with them, and economic and social crises in these areas stress the respective health systems.

Malnutrition is one of the major factors in the development of infectious diseases in the tropics, weakening the body's ability to fight off infections such as DIPHTHERIA or MEASLES. Overcrowding also causes problems, especially in contagious diseases such as TUBERCULOSIS. A vast number of other infectious diseases are due to low standards of public health, food inspection and handling, and lack of sanitary food and water supplies. Diseases associated with contamination by human excrement include TYPHOID FEVER, SHIGELLOSIS, CHOLERA, AMEBIASIS, and TAPEWORM.

Only a few diseases appear to be related to temperature or soil conditions found only in the tropics, such as HOOKWORM or SCHISTOSOMIASIS.

Some tropical diseases are related to a specific insect, such as the mosquito, which can cause such diseases as MALARIA, YELLOW FEVER, SLEEPING SICKNESS, and LEISHMANIASIS. Many of these insect-related diseases, however, are not limited to the tropical areas.

trypanosomiasis   A tropical disease caused by protozoa parasites called trypanosomes. In Africa, trypanosomes spread by the TSETSE FLY cause sleeping sickness; other trypanosomes (spread by beetles) cause CHAGAS DISEASE common in South America.

Cause   African trypanosomiasis is an infection transmitted to man through the bite of the tsetse fly; the protozoa enter the skin through the saliva of the insect.

Symptoms   Symptoms of Rhodesian trypanosomiasis begin two weeks after the bite of the fly, with an inflammation of the skin at the bite site. Fever develops followed by skin rashes; scattered areas of puffy, painful skin; enlarged and painful lymph nodes; and anemia. Later, the person becomes depressed, with tremors, lack of appetite, disturbed speech, and fatigue. The fatigue becomes more pronounced until the person spends almost all his time sleeping; death eventually occurs.

Gambian trypanosomiasis starts six months to several years after the bite of the fly and develops very slowly.

Treatment   If untreated, most cases are fatal; drugs to treat the disease are very toxic and must be used with great caution. However, if treatment is begun early, the prognosis is good. If not treated soon enough, irreversible brain damage or death is common.

Prevention   It is important to take precautions against the tsetse fly. Some drugs are

---

PREVENTION OF TROPICAL DISEASES

Personal protection is the first line of defense against these diseases. For travelers heading to the tropics, the national Centers for Disease Control and Prevention advises that the following guidelines be adhered to.

At least six weeks before departure:
- Get current health information from the CDC on regions to be visited (other sources may include local health departments, physicians, or travel agencies).

In the tropics. . .
- Avoid rural areas when possible.
- When outdoors wear a hat, long-sleeved shirt tight at the wrists and tucked in at the waist, long pants tight at the ankles and tucked into socks, and shoes covering the entire foot.
- On clothing, use a repellent containing permethrin (the Environmental Protection Agency recommends applying this repellent to clothing before wearing, let clothing dry thoroughly first).
- On skin, use a repellent containing DEET (no higher than a 30 percent concentration). Follow instructions carefully; there have been rare cases of toxicity and death with higher concentrations of DEET.
- If accommodations are not well screened or air conditioned, use a bed net sprayed with permethrin repellent and tuck it under the mattress.
- For areas with *Leishmania*-infected sand flies, use a bed net with 18 or more holes per inch.
- Spray screen with permethrin.
- Use aerosol insecticides to clear rooms of insects. Follow instructions carefully.

available for use in preventing the infection, but these are potentially toxic and should be used only for people at high risk.

tsetse flies A type of large brown African fly that uses its proboscis to inflict a painful bite. Tsetses spread the parasitic disease known as SLEEPING SICKNESS.

TSS See TOXIC SHOCK SYNDROME.

tsutsugamushi disease Another name for scrub typhus. (See TYPHUS, SCRUB.)

tuberculin test A skin test (tine test) used to determine whether or not a person has been infected with tuberculosis; the test is used to diagnose suspected cases of TUBERCULOSIS and prior to vaccination against the disease.

During the test, the skin is first disinfected and a small dose of tuberculin (a protein extract of the tuberculosis bacilli) is introduced into the skin. The preferred method is the Mantoux test, where the extract is injected between skin layers with a needle.

After a few days, the skin is inspected at the site; if the skin is unchanged, the reaction is negative, indicating the person has never been exposed to tuberculosis and has no immunity. Skin that becomes hard and raised after the injection indicates that the person has been exposed to tuberculosis, either through vaccination or infection.

tuberculosis A respiratory disease spread from person to person through the air (once known as "consumption," "scrofula," "phthisis," or "wasting"), infecting half the world's population. TB usually affects the lungs, although it can also target other parts of the body (such as the brain, kidneys, or spine). It was once the leading cause of death in the United States.

People with TB infection but not the disease have the bacteria that cause the infection within their bodies, but the germs are inac-

tive. They cannot spread the bacteria to others, but they may develop TB later on. Because of this, they are often treated to prevent them from developing the disease.

In 1993 the World Health Organization declared a "global TB emergency" because of the massive TB epidemic that is spreading around the world. In its 1996 report on TB, the WHO concluded that worldwide, the disease is the leading killer of women and the leading killer of HIV-positive patients. (Among those with HIV, 1 in 10 per year will develop active TB.)

TB kills more adults than all other infectious diseases combined and leaves more orphaned children than any other infectious disease. In 1995, more people died of TB than in any other year in history. If current trends continue, at least 30 million people will die from TB in the next 10 years. TB already kills more people than AIDS, MALARIA, and TROPICAL DISEASES combined. For every person who died in 1995 of the EBOLA virus, more than 12,000 people died of TB.

About 8 million new cases of TB occur each year; the number of cases reported in the United States has increased each year since 1985. In 1993, there were 215,313 cases reported in this country. Between 10 to 15 million Americans are infected with the TB germ; these people may develop TB sometime in the future. In industrialized countries, the steady drop in TB began to level off in the mid-1980s and then began to increase. This may be due in part to immigration from countries with a high rate of TB.

Of most concern is that cases of TB resistant to more than one drug have been reported in 17 states in the United States since 1989. More than 50 million people around the world may already be infected with drug-resistant TB. Because of this, it is essential to treat TB patients with a recommended four-drug regimen of isoniazid, rifampin, pyrazinamide, and ethambutol or streptomycin, since it is less likely that bacteria can become quickly resistant to multiple drugs at the same time.

History Tuberculosis has been the scourge of the world since the dawn of time—evidence of the TB bacteria has been found in neolithic skeletons from 4500 B.C. and was described in the Hammurabi Code, circa 2000 B.C. Hippocrates described "consumption" (or *phthisis*, in Greek) as the most widespread disease of his time, noting that it was almost always fatal and warning other doctors that if they visited patients in the last stages of the disease, the inevitable deaths might ruin their reputations.

Historians think that TB evolved in the Middle East some 8,000 years ago, from cattle to humans, and could have entered the Americas by human migration from Asia across the Bering Sea.

By the 17th century, doctors were closing in on this dread disease. Sylvius identified actual tubercles in his 1679 *Opera Medica,* noting the consistent change in the lungs of consumptive patients and the inevitable progression to lung abscess. Other 17th-century physicians described the infectious nature of the disease; the Republic of Lucca in Italy required disinfection be carried out after the death of a consumptive.

Up until the 18th century, English citizens thought that the "king's evil" could be cured by the King's touch. But it became a serious problem in England during the Industrial Revolution, when it killed one out of every five London natives. The astonishing idea that TB could be caused by "minute living creatures" was discovered by the 18th-century English physician Benjamin Marten, who decided that it was possible to catch the disease by sharing the same bed, eating utensils, or breathing the same air. However, he wrote in his publication *A New Theory of Consumption* that he didn't think simply talking to a person with consumption on a casual basis was enough to transmit the disease.

Not until scientists introduced the idea of putting patients in a sanatorium was there much of a breakthrough in the treatment of TB. Botany student Hermann Brehmer went to the Himalayas to pursue his botany studies while trying to cure his disease; when he did actually succeed in curing himself, he returned home to study medicine in 1854. He built an institution in Gorbersdorf, where patients could breathe clean air and eat healthy food; his hospital became the touchstone for future sanatoriums. The sanatoriums also were a means of isolating the sick from the healthy.

By 1865, French physician Jean-Antoine Villemin discovered that TB could be passed from humans to cattle and on to rabbits, which proved there was a specific microorganism; 20 years later the great German bacteriologist Robert Koch developed a staining technique that allowed him to actually see and identify the *Mycobacterium tuberculosis.* The word *tubercule* means "a small nodule or growth." But it was not until World War II that drugs that could cure the disease were developed.

Actually, sulfonamide and penicillins were not very effective against TB; in 1940, scientists isolated an effective anti-TB antibiotic—actinomycin—but it was too toxic for humans or animals. Three years later, scientists discovered that streptomycin could control the disease without causing serious side effects. On November 20, 1944, the antibiotic was administered for the first time to a critically ill patient. Almost at once, the disease was stopped, the bacteria disappeared, and the patient rapidly recovered. While the new drug had side effects (especially in the inner ear) it was the first drug that really had an effect on TB.

Over the following years, scientists continued to develop better anti-TB drugs, important, because within a few months TB germs resistant to streptomycin began to appear.

Cause TB is caused by three species of mycobacteria: *Mycobacterium tuberculosis, M. bovis,* and *M. africanuum.* When a person breathes in the bacteria, they can settle in the lungs and grow; from here, they can travel through the blood to other parts of the body (such as the kidney, spine, or brain). TB in the lungs or throat is mildly infectious, but the bacteria in other parts of the body are not usually contagious.

TB bacteria are sprayed into the air when a person with the disease of the lungs or throat coughs or sneezes. When another person inhales air that contains TB germs, the person may become infected. People with active TB are most likely to spread it to those they spend time with every day (such as family members or coworkers). The degree of contagiousness is directly related to the number of bacilli expelled into the air. Patients are more likely to be infectious if they have TB in the lungs or larynx, have a cavity in the lung, and cough a lot. Contagion potential is also related to patient behavior, such as failing to cover the mouth when coughing.

Although TB is infectious, it is not highly infectious and is not nearly as contagious as MEASLES or WHOOPING COUGH. Letting fresh air blow through a room will eradicate most of the infectious germs exhaled by a sick patient every day. The bacteria are also sensitive to ultraviolet rays, which means that infection rarely occurs outside in daylight. Indeed, only half of the people who live with an infected patient will contract the disease themselves.

People with TB are most likely to transmit the disease before it has been diagnosed and treated, and at least 12 weeks must pass before a person who has been exposed to the disease will test positive. The infectious state seems to decrease quickly once treatment begins; those who have been treated for two to three weeks, whose symptoms have improved, and who have three consecutive negative sputum tests can be considered non-infectious.

Most people who breathe in the bacteria and become infected are able to fight off the disease; the bacteria become inactive, but they remain alive in the body and can become active later. This is called TB *infection.* People with TB infection have no symptoms, don't feel sick, and can't spread the disease. However, they usually have a positive skin test for TB, and they can develop the disease later in life if they don't receive preventive treatment. Many people who have the infection never develop the disease, however. In these people, the bacteria remain inactive for a lifetime.

Scientists have recently discovered how TB microbes manage to remain dormant in the lungs for so long before developing into active disease. It appears that TB bacteria contain a gene that regulates dormancy. When the bacterium is under stress (as it is in the lungs), the gene becomes dormant in order to protect itself. If this is true, scientists could then manipulate the bacterium so as to trigger a dormant state in drug-resistant microbes.

Because infants and young children don't have very strong immune systems, they are susceptible to TB, as are those with impaired immune systems. This includes patients with HIV infection; substance abusers; diabetics; those with cancer of head and neck, leukemia, severe kidney disease, or low body weight; and people undergoing medical therapies such as corticosteroid treatment or organ transplant.

Symptoms The illness does not cause symptoms at first. TB growing in the lungs may cause chest pain or a bad cough that lasts longer than two weeks. The patient may cough up blood or phlegm from the lungs. Other symptoms include fatigue or weakness, weight loss, appetite loss, chills, and fever.

Diagnosis The disease is diagnosed with a tuberculin skin test to determine if a person has the TB organism. It cannot separate those who have active disease from those who don't. For this skin test, a small amount of fluid (tuberculin) is injected within the skin in the lower part of the arm. Two or three days later a health care worker looks for a reaction on the arm.

A positive reaction usually means that the person has been infected with the TB germ, but not necessarily that they have an active infection. Other tests (chest X ray and sample of phlegm) are necessary to identify active disease. (See TUBERCULIN TEST.)

People should be tested for TB if they have spent time with someone with infectious TB, have HIV, come from a country where TB is common (most countries in Latin America, the Caribbean, Africa, and Asia except for Japan). Others at high risk are those who inject drugs or who live in places in the United States where TB is common (homeless shelters, migrant farm camps, prisons, and some nursing homes) or who are health care workers.

Because it may take several weeks after infection for the immune system to react to the TB skin test, it may be necessary to be retested 10 to 12 weeks after the last exposure to TB. If the reaction to the second test is negative, there is probably no TB infection present.

The skin test is mandatory in some states and countries for immigrants and students from Africa, Asia, and Latin America, as well as for personnel in schools, hospitals, prisons, food handlers, group homes, child care centers, and substance abuse centers. Skin tests are also recommended for elderly people. At the moment, screening of children entering kindergarten or day care centers is not required in all school districts, but the CDC recommends that schoolchildren be tested for TB to ensure that all U.S. citizens are tested at least once in their lives.

A new test can now identify the TB organism much more quickly than in the past. The new test can confirm a TB diagnosis in just six hours, as opposed to the current two to six weeks required to confirm TB bacteria in culture. This new test is under consideration for approval by the U.S. Food and Drug Administration. The new test appears to have a low rate of false positives, which has been a problem with other tests in the past.

Treatment   Up to the 1700s it was thought that the touch of a king or queen would cure TB; today, scientists know that TB is cured by taking several drugs for up to nine months long. If patients stop taking the drugs too soon, or if they don't take the drugs correctly, the TB organisms may become resistant. TB that is resistant to drugs is harder to treat.

Patients who have signs of TB should be isolated and tested promptly. After the development of streptomycin, other drugs became available: isoniazid (1952), pyrazinamide (1954), cycloserine (1955), ethambutol (1962), and rifampin (rifampicin 1963). Aminoglycosides (capreomycin, viomycin, kanamycin, and amikacin) and the newer quinolones (ofloxacin and ciprofloxacin) are used in drug-resistant situations.

Within a month after treatment begins, the patient should feel well, regain weight, and have no fever. Coughing should have slowed down, and there should be improvements on X rays. If the disease was severe, however, complete end of treatment may not occur for a year.

If there is no improvement within three months, a change in therapy may be needed. Relapses usually occur within six months after treatment ends and are usually due to patients who don't follow correct drug procedures.

When TB becomes active again in a patient who had been treated before, there is a very good change that these bacteria will be drug resistant. If the microorganism is resistant to standard drugs, it may be necessary to use more toxic drugs, such as ethionamide, protionamide, pyrazinamide, cycloserine, capreomycin, or viomycin.

Prevention   Some people who have the TB germ but not active disease are more likely than others to develop an active case. These high-risk individuals include those with HIV infection, those who were recently exposed to someone with TB disease and those with certain medical conditions.

For patients who have TB germs but not the active disease, the Centers for Disease Control recommend taking isoniazid for up to 12 months. Isoniazid may cause liver problems in certain people (especially the elderly and those with liver disease), so patients taking this drug are carefully monitored.

Some people are given preventive therapy if their skin test is negative; this is often done with infants, children, and HIV-infected people who have recently spent time with someone with infectious disease.

Side effects to isoniazid include appetite loss, nausea and vomiting, yellow skin or eyes, fever for more than three days, stomach pain, and tingling in fingers and toes. *Drinking alcoholic beverages while taking isoniazid is dangerous.*

There is a vaccine for TB disease that is used in many countries but is not widely used in the United States. This vaccine does not completely prevent people from getting TB. Those who have been vaccinated with BCG can be given a tuberculin skin test; although the vaccine can cause a positive reaction to the test, it is more likely that a positive reaction is caused by TB infection if the reaction is large and the person was vaccinated a long time ago. It may also be positive if the person has been around someone with TB disease or the person is from a country where TB is common.

While there is some question as to how effective the BCG vaccine really is against adults, the World Health Organization recommends its use in newborns in developing countries, because it appears to offer some protection in children.

A new TB vaccine from "naked" DNA might work better with less risk of infection than the current BCG vaccine. The traditional BCG vaccine is made from an altered, weakened form of the disease that infects cows. But researchers in 1996 reported that they had made a new vaccine out of a gene taken from the human version of TB. The use of one gene (known as "naked DNA") instead of the many genes contained in TB DNA, appears to be as effective as the earlier cow vaccine. However, trials in humans are still a long way off.

Unlike traditional vaccines, which stimulate the human body to produce disease-fighting antibodies, naked DNA vaccines are incorporated by the cells and the immune response begins there. There is also a lower risk of infection with this new vaccine. While this did not occur often with the old vaccine, it did happen in certain rare cases.

Scientists also have recently discovered it is possible to transmit TB on an airplane. In the spring of 1994, a woman on an $8^1/_2$-hour United Airlines flight from Chicago to Honolulu infected four passengers sitting near her; all tested positive for the disease, but none have yet become ill. A few days later, the woman died from TB. Because this showed transmission is possible on airlines, the Centers for Disease Control and Prevention recommended that when airlines learn that a passenger or crew member has traveled with the disease (especially on long flights) they should contact passengers and crew members and inform them. The CDC pointed out that only those passengers sitting near the woman were infected; others sitting farther away breathed air that passed through the plane's filtration system.

Health care workers who care for TB patients should wear a HEPA filter respirator, collect specimens in a well-ventilated area (if possible, outdoors), and participate in a TB screening and prevention program.

The U.S. government issued new guidelines in 1994 for prisons, hospitals, nursing homes, and medical and dental offices to curb the spread of drug-resistant TB. The standards require better ventilation, more efficient masks for workers, and use of ultraviolet light to kill germs.

tuberculosis, skin This condition is caused by direct inoculation of *MYCOBACTERIUM TUBERCULOSIS* into a wound in people not previously exposed. It is rare in developed countries.

Symptoms In the localized form of the disease, an inflammatory nodule called the tuberculous chancre is accompanied by inflammation of the lymph nodes and vessels. In immune (or partly immune) patients skin lesions are characterized by patchy lesions with small yellowish nodules on the face. In scrofuloderma, tuberculosis of lymph nodes or bone spreads to the skin, causing ulcers and fistulas underneath ridges of blue skin.

In the disseminated form of the disease, bacteria cause "miliary tuberculosis" in the skin, causing necrotic papules on the face and extremities, with a small dead core that forms chickenpox-like scars.

Treatment Administration of standard antituberculosis drugs for 6 to 12 months is effective.

tularemia An infectious disease of wild animals occasionally transmitted to humans, characterized by a red spot at the skin site of infection, eventually forming an ulcer.

Hunters or others who spend a great deal of time outdoors are at greater risk for exposure, since humans may contract the disease through direct contact with an infected animal (such as rabbits, squirrels, or muskrats).

The disease is found only in North America (a few hundred cases yearly), some parts of Europe, and Asia. There are between 150 and 300 cases a year, primarily in Arkansas, Missouri, and Oklahoma.

Cause The bacteria *Francisella (Pasteurella) tularensis* enters the body through a cut or scratch in the skin, or it may also be acquired following a bite from a tick, flea, fly, louse, or (rarely) by eating infected rabbit meat.

Less common means of spreading tularemia include drinking contaminated water, inhaling dust from contaminated soil, or handling contaminated pelts or paws of animals.

Symptoms Between 2 and 10 days after contact, symptoms suddenly appear. In addition to the skin lesion, symptoms include enlarged lymph nodes, chills, fever, headache, muscle pains, fatigue, and malaise. Sometimes the eyes, throat, digestive tract, and lungs are affected.

Treatment Antibiotics (such as streptomycin or tetracycline) treat the disease with a less than 1 percent fatality rate; untreated, it can be fatal in 5 percent of cases. The disease confers immunity, although occasional reinfection has been reported.

Prevention A vaccine is available for those at high risk, such as hunters, trappers, game wardens, or lab workers. Rubber gloves should be worn when skinning or handling animals (especially rabbits). Wild rabbit and rodent meat should be cooked thoroughly before eating.

tumbu fly bites These fly bites cause myiasis (skin infestation with fly larvae) in South Africa. (See MYIASIS, CUTANEOUS.)

tungiasis A skin infection caused by a burrowing flea found in Africa, the West Indies, and South America.

Cause The female flea burrows under the skin, sucks her victim's blood, swells, and then ejects her eggs.

Symptoms A localized skin rash appears with lesions containing the live fleas.

Treatment Ethyl chloride spray will kill the flea when applied to the lesion where they are located. To remove live fleas, tweezers should be used after applying alcohol. Corticosteroid and antibiotic creams are effective. Exercise or excess warmth should be avoided.

Prevention Avoid contaminated areas and disinfect clothing, bedclothes, and furniture if necessary.

Complications Complications may be fatal, and include skin ulcers, GANGRENE, and blood poisoning (SEPTICEMIA).

typhoid fever   A serious bacterial infection of the intestinal tract and sometimes the bloodstream, also known as enteric fever. It is caused by eating food or drinking water contaminated with *Salmonella typhi.* An almost-identical disease called PARATYPHOID FEVER is caused by a related bacterium.

Typhoid fever today is an uncommon disease in the United States. In 1942 there were 4,000 reported cases, but since 1964 fewer than 500 cases have occurred each year, mostly imported from Mexico or India. In a 1989 outbreak, 67 guests in a New York resort hotel got typhoid from drinking contaminated orange juice. The juice was probably tainted by a Central American employee who prepared the juice, but who had left the hotel before he could be tested. (Typhoid fever is still common in Latin America, Africa, and Asia.)

Before the advent of antibiotics, 12 percent of victims died. Today, fewer than 10 percent of cases are fatal; these occur in malnourished people, infants, and the elderly. About 3 percent of those who recover from a mild illness become chronic carriers. There are about 2,000 of these carriers in the United States, almost all of them elderly women with gallbladder disease. Carriers are infectious for years unless the gallbladder is removed or they are treated with antibiotics. See also DIARRHEA AND INFECTIOUS DISEASE.

History   Thomas Willis first described typhoid fever in 1643; typhoid fever was often confused with "typhus" fever until the two were distinguished in 1837, and the name *typhoid* fever—meaning "typhus-like" was coined.

The most famous typhoid patient of all was Typhoid Mary, a cook in New York City who was the first known typhoid carrier in the United States. Although she was healthy, she was infected with typhoid bacteria, which she shed in feces. Her improper hand washing allowed the bacteria to contaminate the food she prepared for others. Between 1900 and 1915, she passed the disease to at least 53 people, 3 of whom died. Because she refused to stop working as a cook, she was forcibly confined to a hospital by public health authorities. She lived in that hospital for more than 20 years, until she died.

Cause   Typhoid fever is caused by the bacterium *Salmonella typhi,* a species of *Salmonella.* While the common *Salmonella* species in the U.S. live in animals and infect humans via contaminated food (chicken, eggs, etc.), *S. typhi* lives in the intestinal tract of humans. Once ingested, the bacteria lodge in the lower small intestine, where they multiplies and invade the bloodstream.

The disease is contracted from food or water that has been contaminated by the feces of patients or carriers, or from intimate contact with an infected person. It occurs in developing countries by eating shellfish taken from contaminated beds, eating raw fruits, or drinking tainted water supplies. It can also be contracted from food left outdoors accessible to flies. Anyone can get typhoid fever, but the greatest risk is to travelers visiting countries where the disease is common.

People are infectious as long as the bacteria are being shed in feces (usually three to four weeks), but some may remain infectious up to three months. To be considered a noncarrier, a patient must have stool cultures every week until there are three negative cultures in a row.

The most important modern source of the typhoid bacillus (found throughout the world) is the typhoid carrier; these carriers at times contaminate water, milk, or food and set off typhoid epidemics.

Symptoms   Between 8 and 14 days after ingesting bacteria, symptoms of fever, headache, joint pains, sore throat, and constipation begin. There may be appetite loss and abdominal pain. Most people have a mild illness and recover without antibiotics. Untreated, the fever will continue to rise for two or three days, remain high for up to two weeks (103 to 104 degrees F) and then fall.

Nosebleed and BRONCHITIS are often present. At the height of the fever, the patient appears extremely ill and can be delirious.

Relapses occur in 10 percent of untreated patients, and 20 percent of treated patients about two weeks after the fever abates. If the fever returns, antibiotics must be restarted. Some patients notice rose spots on chest and abdomen during the second week.

Infection confers some immunity, but not enough to protect a patient if there are large numbers of bacteria ingested a second time.

Diagnosis   The diagnosis is confirmed by obtaining a culture of typhoid bacteria from a sample of blood during the first week; feces and urine tests reveal the bacillus during the second.

Complications   Patients with serious cases can go on to experience frothy, bloody diarrhea in later stages and become apathetic. It can inflame the intestines and in severe cases, intestinal ulcers can perforate, causing severe infections. This can also lead to severe intestinal bleeding, which kill 25 percent of untreated victims.

Treatment   Antibiotics can shorten the disease and reduce chances of complications and death. Otherwise, it can take months to recover. Doctors may prescribe chloramphenicol, ciprofloxacin, ceftriaxone, or cefoperazone. In addition, patients need bed rest and good nutrition. Aspirin, enemas, or laxatives should not be given.

Gloves should be worn when nursing a typhoid patient, and rigorous hand washing is critical. Because the germ is passed in the feces of infected patients, only those with active diarrhea who can't toilet themselves (infants and some handicapped people) should be isolated.

With early diagnosis and proper treatment, the outlook is usually excellent. Permanent immunity usually follows an attack of typhoid, although relapses are common if the disease is not fully eradicated by thorough antibiotic treatment.

Prevention   Typhoid fever is a reportable disease. An oral vaccine (Ty21a) licensed in 1990 causes fewer side effects than the older injectable vaccine. This new version provides between 70 and 90 percent protection and is recommended for anyone older than six who is traveling off tourist routes (or for a long time) in Latin America, Asia, or Africa. Two even more effective vaccines are now being tested.

The oral vaccine includes four capsules taken every other day for three doses. All doses must be taken to provide maximum protection. The capsules should be kept refrigerated until they are taken with a cool liquid a half hour before a meal. Antibiotics or the antimalarial drug mefloquine should not be taken at the same time. The entire four-dose series should be repeated every five years for those who need protection.

There are few side effects with this drug, although some people notice nausea, vomiting, cramps, and skin rash. The older injected vaccine caused fever, headache, and local pain and swelling in about one third of patients. A new injected vaccine called Typhim Vi is available in Canada and the United States that is equally effective with few side effects. It is approved for children over two and adults. It should be taken two weeks before travel to allow immunity to develop.

Further preventive measures for travelers include drinking only pasteurized milk products, boiled or bottled water or carbonated beverages, eating only cooked food or fruit that is peeled by the diner, eating shellfish boiled or steamed at least 10 minutes, and controlling flies with screens and sprays.

Most infected people may return to work or school when they have recovered, as long as they wash their hands after toilet visits. Children in day care must obtain the approval of the local or state health department before returning to school. Food handlers may not return to work until three consecutive negative stool cultures are confirmed.

typhus   Any of a group of infectious diseases with similar symptoms, caused by rickettsiae (microorganisms similar to bacteria) that are spread by insects. (See also RICKETTSIAL INFEC-TIONS.)

In the past, epidemic typhus was the most significant type of this disease, which was spread by body lice. Epidemics of this type of typhus swept across the country, killing hundreds of thousands of people during war, famine, and natural disaster. It is rare today, except in some areas of Africa and South America.

Cause   Typhus is caused by rickettsiae; in epidemic typhus, they are ingested by lice from the blood of infected patients. The lice deposit feces containing the rickettsiae on other people's skin; when the person scratches the skin, the microorganisms enter the bloodstream.

Endemic (or murine) typhus is found in rats; about 50 cases occur in the United States each year, spread to humans through the bite of fleas. Scrub typhus is spread by mites in India and Southeast Asia. ROCKY MOUNTAIN SPOTTED FEVER is another disease similar to typhus.

Symptoms   Epidemic typhus is character-ized by a measles-like rash, severe headache, back and limb pain, high fever, confusion, prostration, weak heartbeat, and delirium. Untreated, the patient may die from blood poisoning, heart or kidney failure, or pneu-monia. Other types of typhus have similar symptoms and complications.

Diagnosis   Particular types of typhus are diagnosed by tests that detect certain blood products produced in reaction to the rick-ettsial organisms.

Treatment   Antibiotic drugs treat typhus fever; other treatment is aimed at relieving the rest of symptoms. It may take a long time to recover from the disease, especially among the elderly.

Prevention   Epidemic typhus may be pre-vented by vaccination and control of infesta-tions via insecticides. Other types of typhus may be prevented by wearing protective clothes to prevent tick, mite, and flea bites.

typhus, endemic flea-borne   A mild type of TYPHUS that is less severe than louse-borne typhus (see TYPHUS, EPIDEMIC LOUSE-BORNE) and occurs around the world, usually in places where people and mice live in the same buildings. It is found in the United States along the southern Atlantic and Gulf coasts.

Cause   Endemic flea typhus is transmitted to humans through the bite of an infected rat flea (*Xenopsylla cheopsis* in the order Siphonaptera), which leaves feces while suck-ing blood. It's also possible to inhale infected flea feces.

Symptoms   Between one and two weeks after a flea bite, symptoms of fever and rash on the trunk appear, lasting up to about two weeks.

Treatment   Antibiotics treat this disease, which is rarely fatal.

Prevention   The disease can be prevented by controlling rats and the fleas they carry.

typhus, epidemic louse-borne   An infectious form of TYPHUS caused by a parasite of the body louse (*Pediculus humanus*), found in mountainous regions of Mexico, Central and South America, the Balkans and eastern Europe, Africa, and many parts of Asia.

Cause   The more crowded the conditions, the more likely the disease will be transmitted from person to person because of a heavy infestation with lice. When a louse sucks the blood of someone infected with the parasite, the parasite enters the louse and grows. When the infected louse then bites another person, the infected louse feces is rubbed into a wound or the eye of the human host.

Symptoms   Within 10 to 14 days after infection, symptoms appear suddenly, includ-ing headache, aches, pains, and chills. A fever follows these signs, and a rash appears over the body except for the face, palms of the hands, and feet. The flulike symptoms can worsen into delirium and stupor that can lead to coma and death if untreated.

Treatment Drug therapy can effectively cure typhus. The fever can be reduced with tepid baths or cool temperatures. Isolation is required until all lice have been removed from the patient.

Prevention Anyone who has had contact with the patient must be quarantined for 15 days. Immunization, louse control, and good personal hygiene are effective ways of protecting against typhus. No typhus cases are known to have occurred in an American traveler since 1950, and no typhus vaccine is available in the United States. The risk to a U.S. traveler of contracting typhus is very small. See also TYPHUS, SCRUB; TYPHUS, ENDEMIC FLEA-BORNE.

typhus, scrub A mite-borne disease also known as tsutsugamushi disease, tropical TYPHUS, or mite-borne typhus found in south-east Asia, the western Pacific, and Australia. It is most often found in scrubby land, forest clearings, or other mite-infested areas.

Cause The infected parasites of rodents are transmitted by mites that spend most of their life on vegetation, where they can bite humans and transmit the infection.

Symptoms One to three weeks after the mite bite, the victim feels tired and chilled, with a severe headache and backache. At the mite-bite site, a small swelling is followed by blisters and then by a black flat scab. Fever gradually rises over one week, followed by a rash over the trunk. If untreated, other symptoms including heart problems and delirium may follow, and the disease may be fatal.

Treatment With appropriate treatment, recovery is quick and complete.

Prevention Avoiding mites can prevent the disease, as can applying a miticide in outdoor and indoor living areas. Insect repellent on clothing and skin can provide some protection.

ulcers and infectious disease See *HELICOBAC-TER PYLORI*.

Universal Blood and Body Fluids Precautions
See UNIVERSAL PRECAUTIONS.

universal precautions An approach to hospital infection control designed to prevent transmission of blood-borne infections such as AIDS and HEPATITIS B in health care settings.

The precautions were first developed in 1987 by the U.S. Centers for Disease Control and in 1989 by the Bureau of Communicable Disease Epidemiology in Canada.

The guidelines include specific recommendations for use of gloves and masks and protective eyewear when there is the risk of contact with blood or body secretions containing infected blood. See also HOSPITAL-ACQUIRED INFECTIONS.

upper respiratory infections See RESPIRATORY TRACT INFECTIONS.

urethritis Inflammation of the urethra usually caused by one of a variety of infectious organisms, the best known of which is the bacterium that causes GONORRHEA.

Cause Nonspecific urethritis may be caused by one of a number of different types of microorganisms, including BACTERIA, YEASTS, or CHLAMYDIA. Bacteria may spread to the urethra from the skin or rectum.

Symptoms A burning sensation and pain when urinating that can be severe. The urine may be stained with blood; if gonorrhea is the underlying cause, there may be a yellow pus-filled discharge. The infection may be followed by scarring that narrows the urethra, which can make urinating more difficult.

Treatment Treating the underlying infection will cure the urethritis. Gonorrhea is usually cured by PENICILLIN or other antibiotic. Treatment of nonspecific urethritis depends on what organism is causing the infection. If the urethra is scarred (urethral stricture), a physician may try to stretch and widen the tube under anesthesia.

urinary tract infection (UTI) This condition, also known as a bladder infection, is the most common bacterial infection in adult women and the most common medical problem of pregnancy. Most of the time, the problem is caused by fecal bacteria in the bladder, usually *ESCHERICHIA COLI. Gardnerella* (which causes VAGINITIS in women) may also infect the urinary tract.

Women most likely to get UTIs are older or who are sexually active. A woman with a UTI is not infectious to others. UTIs in men are uncommon and may indicate that there is an abnormality in the urinary tract.

Cause The bacteria that cause UTI usually originate in the rectum of vagina, and then move up into the bladder. Because the urethra in women is so close to other body openings, bacteria can more easily contaminate the urinary tract. This happens most often during sexual intercourse; one study found that 75 percent of women with UTIs reported having sex within 24 hours before the start of the infection. The bacteria do not come from a woman's partner, however, but originate within the woman's own body.

UTIs are 14 times more likely to occur in women because of their shorter urethra, their failure to empty their bladders as fully as men, and because the opening of the urethra in women is always contaminated by germs from the vagina and anus.

While most women have a natural defense mechanism in the walls of the bladder that interferes with bacterial growth, some women appear to lack this mechanism. In addition, as women age and their estrogen levels fall, they are more prone to thinning of mucous membranes and more frequent UTIs.

Symptoms   Burning and pain during urination plus the frequent urge to urinate even when the bladder is empty. It is also possible to have a UTI with no symptoms. Untreated, a UTI could lead to a serious kidney infection. It usually takes 24 hours for the bacteria to reach the bladder before symptoms appear.

Diagnosis   While some physicians may start treatment without testing for bacteria, a urinalysis—and usually a urine culture—should always be performed. Culture results take between 24 to 48 hours. It is possible to have a high degree of bacteria in the urine without having any pain or symptoms.

Treatment   There are many different antibacterials available to treat UTIs. Plenty of fluids will help to flush the bladder and dilute the urine; water, fruit juice, or caffeine-free soft drinks are best choices. While many women can successfully prevent infections by drinking cranberry juice, which increases the acidity of the urine and interferes with bacterial growth, cranberry tablets are now available for the same purpose.

For those women with recurrent UTIs, the antibiotic will be prescribed for up to 10 days together with a pain reliever.

Kidney infections are treated with a variety of antibiotics over a longer period of time. A relapse within 10 days could indicate the presence of kidney stones or kidney disease. Those with a severe kidney infection, or pregnant women, are usually hospitalized and given intravenous drugs.

Complications   Untreated UTIs can lead to kidney infection (especially in pregnant women), with high fever, chills, severe flank pain, and painful urination. There may also be nausea and vomiting.

Prevention   There is no sure way to prevent UTIs, but there are ways to reduce the risk. Women should completely empty the bladder as often as possible (at least once every three hours) and after sex. It is important to wipe from front to back after a bowel movement to avoid contaminating the urethra. A properly fitting diaphragm will not press against the urethra, which could interfere with complete emptying of the bladder. It may help to cut down on caffeinated drinks (cola, coffee, or tea), which can irritate the bladder.

vaccine A tiny dose of a specific protein of the organism that causes disease, given to prevent that disease. When a person is vaccinated, the vaccine helps build protective substances in the body to fight off any invasion by the disease-causing organism.

At present, there are vaccines for ANTHRAX, some types of PNEUMONIA, CHICKEN POX, DIPHTHERIA, GERMAN MEASLES, MEASLES, HEPATITIS A, and HEPATITIS B, INFLUENZA, LYME DISEASE (for dogs), MALARIA, MUMPS, WHOOPING COUGH, PLAGUE, POLIO, Q FEVER, RABIES, SMALLPOX, TETANUS, TUBERCULOSIS, TYPHOID, and YELLOW FEVER.

Despite the fact that immunization is required by the time a child reaches school age, far too many U.S. children are still not vaccinated. From time to time, there are epidemics among those who are not, such as the 1990–91 epidemic of measles that swept through the Philadelphia area. Measles infected almost 56,000 Americans between 1989 and 1991, killing 166 of them. Most were babies, young children, and teens. Today, more and more vaccines are required for children; within the next few years, there may be one vaccine that protects against six diseases.

For some time there has been controversy over the safety of the DPT vaccine, which has recently been replaced with the safer DTaP.

Those who believe they were injured by a vaccine may have compensation through the VACCINE INJURY COMPENSATION PROGRAM passed by Congress in 1986.

The doctor must keep a record of what vaccines were given, together with the date, manufacturer, lot number, and signature of person giving the vaccine. Patients will be given an information booklet, and parents must sign a

---

WHO SHOULD NOT BE VACCINATED

- anyone who has had a serious allergic reaction to a previous shot
- anyone with a severe allergy to eggs should not receive MMR, flu, or yellow fever vaccines, except under special medical situations
- anyone with a high fever or serious illness

RECOMMENDED IMMUNIZATION SCHEDULE FOR ADULTS BY AGE, HEALTH, JOB

All ages
- Td (tetanus, diphtheria) every 10 years.
- Anyone born after 1957 should have two doses of measles vaccine given at least one month apart. Most high schools and colleges now require this.

Adults over age 65
- Td every 10 years.
- Influenza vaccine every fall.
- One dose pneumococcal pneumonia vaccine (with booster every six years for transplant patients or those with chronic kidney failure or no spleen).

Health care/public safety workers
- Hepatitis B vaccine (three-dose series).
- Influenza vaccine every fall.
- MMR (unless proof of immunity) or birthdate before 1957.

Medical or research lab workers
- Inactivated polio vaccine for those who haven't received three doses of OPV.
- Plague vaccine for anyone working with plague (three-dose series; booster every one to two years).
- Anthrax vaccine for anyone working with anthrax bacteria.
- Rabies vaccine for anyone testing or isolating rabies virus.

RECOMMENDED IMMUNIZATION SCHEDULE FOR ADULTS
BY AGE, HEALTH, JOB *(continued)*

Veterinarians or small animal handlers
- Rabies vaccine and blood test every two years, with booster if needed.
- Plague vaccine for those in western states (three-dose primary series; boosters every one to two years).

Field personnel
- Plague vaccine (three-dose primary series; boosters every one to two years).
- Rabies vaccine and blood tests every two years, with booster if needed.
- Anthrax vaccine for those in contact with imported animal hides, furs, bonemeal, wool, animal hair (especially goat), and bristles.

Homosexually active males or anyone with multiple partners
- Hepatitis B vaccine (three-dose series).
- Flu.
- Tb.

Injection drug users
- Hepatitis B vaccine (three-dose series).
- Td vaccine.

Developmentally disabled residents of institutions
- Hepatitis B vaccine (three-dose series).
- Influenza vaccine every fall.

Household contacts of Hepatitis B carriers
- Hepatitis B vaccine (three-dose series).

Pregnant women
- Booster of Td if more than 10 years have elapsed.
- Hepatitis B if woman is at risk of exposure because of lifestyle or household contact with carrier.
- Influenza vaccine if there are medical conditions that increase risk of flu.
- Yellow fever and polio vaccines should be given only if she is traveling to areas where

there is high risk of exposure and travel can't be postponed until after delivery.
- Pregnant women who aren't immune to measles, mumps, or rubella should receive these live virus vaccines immediately after delivery.

People with weakened immune systems
- Influenza vaccine every fall.
- Pneumococcal vaccine; one dose (booster in six years).

HIV infected patients
- Influenza vaccine every fall.
- Pneumococcal vaccine; one dose (booster in six years).
- MMR vaccine (two doses).
- Hib (primary series).
- eIPV (inactivated polio vaccine) if not immune.

Hemodialysis and kidney transplant patients
- Influenza vaccine every fall.
- Pneumococcal vaccine; one dose (booster in six years).
- Hepatitis B vaccine (three-dose series).

Those with abnormal or absent spleens
- Pneumococcal vaccine.
- Meningococcal vaccine.

Clotting disorder patients who receive factor VIII or IX
- Hepatitis B vaccine (three-dose series).

Alcoholics
- Pneumococcal vaccine.
- Flu.
- Dt.

Patients with chronic lung, heart, kidney disease, diabetes, sickle-cell anemia
- Influenza vaccine every fall.
- Pneumococcal vaccine.

consent form before the child is vaccinated. Most doctors offer immunization record forms for parents to keep track of all shots. School and day care programs require proper, up-to-date vaccinations.

Vaccine Injury Compensation Program A special program, passed by Congress in 1986, that provides compensation for children who have adverse results after receiving vaccines. All claims are reviewed by medical staff, and awards are decided by a group of attorneys of the U.S. claims court. The program is paid for by a surtax on all vaccines, and it applies to DPT, MMR, OPV, and Td vaccines.

To report an adverse event after a vaccine, call the doctor where your child received the shot to report any reactions. Give complete information about what happened and when it occurred. Your doctor should report any unusual or serious reactions to the Vaccine Adverse Events Reporting System at (800) 822-7967.

For more information about the compensation program, call (800) 338-2382. For more information on filing a claim, contact the U.S. Court of Federal Claims, 717 Madison Place, NW, Washington, DC 20005 or call (202) 219-9657.

In Canada, the province of Quebec is the only one with a vaccine injury plan.

vaccinia   A viral cattle disease ("cowpox") inoculated in humans to produce an antibody against SMALLPOX. Vaccinia is the source of the word *vaccine.*

vaginal infections   Any infection of the vagina caused by bacteria or yeast. Together with a physical exam and history, lab tests are needed to examine vaginal fluid microscopically. Some vaginal infections cause VAGINITIS, an inflammation of the vagina that may include discharge, irritation, and itching.

Some of the most common vaginal infections are bacterial VAGINITIS, TRICHOMONIASIS, and VAGINAL YEAST INFECTION.

vaginal warts   See WARTS.

vaginal yeast infection   A type of infection (also known as CANDIDIASIS) that infects the vagina.

Cause   These vaginal infections are caused by yeast, which lives normally in the vagina; however, when certain conditions upset the delicate balance, a vaginal yeast infection can occur. These conditions include

- diabetes (the high sugar content in urine helps yeast grow)
- obesity (thick folds of fat favor yeast, which grow in warm moist environments)
- pregnancy (hormone balance changes that are favorable to yeast)
- antibiotics (kill off bacteria, allowing yeast to grow)
- steroids (disturb immune system)

Yeast infections commonly occur after a woman has been taking antibiotics for a different infection. Penicillins, tetracyclines, and cephalosporins are particularly associated with this problem.

There is conflicting evidence as to whether birth control pills are associated with infections.

It is not clear whether a woman can give infections to her sexual partner; some studies suggest male partners of women with infections have positive cultures for yeast, but without symptoms. It is possible to pass the infection to a newborn during delivery, causing THRUSH in the baby in the first few weeks of life.

Symptoms   White, thick, cheesy discharge that can cause severe itchiness and uncomfortability; the vulva or vagina may be red and swollen. Some infections are mild, with only slight itchiness and redness. The outer lips of the vulva may feel dry or scaly.

Diagnosis   A vaginal culture is the most accurate test.

Treatment   Creams and suppositories are available over the counter to cure yeast infections. They are inserted into the vagina for two to seven nights, depending on the brand. If there is no improvement in three days, a doctor visit is called for, since the condition could be caused by something other than a yeast infection.

Pregnant women should wait until they have passed 14 weeks of pregnancy before inserting vaginal antifungal yeast infection medicine.

If one course of medicine doesn't work, the doctor may try a different drug; if this fails, ketoconazole pills may be prescribed, which will eradicate yeast in most women with a chronic problem.

Because yeast grows best in dark, moist places, the area should be kept open to air as much as possible. This means avoiding underwear, and wearing a loose dress or nightgown. When underwear must be worn, it should be white 100 percent cotton, with no pantyhose or tight-fitting pants.

vaginitis (vaginosis)   Any mild infection or inflammation of the vagina. It may be called bacterial vaginosis or nonspecific vaginitis when a specific organism (such as TRICHOMONAS) is not identified.

Cause   The bacterium *Gardnerella vaginalis* has been associated with vaginosis, although recent studies suggest a mixture of bacteria may be associated with the illness. Most of these bacteria are normally found in the vagina, but in vaginitis the numbers are much higher than normal.

It is not clear how women get vaginitis, although women who are sexually active and those who have more than one partner have higher rates of disease. Women in their teens and twenties have more infections than older women. While it may be related to sexual activity, it is not passed directly from one person to another.

Symptoms   Gray or frothy vaginal discharge with a foul or fish-smelling odor. It rarely causes itch, burning, or irritation. Some studies suggest an increased risk of preterm labor in women with untreated disease. Pregnant women may also experience discomfort and spotting during pregnancy, but you can't give vaginosis to an unborn baby or at delivery.

Diagnosis   Inspection of vaginal discharge or microscope investigation.

Complications   There are no complications. However, recent studies show that pregnant women with vaginosis are 40 percent more likely to give birth to premature, low-birth-weight babies than are uninfected pregnant women. *Scientists recommend that pregnant women mention any symptoms of vaginal infection to their doctors and get treatment if they have bacterial vaginosis.*

Treatment   Vaginosis is easily treated with the antibiotic metronidazole (Flagyl), which is also used to treat TRICHOMONIASIS. A woman should not take metronidazole during the first 14 weeks of pregnancy.

Sexual intercourse should be avoided during treatment because it may worsen symptoms. Douching is not recommended, since it upsets normal flora in the vagina and will make symptoms worse. Patients should bathe or shower daily with plain soap and water. Bubble baths and bath salts or oils should be avoided until the infection clears.

vaginosis   See VAGINITIS.

valley fever   The common name for COCCIDIOIDOMYCOSIS (or "cocci" for short).

vancomycin-resistant enterococci (VRE)   A bacterium that may infect many patients in intensive-care units and are resistant to most antibiotics available—and represent an increasing public-health concern.

Enterococci normally live in the stomach and intestines and on the skin; generally, they do not cause disease, but they can cause infections (especially in patients weakened by another illness). What makes this particular bacteria so dangerous is that many strains are able to resist antibiotic treatment, including penicillins, cephalosporins, and aminoglycosides. As a result, for many years doctors relied on vancomycin to treat serious enterococcal infections. In the late 1980s, however, strains of enterococci began to appear that resisted even this drug of last resort. They now cause 10 percent of all HOSPITAL-ACQUIRED INFECTIONS. VRE were first documented in Europe in the 1980s and are now emerging as a new threat to patients in the United States.

In 1993, infection with enterococci bacteria occurred in about 3 or 4 cases per 10,000; of these, about 14 percent were resistant to vancomycin. As many as 73 percent of patients who contract VRE die.

Recent information suggest that in the United States, VRE are most commonly found in teaching hospitals and hospitals with more than 500 beds. Reports also suggest that it is rare for a patient who has not been in a hospital to have VRE. However, in Europe, VRE can be found in waste waters and in the feces of both nonhospitalized patients and healthy volunteers.

In one recent study reported in the British medical journal *Lancet,* researchers found that of 38 patients admitted to intensive care, 9 brought the infection with them, 12 became infected in the unit, and 1 person who had one strain of the bacteria on admission developed a second different variety while hospitalized. Of these 13, 11 were infected by a strain that had spread from another patient.

There is no proven treatment for VRE; the infection is transmitted by hands. Chlorhexidine (but not regular soap) kills the bacteria.

Guidelines published by the Centers for Disease Control and Prevention suggest hospital labs periodically test patients for VRE and isolate those patients who are infected. Health care workers who treat these patients should wear protective clothing. Because VRE can live on dirty telephones, walls, and patient charts, hospitals should improve simple housekeeping, according to the CDC.

varicella   See CHICKEN POX.

varicella-zoster immune globulin (VZIG)   An immune globulin obtained from the blood of normal people with high levels of varicella-zoster-antibodies. The immune globulin can be administered to anyone exposed to CHICKEN POX to prevent or modify symptoms of the infection.

varicella-zoster virus (VZV)   A member of the family of herpes viruses, which causes the diseases varicella (CHICKEN POX), and herpes zoster (SHINGLES). When the virus enters the upper respiratory tract of a nonimmune host, it produces skin lesions of chicken pox. The virus then passes from skin to sensory ganglia, where it establishes a latent infection. When the patient's immunity to HSV fades away, the virus replicates within the ganglia and results in shingles (herpes zoster).

The virus is highly contagious and may be spread by direct contact or droplets. Dried crusts of the skin lesions do not contain the virus.

variola   Another name for SMALLPOX.

venereal disease   Another name for SEXUALLY TRANSMITTED DISEASE that got its name as a reference to Venus, goddess of love.

venereal warts   See WARTS, GENITAL.

vibrio   Any bacterium that is curved and capable of unconscious movement, with a tail that makes them good swimmers. Vibrio includes bacteria that belong to the genus *Vibrio.* These include *V. cholerae* (the cause of CHOLERA), *VIBRIO PARAHAEMOLYTICUS* (the cause of a type of seafood poisoning); *V. alginolyticus* and *V. vulnificus* can infect wounds received in warm salt water; *V. vulnificus* can cause blood poisoning if swallowed, especially in people with impaired immune systems or liver problems; *V. vulnificus* has been identified in raw Gulf Coast oysters and has been responsible for at least 13 fatalities since 1992.

Several other marine vibrios have been implicated in human disease. Some may cause wound or ear infections and others cause GASTROENTERITIS. These include *V. alginolyticus*, *V. carchariae*, *V. cincinnatiensis*, *V. damsela*, *V. fluvialis*, *V. furnissii*, *V. hollisae*, *V. metschnikovii*, and *V. mimicus*. See also VIBRIO PARAHAEMOLYTICUS GASTROENTERITIS; DIARRHEA AND INFECTIOUS DISEASE; TRAVELER'S DIARRHEA.

Vibrio cholerae The species of comma-shaped bacillus that causes CHOLERA. See also VIBRIO.

Vibrio parahaemolyticus A type of bacterium often isolated from ocean fish and shellfish that can cause a type of food poisoning. See also VIBRIO PARAHAEMOLYTICUS GASTROENTERITIS; VIBRIO.

Vibrio parahaemolyticus gastroenteritis A type of food poisoning caused by eating fish or shellfish contaminated with the bacteria *V. parahaemolyticus*. Sporadic outbreaks of this type of gastroenteritis have occurred in the United States. It is also very common in Japan, where large outbreaks regularly occur. See also DIARRHEA AND INFECTIOUS DISEASE; ANTIDIARRHEAL DRUGS; TRAVELER'S DIARRHEA; SHELLFISH POISONING, DIARRHEIC.

Cause The disease occurs when the bacterium attaches itself to a person's small intestine and secretes an as-yet-unidentified toxin. Infections with this organism have been associated with eating raw, improperly cooked contaminated fish and shellfish, especially during the warmer months. Improper refrigeration of contaminated seafood allows the bacteria to flourish, increasing the chance of infection.

Symptoms Between 4 and 96 hours after ingestion, the victim may experience diarrhea, abdominal cramps, nausea and vomiting, headache, fever, and chills. The illness is usually mild, although some cases require hospitalization.

Diagnosis The organism can be cultured from stool.

Treatment Symptomatic, including plenty of clear fluids. In most cases, the infection will clear up of itself.

Vincent's disease Also known as trench mouth, this is a painful bacterial infection and ulceration of the gums, known medically as acute necrotizing ulcerative gingivitis. The condition is relatively rare.

Cause Vincent's disease is caused by abnormal growth of microorganisms that are usually harmlessly found in pockets in the gums. Predisposing factors include poor dental hygiene, smoking, throat infections, emotional stress, and impaired immune system. It is usually preceded either by gingivitis or periodontitis (gum infections).

Symptoms Over several days, the gums become sore and inflamed, bleeding at the slightest pressure. Ulcers which bleed spontaneously develop on the gums between the teeth. This is accompanied by bad breath, foul taste, and sometimes swollen glands. As the disease worsens, the ulcers spread along the gum margins and into deeper tissues. Sometimes, the infection spreads to the lips and the lining of the cheeks, causing tissue destruction.

Treatment Mouthwash containing hydrogen peroxide may help relieve pain and inflammation. After a few days, when the gums are less painful they can be scaled to removed hardened mineral deposits and plaque from the teeth. In severe cases, antibacterial drugs may be prescribed to treat the infection.

viral infections One of the most important types of infectious diseases that are caused by a virus, the smallest known kind of infectious

VIRUS TYPES

Family	Examples of Diseases
Adenoviruses	Respiratory and eye infections
Arenaviruses	Lassa fever
Coronaviruses	Common cold
Enteroviruses	Viral meningitis
Herpesviruses	Cold sores, genital herpes, chickenpox, shingles, glandular fever, congenital abnormalities
Orthomyxoviruses	Influenza
Papovaviruses	Warts
Paramyxoviruses	Mumps, measles, rubella
Picornaviruses	Polio, viral hepatitis types A and B, respiratory infections, myocarditis
Poxviruses	Cowpox, smallpox, molluscum contagiosum
Retroviruses	AIDS, degenerative brain disease, possibly cancer
Rhabdoviruses	Rabies
Togaviruses	Yellow fever, dengue, encephalitis

agent. About half to a hundredth the size of the smallest BACTERIA, viruses also have a much simpler structure and method of multiplication.

Scientists debate whether viruses are really living organisms or just collections of large molecules capable of self-replication under favorable conditions. They take over cells of other organisms, where they proceed to make copies of themselves. Outside living cells, viruses are inert and not capable of metabolism or other activities typically found in living organisms.

It is believed that there are more viruses than any other type of organism, and they parasitize all recognized lifeforms (mammals, birds, reptiles, insects, plants, algae, and even bacteria).

Viral infections may be mild (such as WARTS or the common cold) or they can be extremely serious, including RABIES, AIDS, SMALLPOX, POLIOMYELITIS, and most likely, at least some forms of cancer. There are no specific cures for viral diseases, although it is possible to treat their symptoms.

However, it is possible to prevent some of the viral diseases through vaccination, including smallpox, measles, and polio.

virucide   Any agent that can destroy a VIRUS.

virus   The smallest known type of infectious agent. These tiny parasitic microorganisms are much smaller than bacteria, and they don't have any independent metabolic activity. Viruses are about half to a hundredth the size of the smallest bacteria, and they lack bacteria's complex structure.

A virus includes a core of nucleic acid (genetic material RNA or DNA), surrounded by a layer of protein—really just a movable bit of genetic information. Viruses lack the ability to independently reproduce unless they enter a living cell and take over that cell's reproductive apparatus, directing the cell to manufacture viral components instead of its normal ones. The damage that results from this takeover produces the symptoms of viral disease. Scientists believe viruses began as bits of genetic material that escaped from cells, eventually acquiring the ability to move from one organism to the next.

More than 200 viruses have so far been identified as causing human disease, and they have been divided into at least 20 types, including ADENOVIRUS, ARENAVIRUS, CORONAVIRUS, ENTEROVIRUS, herpesvirus, poxvirus, picornavirus, RHINOVIRUS, and RETROVIRUS. They are responsible for an astonishingly wide variety of diseases, ranging from the mild common cold or WARTS to extremely serious illnesses such as AIDS and RABIES. The number of viruses probably exceeds the number of types of all other organisms, and they invade all other types of life-forms—mammals, birds, reptiles, insects, plants, algae—even bacteria. While not all viruses cause disease, many do.

They enter the human body by a variety of ways: They are swallowed, inhaled, or taken into the skin via a puncture (such as an insect bite). They may enter directly via the mucous membranes of the genitals during sexual intercourse and by the conjunctiva of the eye during accidental contamination. Once inside the body, some viruses enter the lymph nodes near where they entered; some invade the white blood cells. Many pass into the blood, spreading throughout the body within a few minutes. From there, they may invade the skin, brain, lungs, or liver.

When they invade the cells, they may disrupt or destroy cellular activities; this can cause serious disease if vital organs are involved. The body's immune system rallies to fight off the viral attack, leading to symptoms of fever and fatigue.

The healthy immune system is able to fight off a viral attack fairly quickly in many cases, within a few days to weeks. Often, the immune system is so sensitized by this attack that a second illness from the same virus is rare (such as in MEASLES). However, some viruses attack so fiercely and fast that serious damage or death may occur before the immune system can muster its defenses (as in the case with polio or rabies). Other times, a virus can hide from the immune system, leading to a chronic infection. This is what happens with many HERPES infections, such as genital herpes and SHINGLES. In the case of the AIDS virus, the weakened immune system opens the door to many OPPORTUNISTIC INFECTIONS.

The name *virus* comes from the Latin word for "poison," first used during the late 19th century for any infectious microbe that caused a disease. It was not until 1892 that Russian bacteriologist Dmitri Ivanovski discovered the sap of a tobacco plant with tobacco mosaic disease could be filtered through a bacteria-trapping filter and still produce the disease. After several other scientists discovered other filter-passing agents, Dutch botanist Martinus Beijerinck named this organism that was able to pass through bacteria filters a *filterable virus.* The two-word term was used for many years, eventually shortened to *virus.* The first human virus was identified by name in 1901 by U.S. army surgeon Walter Reed, who showed that YELLOW FEVER was caused by a filterable virus. Still, it was not until 1927 that its viral heritage was fully understood.

Unlike bacteria, which are easily killed by antibiotics, it's not as easy to design a drug that will kill a virus without killing its host cell. Still, scientists have made progress, such as in the antiviral drugs used to treat herpes infections. INTERFERONS are a group of natural substances produced by infected cells that protect uninfected cells from viral attack. Some interferons are now produced artificially and are being studied against a wide variety of viral infections.

Far easier than curing a viral infection once it occurs is vaccination—protecting against infection before it occurs. Highly effective vaccines are available to prevent a wide variety of viral infections, including polio, measles, MUMPS, RUBELLA, HEPATITIS B, yellow fever, and rabies. The SMALLPOX vaccine has resulted in the total eradication of that disease from the face of the earth.

vulvovaginitis Inflammation of the vulva and vagina usually due to the infections CANDIDIASIS or TRICHOMONIASIS.

Cause YEAST INFECTIONS are the cause of the inflammation.

Symptoms Profuse infected vaginal discharge.

Treatment Antifungal or antibiotic drugs.

warts Generally harmless small, hard round raised bumps, with a rough surface that usually appear on hands and fingers around the knees or on the genitals.

Common warts are the ones that appear on backs of hands, fingers, and knees, usually about a quarter inch in size. Sometimes a few of these bumps run together, but they usually appear separately. Tiny black specks in the wart are caused by tiny clots of blood. Common warts usually appear in places that are often injured, such as the face, hands, knees, and scalp (especially in young children).

Digitate warts are dark-colored growths with fingerlike projections.

Filiform warts look like long, slender growths that occur on the eyelids, armpits, or neck and are usually found in overweight middle-aged people.

Flat warts are small (about $1/16$ inch) tan, flat, round, and grouped together on the face, wrists, backs of hands, and shins. They may itch.

Plantar warts are flat, rough warts that appear on the soles of the feet. They occur alone or in groups and are flat because of the pressure of the rest of the body placed upon them.

Cause Warts are caused by one of the more than 58 types of HUMAN PAPILLOMAVIRUS (HPV). A person gets a wart by touching someone else's wart, touching something a wart-infected person has touched, or by self-inoculation. People who bite on their own warts can spread them to other areas of their own bodies. The incubation period between first infection and the appearance of the wart averages between two to three months, but it may be as long as 20 months. The person is infectious as long as the wart appears.

Diagnosis Most warts are diagnosed by appearance; rarely, a doctor may biopsy a piece of wart to make a diagnosis.

Treatment More than 65 percent of warts disappear on their own within two years. There is no specific medication to kill the virus, although different treatments can eradicate the wart itself. Over-the-counter removal preparations include topical medications containing salicylic acid, which peels off the affected skin. The virus is killed as well, since it is inside the tissue. The skin should be softened first before applying the medicine; a few times a week, the dead skin should be removed with an emery board.

If the warts don't disappear with this treatment, a dermatologist may apply liquid nitrogen to freeze the wart solid; as it thaws, it forms a blister that lifts off the wart. This takes four to six weeks. Sometimes a blister-producing liquid (cantharidin) or a corroding acid liquid or plaster may be used. Some doctors may use heated electrical needles. Since wart treatment can cause scars, it is best to wait for the warts to disappear on their own.

warts, genital Soft warts that grow in and around the entrance of the vagina, the anus, and the penis. Genital warts are the most common viral SEXUALLY TRANSMITTED DISEASE in the United States, outranking even genital HERPES.

Almost 2 million Americans are treated for genital warts each year, and most cases are diagnosed in women between the ages of 15 and 24. Older women may have the virus, but their immune systems control the outbreaks. Those who are most at risk are people with more than one sex partner and those who do not use condoms.

Cause Eight different types of HUMAN PAPILLOMAVIRUS (HPV) are associated with genital warts. However, only a few (types 16 and 18) are associated with cervical cancer, and these are not usually visible. The different types of warts can only be distinguished in a research lab. The virus is transmitted during unprotected sex with an infected partner. A person is infectious when visible warts are present in the genital area; however, even if the warts have disappeared, the virus may still be present in the body.

Symptoms Genital warts are pink to gray, soft, raised, or flat, and may cause itching, burning, or bleeding around the genital area. They may appear alone or in clusters, ranging in size from pinpoint to a small mass. Men usually notice the warts on the penis, although they can also appear in the anus or the urethra. Men may completely miss small warts. Women may find warts on the vulva, vagina, or anus; occasionally they may occur on the cervix. Incubation period is unknown. The warts won't be painful, but they can grow and block the openings of the vagina, anus, urethra, or throat.

Complications Pregnant women with genital warts may have problems during delivery because hormonal changes can cause the warts to grow in size and number. Occasionally, babies exposed to warts in the birth canal develop warts in the throat and a few develop warts on the genitals or eyes. Warts may also multiply and grow larger among those with weakened immune systems or diabetes.

Two or more strains of the HPV strain have been associated with a higher risk of cervical cancer, especially among women with persistent warts and many sex partners. However, most women who have genital warts are not considered to be at increased risk for developing cervical cancer. The association between this type of cancer and HPV is not well understood.

Diagnosis A doctor can diagnose the condition from the wart's appearance; a magnifying glass may be needed to find small warts. Odd-looking warts may require biopsy. A Pap smear will identify warts on the cervix or those deep inside the vagina.

Treatment There is no cure that will remove all traces of the HP virus from the body. Instead, treatment aims at removing or shrinking the warts, whether by freezing, using a topical solution, or laser or conventional surgery. Unfortunately, warts often reappear after treatment.

Podophyllin topical solution is applied by a doctor to external warts only (it shouldn't be used in the cervix, rectum, or while pregnant). The solution must not touch the surrounding skin, as it can be irritating. If there are no results after four weeks, another treatment method should be used. Podofilox 0.05% is a prescription topical solution that can be applied by the woman for external warts. It works by killing wart tissue.

Cryotherapy freezes the wart off; it is sometimes used for cervical or rectal warts. Laser therapy is performed in a doctor's office and is sometimes used for cervical warts.

Electrosurgery is also performed in a doctor's office, but this is used for rectal warts. As a last resort, a doctor may turn to surgical removal if the warts are very large or causing problems. Still, 20 percent of the time warts grow back after this treatment.

Prevention Infected partners should avoid sex when the warts are large, bleeding, or painful. A doctor should be consulted if warts block rectal openings or if there is trouble urinating.

All women with anogenital warts need a Pap test every 6 to 12 months to detect early signs of cervical cancer. Young girls with cervical HPV should have regular Pap tests to treat any changes in the cervix. Most cervical problems take care of themselves, but those with a positive Pap test should seek medical help regularly to monitor the changes.

Anyone who has genital warts or who has been diagnosed in the past should always use a condom during sexual intercourse. At present, there is no way to prevent the disease. Physicians at the University of Rochester Medical Center are beginning the world's first test in humans of a potential vaccine to protect against the virus.

For more information, contact the American Societal Health Association, P.O. Box 13827, Research Triangle Park, NC 27709; phone (919) 361-8400; fax (919) 361-8425.

water, contaminated   Water can be a source of infection if it contains infective or parasitic organisms and is drunk, swum in, or comes into contact with food. Throughout the world, tainted water is a major source of the spread of infectious disease, including viral HEPATITIS A, DIARRHEA, TYPHOID FEVER, CHOLERA, AMEBIASIS, and some types of worm infestation. Water can become contaminated by feces (either human or animal) that contain infective material in rivers, lakes, reservoirs, or wells. Contamination can also occur via untreated sewage or leakage between sewage and water supplies.

The risk of waterborne infection in the United States is far less than in the Third World because of adequate sanitary facilities, sewage treatment and disposal, and the sterilization and testing of municipal water supplies. This does not mean that all U.S. drinking water is safe, however. The CRYPTOSPORIDIOSIS parasite is believed to infect millions of Americans each year through tainted tap water. In 1993, more than 400,000 Milwaukee residents became ill after drinking contaminated tap water. Those infected reported nausea, severe abdominal cramps, diarrhea, and low-grade fever. Some deaths were reported. The parasite, which is not killed by chlorination, can also be found in

pools, lakes, rivers, hot tubs, ice cubes, and on fruits and vegetables. Symptoms usually strike 2 to 10 days after exposure. Similarly, the microorganism called *Cyclospora* can cause many of the same symptoms in those who drink tainted water or food.

Recent research determined that pregnant women in the United States who drank more than five glasses of tap water a day had higher levels of miscarriage.

To avoid infection outside the United States, travelers should use bottled or canned water and drinks of well-known brand names. Ice should not be put into drinks. Rainwater is usually free from infective organisms if it not allowed to stand for a long period before drinking.

Water that may be tainted should be boiled before drinking for five minutes, since this will kill any infective organisms. Alternatively, the water can be filtered and then sterilized chemically. Various filters can remove bacteria and other infective organisms as well as inanimate particles. Chemical sterilization methods use pills containing chlorine or iodine; water should be left for 20 to 30 minutes after chemical treatment before being used.

Swimming in polluted water may lead to an EAR INFECTION. Swimmers who inadvertently swallow water may contract a disease transmitted in polluted drinking water. This is why swimmers should avoid swimming in polluted rivers or in the ocean near large coastal resorts. In tropical countries, swimming in rivers, lakes, or ponds is not recommended because of the risk of SCHISTOSOMIASIS, a serious disease caused by a river fluke that can burrow through the swimmer's skin. SWIMMER'S ITCH is caused by a similar type of fluke. Outbreaks of swimmer's itch have occurred in the United States.

Finally, fish and shellfish that live in polluted water may accumulate infective organisms in their own bodies and, if improperly cooked, can pass on infections to consumers.

Waterhouse-Friderichsen syndrome A very rare (but serious) condition caused by an overwhelming infection of the bloodstream. The condition is almost always fatal unless it is immediately treated in a hospital with intensive care.

Cause Bacteria of the meningococcus group are the cause of this disease, and therefore MENINGITIS is often associated with this syndrome.

Symptoms The onset of symptoms with this syndrome is abrupt; within hours, the victim sinks into a coma as blood pours into the adrenal glands, leading to acute adrenal failure and shock. Rapidly enlarging purple spots appear on the skin.

Treatment Emergency treatment includes vasopressor drugs, intravenous fluids, plasma, and oxygen. No sedatives or narcotics are given. Specific treatment for BACTEREMIA is intensive antibiotic therapy given until symptoms subside.

Weil's syndrome A severe form of LEPTOSPIROSIS, an infectious disease caused by organisms of the genus *Leptospira*. Weil's syndrome was named after German physician Adolph Weil, who identified this syndrome as a type of "infectious jaundice" in 1886.

Cause The organisms are transmitted to human beings via the urine of a wide variety of wild and domestic animals, including rats, mice, deer, dogs, bats, foxes, rabbits, pigs, goats, birds, frogs, snakes, fish, raccoons, and so on. The germs attack humans by entering the skin.

Symptoms Weil's syndrome can lead to liver and kidney problems, vomiting, and MENINGITIS.

Treatment It can be treated with antibiotics but not prevented.

Whipple's disease A rare intestinal disorder that causes (among other things) abnormal skin pigmentation, found most often among middle-aged men. People with the disease become severely malnourished.

Cause Unknown, but probably due to an unidentified bacterial infection.

Symptoms In addition to the above symptoms, there is malabsorption, diarrhea, abdominal pain, progressive weight loss, joint pain, swollen lymph nodes, anemia, and fever.

Diagnosis Jejunal biopsy.

Treatment Antibiotics (penicillin and tetracycline) for at least one year.

whipworm infestation (trichuriasis) Whipworms are parasitic roundworms of the species *Trichuris trichiura* that infect the intestinal tract. Adults worms are 30 to 50 mm long and look somewhat like a whip. The eggs are remarkably hardy and may resist freezing; they can remain alive in the environment for years. About 2 million people in the United States are affected, primarily children and institutionalized patients.

Cause Whipworm infection occurs when a person comes in contact with and ingests whipworm eggs in fecal-contaminated soil. Whipworms are small worms about 1 or 2 inches long that can live in the intestines for up to 20 years. The eggs hatch, and the whipworm embeds itself into the mucous membrane. While the worms live in the large intestine (predominantly in the cecum) and appendix, they may infest the colon as well.

Symptoms Light infestation causes few symptoms, but a heavier worm load may cause bloody diarrhea that appears to contain mucus.

Diagnosis Examination of stool can reveal the presence of whipworm eggs.

Treatment Mebendazole can kill the worms, although a serious case may require more than one treatment. Recovery is complete.

Complications In very severe cases, dehydration and anemia as a result of the bloody diarrhea can occur. Rarely, rectal prolapse can occur.

Prevention Good public health practices, including covered sewers and safe garbage disposal, can reduce the incidence of whipworms.

Whitmore's disease The common name for melioidosis, an uncommon bacterial infection of rodents caused by *Pseudomonas pseudomallei*, which is endemic in southeast Asia and Australia.

Cause The disease is also found in pigs, cattle, sheep, and horses. The exact mode of transmission in unknown, but it is thought to be acquired by humans through breathing in the bacteria or through contact with broken skin. The bacteria are also found in soil and water (especially rice paddies).

Symptoms The exact incubation period is not known; it may be months or years. There may be no symptoms at all. If there are, in humans, the disease takes three forms—an acute septicemic (blood poisoning) with diarrhea; a typhoidal form with local abscess formation and severe hives; and a chronic form.

Treatment ABSCESSES must be surgically drained; antibiotics are administered (tetracycline with chloramphenicol, piperacillin, gentamicin, or doxycycline).

whooping cough The common name for "pertussis," an acute infection of the upper respiratory tract featuring violent, loud bouts of coughing that end in a whoop. Vomiting usually occurs at the end of the coughing spell. Most serious in young children, whooping cough is highly contagious and will infect virtually all susceptible people who come in contact with the bacterium.

Before the vaccine was available in the 1940s, hundreds of thousands of children suffered from whooping cough each year, and many thousands died—more every year than from all other infectious diseases combined. Today, the disease infects only about 3,000 to 5,000 American children a year and kills less than 20 of them. Because the disease can be deadly in infants, babies should be isolated from anyone with whooping cough.

But while the number of cases has declined since the introduction of the vaccine, it is far from eradicated. In the fall of 1992, more than 200 Massachusetts children between the ages of 10 and 19 became ill; all had attended two schools in the same area. All had been vaccinated as young children, but their immunity had worn off.

Whooping cough affects people of all ages all over the world, and is a common cause of death in the developing countries. The disease is most serious in babies, who may often develop pneumonia; babies younger than three months of age get the worst cases. Seventy percent of deaths occur in young babies (about 1 in 200 infected babies will die).

The most infectious time is at the beginning of the illness.

Doctors must report any suspected or confirmed cases of whooping cough to the health department. If the child attends school or child care, the parent must notify the principal so staff and other children can be given preventive medicine.

Recent studies have suggested that more and more adults are contracting whooping cough, either because they were never immunized or because immunity has eroded. In one study, 23 percent of adults who went to hospital emergency rooms with complaints of a cough lasting more than one month were found to have whooping cough. Because many physicians think of pertussis as a disease of childhood, it is often overlooked in diagnosing persistent coughs in adults. In fact, new studies show that whooping cough may strike repeatedly throughout life. Data suggest that by age 20 everyone, even in the United States, has developed whooping cough.

Cause The disease is caused by a rod-shaped bacterium called BORDETELLA PERTUSSIS, which produces a toxin that invades the lining of the throat, windpipe, and bronchial tubes. The tissue damage causes very thick mucus production that is irritating, leading to severe coughing spells as the victim tries to expel the mucus. The thick mucus often leads to PNEU-MONIA. A similar but less common bacterium called *B. parapertussis* may cause a milder form of the disease.

The disease is spread during coughing, which spews the bacteria outward for several feet. These bacteria can survive on tissue or bed covers for a short time; the disease can also be passed on when another person touches these items. Whooping cough is infectious enough so that it will be spread to everyone in the household from one infected patient.

Symptoms Whooping cough occurs in three stages in children; the first stage starts slowly with coldlike symptoms (sneezing, red or sore eyes, and a low-grade fever) and an irritating dry cough for one or two weeks. This is the period when the patient is most infectious.

These initial symptoms are followed by intense, violent spasms of repeated coughing with no time to breathe between spasms. There is a repetitive series of 8 or 10 rapid coughs on one breath that often end in gagging or vomiting. The coughs may end in a characteristic "whoop" as the patient tries to take a breath. (Babies under six months of age will choke but won't make the whooping sound; these youngest patients can become very sick.) The infected person may appear blue, with bulging eyes and a dazed, apathetic expression. Infants may experience temporary apnea (cessation of breathing) after a coughing spasm. The periods between coughing are comfortable; there is little fever. This stage may last about two weeks.

The final stage dwindles down into a chronic cough for three to four weeks; some children experience a cough of more than two months.

Adults can get whooping cough, although there is not usually a whoop and the cough is milder. Public health experts suggest that whooping cough should be suspected in anyone who has a cough lasting more than seven days. Some adults may be infected without symptoms; these adults are capable of spreading the disease to children.

Complications A child with the disease may have an ear infection or pneumonia. About 1 in 500 infants younger than six months may develop seizures, coma, or brain damage. The chronic cough may cause nosebleeds and bleeding from blood vessels on the surface of the eyes; recurrent vomiting can cause dehydration and malnourishment.

Diagnosis The disease is diagnosed by identifying the bacterium in a culture grown from a nasal swab taken in the early stages of the illness. There are two tests, neither of which is 100 percent accurate, and there are many false negatives. The rapid test gives results in a few minutes; a blood test done in mid-disease may identify the bacterium or detect antibodies.

Treatment If the illness is recognized early enough, antibiotics such as erythromycin or clarithromycin are often given; they may shorten the duration of illness and the period of contagiousness, although they are not particularly helpful once the severe coughing stage of the illness has begun.

Patients should be kept warm, given small, frequent meals and plenty to drink and protected from things that produce coughing (such as drafts or smoke). An infant or child who becomes blue or keeps vomiting after coughing needs to be admitted to the hospital.

Prevention Administration of the pertussis vaccine, which is usually given as part of the DPT (diphtheria-pertussis-tetanus) vaccine in infancy and childhood, will prevent the disease. It is usually given in combination with DIPHTHERIA and TETANUS vaccines to children at two, four, and six months of age in the United States. A booster dose is given at age five.

The pertussis vaccine is made from killed whole pertussis cells or a whole bacterium; some babies have no side effects after whole-cell pertussis immunization. About half suffer from swelling and pain in the arm, fever, crankiness, drowsiness, or poor appetite for a day or two after the shot, but treatment with acetaminophen before the vaccination helps reduce the side effects.

The pertussis part of the DPT vaccine was controversial, however, because some parents and scientists believed a few children developed more serious side effects, including seizures, brain damage, or death. Very rarely (about 1 in every 100,000) a baby may have a severe reaction with high-pitched screaming or seizures. About 1 in 300,000 may suffer permanent brain damage. Because of these very small risks, the vaccine is not given to an infant who has a history of seizures, who has a feverish illness, or who has suffered a previous reaction to the pertussis vaccine.

In developed countries, most infants are vaccinated in the first year of life, but the vaccine is not completely effective in preventing the illness and not all children are suitable for vaccination. For this reason, epidemics still occur. It is estimated that between 20,000 to 30,000 cases still occur each year in the United States, although not all cases are reported.

In 1981, the Japanese developed an acellular vaccine that produces fever and milder side effects; this vaccine is made of only a few parts of the pertussis cell. Japan has been giving the new vaccine to infants since 1989; it was recently approved in the United States for the primary series given to infants.

The vaccine is given in an infant's thigh muscle or a child's arm muscle. The vaccine is not given to anyone older than seven because the disease is usually milder in older children and adults, and it is believed that reactions are worse in this age group (although no studies prove this).

Anyone who has had an allergic reaction after the shot should not again be vaccinated for this disease, nor should anyone who experiences any major unresponsiveness or change in consciousness within seven days.

Other patients who should not be given further doses of the vaccine include those who have had persistent uncontrollable crying for more than three hours, a fever higher than 105 degrees F not caused by another illness, or collapse *unless* there is a serious outbreak in the patient's area.

If the percentage of vaccinated children drops significantly (as it did in the United Kingdom in the 1970s), the number of children who contract the disease skyrockets. Because the illness is potentially deadly, it is important that all infants suitable for vaccination be treated. The risks of vaccination are far less than the dangers of having whooping cough.

World Health Organization (WHO) An agency of the United Nations that was established in 1948 to oversee international health matters and public health. Its headquarters is in Geneva, Switzerland. Regional offices are located in Europe, Africa, North America, South America, Southeast Asia, the eastern Mediterranean, and the western Pacific (including Australia).

The WHO has fought effectively against certain infectious diseases such as TUBERCULOSIS, MALARIA, and SMALLPOX, which was declared officially eradicated throughout the world in 1980.

It also sponsors medical research programs, organizes a network of collaborating national labs, and provides expert advice to its 160 member states on health service organizations, family health, medicinal drugs, drug abuse, and mental health.

worms See HELMINTH.

Y

yaws One of the world's most prevalent infections, this is a childhood skin disease found throughout the poorer subtropical and tropical areas of the world. Also known as frambesia, pian, or bouba, yaws is not a sexually transmitted disease. It occurs between the Tropics of Cancer and Capricorn, where more than 50 million people have been treated with PENICILLIN in an effort to eradicate the disease. As a result, the incidence of disease has been reduced in many areas, although it still occurs in many communities.

The disease is not believed to have been known in the ancient world. It was first noted in the West Indies after the discovery of America; it is believed that is was brought from Africa to America by the slave trade.

It is very rare in India, and it is almost unknown in Europe, Japan, New Zealand, and Tasmania.

Cause Yaws is caused by the spirochete *Treponema pertenue*, a close cousin of *T. pallidum*, the spirochete that causes SYPHILIS. The relationship between the two diseases is not clear. However, unlike syphilis, yaws appears to be acquired by direct contact with an infected person, not by sexual intercourse.

Symptoms While not a fatal disease, yaws is very disfiguring and often disabling. About a month after infection, symptoms of malaise, low fever, and headache appear. In the primary stage, a highly contagious, itchy red raspberry-like growth appears on the site of the infection. In places where people regularly go barelegged and barefoot, these growths usually appear on the soles of the feet and the lower legs. Scratching spreads the infection, leading to development of more growths on other parts of the skin.

During the next few weeks, the growths develop into blisters, which begin to ooze and then form a crust. Sores then develop. The nearby lymph glands may become swollen, and the joints and bones may ache. There may be an irregular fever. The initial sores may disappear with no other problems except for scarring. More typically, they last for several months.

The secondary stage is the most infectious, usually developing three months after onset of the disease. At this point, areas of rash and sores appear all over the body; as some sores disappear (leaving discolored patches), others enlarge and develop into nodules. These lesions are usually painless (except on the soles of the feet), but they may be very itchy. This stage lasts for three to six months in children, and from six months to a year in adults.

The tertiary stage—characterized by the destruction of large areas of the bones, nose, and joints by the ulcers—may last for years, but it does not always occur.

Treatment A single dose of penicillin will cure this disease. Without treatment, growths heal slowly over about six months, but recurrence is common. About 10 percent of untreated patients experience the tertiary stage.

Prevention There is no way to prevent yaws, but in places where the disease is widespread, proper care of injuries or wounds will lessen the chance of contracting the disease.

yeast infection A skin infection caused by types of fungi, the most important of which is CANDIDA ALBICANS, which causes CANDIDIASIS. *Candida* can normally be found in the mouth, vagina, and large intestine, but for unknown reasons it can sometimes turn against its host—most commonly in those who take antibiotics, oral steroids, and birth control pills, and in diabetics and the overweight.

This type of yeast causes THRUSH (white patches on the inside of the cheeks), cheesy vaginal discharge, or monilial intertrigo (damp red eruptions under the breasts, the foreskin, and under body folds in the obese). It also causes *Candida* paronychia (redness and swelling around the nails).

Candidal infections usually respond to topical broad-spectrum antibiotics or specific preparations designed to fight yeasts (nystatin). See also VAGINAL YEAST INFECTIONS.

yellow fever   A short-acting infectious viral disease that gets its name from its symptom of yellowed skin from jaundice. The three varieties of yellow fever include urban, jungle, and sylvan and can range from mild to fatal. In general, the disease is a risk only for those who travel to sub-Saharan Africa or tropical South America. Eradication of the mosquito from populated areas has greatly reduced the incidence of the disease. It is fatal only about 5 percent of the time.

Still, epidemics of yellow fever can occur when large numbers of susceptible humans and infected mosquitoes coexist. The disease has been known since the time of the first explorations of Africa; every few years since, many thousands of Africans have gotten yellow fever, and as many as half of those infected will die. Nigerian epidemics between 1986 and 1988 killed 10,000 people.

Epidemics of yellow fever end when the dry season comes and the mosquitoes who carry the virus become less abundant. Epidemics have also ended when the surviving human population becomes immune, either through infection or mass vaccination.

History   The disease was considered to be the American PLAGUE, a tropical fever that profoundly affected the development of the New World in the wake of Columbus's arrival. After his visit, the yellow fever virus helped to exterminate entire civilizations on the new continent. Dreadful epidemics in coastal cities such as Philadelphia, New Orleans, and Charleston were devastating to the new settlers as well as the native American populations. In 1793, Philadelphia was struck by a severe yellow fever outbreak that was to kill 4,000 of its citizens (15 percent of the total population of the city) in three months. The outbreak, which was blamed on German and Haitian immigrants, virtually brought the great city to a standstill and was one reason why the former great seaport dropped behind New York City in maritime importance.

In the late 19th century, the origin of the disease was discovered to be the AEDES mosquito, which explained why it was not contagious and why it occurred only during the summer months. The fact that port cities faced the most severe epidemics helps support the theory that ships transported the mosquitoes to the United States. Moreover, the mosquitoes' inability to fly over great distances limited the spread of the disease.

The virus was identified by Adrian Stokes in 1927 at the Rockefeller Foundation's Yellow Fever Research Institute in Lagos, Nigeria. Dr. Stokes was one of four Foundation scientists who died of laboratory infections with yellow fever virus while working at the institute (two others died in labs in Mexico and Brazil).

Cause   The yellow fever virus is included in a group of viruses called flavivirus (from the Latin word *flavus,* meaning "yellow"). This is the same group of viruses that contains St. Louis and Japanese ENCEPHALITIS. There is no difference in the way the three types of yellow fever (urban, jungle, and sylvan) affect victims; the three types differ only in their natural cycles.

Yellow fever virus mostly infects monkeys and mosquitoes, although it sometimes is transmitted via monkeys, who pass it on to humans. In cities ("urban yellow fever"), the disease is transmitted between humans by *Aedes aegypti* mosquitoes. This mosquito is found in the southeastern United States, but no disease has been reported since 1905 in

New Orleans. However, the potential for the disease to spread in this country remains.

Most yellow fever is of the *jungle* type, which is transmitted between monkeys in Africa by forest mosquitoes. Countries reporting cases in 1995 include Angola, Cameroon, Gabon, Gambia, Ghana, Guinea, Mali, Nigeria, Sudan, Zaire, Bolivia, Brazil, Colombia, Ecuador, and Peru and West Africa.

Sylvan yellow fever is transmitted between forest monkeys in South America by treetop-living species of mosquitoes (not Aedes) that only bite humans when they cut down a giant tree, bringing the mosquitoes down to ground level.

While people can't directly transmit the disease to other humans, they can infect mosquitoes from just before fever appears to about five days into the illness. The infected mosquitoes remain infectious for their entire life span. For these reasons, patient isolation and standard blood and body fluid precautions should be taken by caregivers.

Major epidemics can reappear in towns and cities that don't control the mosquitoes. In the forests, the virus cycle is in monkeys and is carried by forest mosquitoes. When monkey populations increase, there are more nonimmune monkeys, and the virus spreads among them. In addition, as the monkey populations increase, more of them venture into farmers' fields, where other mosquitoes become infected and they in turn infect the farmer.

Symptoms   Many people have no symptoms, some have a mild illness and a few (about 5 percent of those infected) become very sick and die. In those who have symptoms, between three and six days after infection there is a sudden fever and headache, backache, with nausea and vomiting. Characteristic signs are pulse slowing as temperature rises and albumin in the urine; in those with serious disease, those signs progress to nosebleeds, bleeding from the mouth, coffee-ground-colored or black vomit due to blood in the stomach, black stool due to digested blood.

In most people symptoms pass in about three days; others experience neck, back, and leg pain; fever; chills; weakness; restlessness; and irritability.

Most people recover because their immune systems are able to fight off the disease and develop antibodies that destroy the virus. Recovery in these cases is slow but complete, without permanent damage. One attack of yellow fever in humans provides lifetime immunity.

Diagnosis   Urine tests will show high level of albumin; blood tests reveal low levels of white blood cells. Antibodies to the virus in blood samples will be conclusive.

Complications   Some patients begin to feel better but after three to nine days progress to the second stage of yellow fever, including liver and kidney damage, jaundice and kidney failure, agitation. The gums bleed, vomit contains blood and stools turn black, and skin and eyes become yellow tinged. Fatal cases proceed to delirium, coma, and death.

Treatment   No drug is effective against the yellow fever virus, so treatment is aimed at lowering fever, maintaining blood volume via transfusion of fluids and avoiding liver damage. In mild or moderate cases the prognosis is excellent: up to 95 percent of patients will survive.

Prevention   Vaccination confers long-lasting immunity and should always be obtained before traveling through affected areas. Although the vaccination is effective for life, international regulations require revaccinations every 10 years. The vaccine is effective beginning 10 days after the first dose. The yellow fever vaccine is given only at approved yellow fever vaccination centers.

Reactions to the vaccine are usually mild. Between 2 and 5 percent of vaccinated patients have mild headaches, low-grade fevers, or other minor symptoms between 5 and 10 days later. Immediate hypersensitivity reactions (including rash, hives, or asthma) are extremely uncommon (less than one in a million). They occur primarily in those with egg allergies.

A yellow fever vaccination certificate is required for entry to many countries. If travel plans include travel to any country in Africa or South America, travelers should get a yellow fever vaccination and certificate before leaving the United States for these locations. For a complete list of yellow fever vaccination requirements for all countries, call the CDC Fax Information Service for International Travelers at (404) 332-4565.

In addition, countries where yellow fever is reported are listed every two weeks in the Summary of Health Information for International Travel ("the blue sheet"), available 24 hours a day from the CDC Fax Information Service for International Travelers or by calling the CDC international travelers' hot line at (404) 332-4559. The blue sheet is also available from state or local health departments. In Canada, information can be found at the Tropical Health and Quarantine Division at the Laboratory Center for Disease Control at (613) 957-8739 or fax (613) 998-6413.

All those who can't be vaccinated for medical reasons must obtain a medical waiver instead of the yellow fever certificate. This will include a doctor's letter stating the reasons against the vaccine; the waiver is obtained from the consular or embassy officials of the country to be visited before leaving the United States. A single injection of the vaccine gives protection for up to 10 years, but children under age one should not be vaccinated.

The World Health Organization must be notified within 24 hours about new cases of yellow fever in areas previously free of the disease, including cases in monkeys.

Yersinia enterocolitica A member of the *Yersinia* genus of small bacteria that cause entercolitis and other diseases. See also YERSINIOSIS.

Yersinia (Pasteurella) pestis A small gram-negative bacterium that causes PLAGUE, transmitted from rodents to humans usually via the flea. *Y. pestis* can live for a long period of time in infected carcasses, soil, or sputum. It is also known as *Pasteurella pestis*. It is named for the 19th-century French bacteriologist Alexandre E. J. Yersin. See also YERSINIOSIS.

Yersinia pseudotuberculosis A member of the *Yersinia* genus of bacteria that causes pseudotuberculosis.

yersiniosis A common but underreported food-borne illness that was first recognized in the United States in 1976, where it was traced to tainted chocolate milk. Infants and children are the most common victims; children with abnormally high iron levels in their blood are particularly susceptible.

While it can occur at any time, most cases appear during the winter in North America.

Cause The disease is caused by eating tainted food or touching sick pets or contaminated people. The illness is caused by two species of rod-shaped bacteria, YERSINIA ENTEROCOLITICA and YERSINIA PSEUDOTUBERCULOSIS both of which are related to YERSINIA PESTIS (the bacterium that causes human PLAGUE). All three belong to the family Enterobacteriacae (which also includes SALMONELLA). The bacteria is found in swine and swine waste, cows, dogs, cats (especially those from animal shelters), poultry, shellfish, ice cream, fruit, and vegetables, but most outbreaks are traced to chocolate milk, milk, mussels, oysters, tofu, pork, and contaminated water.

Because the bacteria can grow even when refrigerated, high-risk foods include undercooked pork, beef that has been vacuum packed or fresh packed, unpasteurized milk, and cheese.

Outbreaks are fairly common among day care centers. Infected pups and kittens can infect small children. The water from un-treated wells, lakes, rivers, and streams may also be a source for the disease.

Symptoms High fever (up to 104 degrees F), nausea and vomiting, bloody or mucousy diarrhea, abdominal pain (similar to appendicitis pain). It is often misdiagnosed as appendicitis. Children may be quite ill and may also suffer headache, sore throat, and loss of appetite. Symptoms usually last up to 10 days, although some children may be ill for a month. It is almost never fatal, however.

Some women experience a skin rash on the front of the legs, together with painful legs. The bacteria may remain in the stool for up to three months afterward.

Diagnosis Stool culture is the best test, although it is not easy to diagnose. Blood tests may detect antibodies a few weeks after the illness appears.

Complications Bone infection, blood-stream infection, and MENINGITIS may follow yersiniosis, but these are rare except in the very old or those with weakened immune systems.

Treatment Antibiotics are effective and should be taken up to seven days; serious illness may require hospitalization with intravenous medication. Analysis of stool samples can determine which antibiotic to use.

Prevention If yersiniosis is suspected, contact the health department with details. Anyone with these symptoms at a child care center should see if others have a similar illness; investigation may be needed if there are many ill children.

abscess A clearly defined walled-off inflammatory area (usually caused by infection) that contains pus.

acute condition A condition that appears suddenly.

antibiotic A drug that kills or slows the growth of bacteria. Antibiotics are used to fight bacterial infections; they have no effect on viruses.

antibiotic resistance The ability of a bacterium to change (mutate) its characteristics so that it is no longer sensitive to a particular antibiotic.

antibody A protein that is manufactured by a type of white blood cell (lymphocyte) to neutralize a foreign protein in the body. Antibodies identify, neutralize, or destroy bacteria, viruses, and other harmful microorganisms.

antigen A substance that can trigger an immune response, causing the production of an antibody as part of the body's defense against infection. Many antigens are not found naturally in the body; they include microorganisms, toxins, and tissues from another used in an organ transplant.

ARC Abbreviation for "AIDS related complex," a collection of signs and symptoms that often appear as HIV infections progress from a no-symptom state to full-blown AIDS.

arthropod Insects and ticks capable of transmitting bacteria or viruses that cause infectious disease in humans.

biopsy Removal and examination of a small piece of tissue.

bone marrow Tissue contained within the internal cavities of the bones.

bubo Enlarged, inflamed lymph node (especially under the arm or in the groin) caused by infections such as plague, tuberculosis, or syphilis.

canker sore A small, painful ulcer, usually found on the mouth or lips.

carbuncle A staphylococcal infection of skin and skin tissue made up of a cluster of furuncles.

carrier A person who harbors the microorganisms that cause a particular disease without experiencing symptoms of infection but who can transmit the disease to others.

chancre An ulcer at the site of infection in the skin caused by disease, such as syphilis or tuberculosis.

congenital Present at birth.

contagious Capable of being transmitted to others.

contagious disease Originally, a disease that was transmitted only by physical contact. Today, it is usually used to mean "communicable disease."

corticosteroid A group of drugs based on the structure of cortisone (a hormone produced by the adrenal glands) with antiinflammatory properties.

culture Growth of microorganisms on artificial media; cultures are used to diagnose a particular bacterium or virus.

curettage The removal of skin tissue with a curet (sharp blade).

disinfection Eliminating most germs on surfaces.

dysentery Bloody diarrhea.

ecthyma A shallow bacterial infection that often causes scarring.

endemic Occurring frequently in a particular region or population.

enteric Pertaining to the intestines.

epidemic A sudden outbreak of infectious disease that spreads rapidly through the population, affecting a large number of people. Narrowly defined, *epidemic* refers to outbreaks in human populations and *epizootic* to outbreaks in animal groups.

exposure   The condition of being subject to an infectious disease as a result of contact with an infected person or contaminated environment.

fungus   Simple parasitic life-forms that make up a plant phylum (including yeasts, rusts, molds, smuts, mushrooms, mildews, etc.).

gram-negative bacteria   A type of bacteria that resist the chemical strain used in Gram's method of identifying microorganisms for characterization purposes. Some of the most common gram-negative bacteria include *Bacteroides fragilis, Brucella abortus, Escherichia coli, Haemophilus influenzae, Klebsiella pneumoniae, Neisseria gonorrhoeae, Proteus vulgaris, Pseudomonas aeruginosa, Salmonella typhi, Shigella dysenteriae,* and *Yersinia pestis.*

gram-positive bacteria   A type of bacteria that retain the violet color of the stain used in Gram's method of staining microorganisms. Some of the most common kinds of gram-positive bacteria are *Bacillus anthracis, Clostridium, Mycobacterium leprae, Mycobacterium tuberculosis, Staphylococcus aureus, Streptococcus pneumoniae,* and *Streptococcus pyogenes.*

Gram's stain   Laboratory staining test used to identify bacteria. A bacterium will either retain or resist a chemical stain depending on what type of cell wall it has. Bacteria that accept stain are "gram-positive," those that don't are "gram-negative."

host   The insect, animal, or human on which a microorganism is able to live and reproduce.

immune disorder   Any temporary or permanent condition that weakens the immune system.

immune globulin   Human blood plasma from many sources that contain protective antibodies to a particular disease.

immune system   The network of cells and proteins that is designed to fight infection in the human body. The system includes the spleen, lymph glands, white blood cells, and antibodies.

immunity   A state of protection against a disease through the activities of the immune system. Natural immunity is present from birth and is the first line of defense against most infectious agents. Acquired immunity is the second line of defense, that develops either through exposure to microorganisms or as a result of immunization.

immunization   The injection of weakened or killed microorganism to trigger the production of antibodies to provide protection against a particular disease (active immunization). Passive immunization is the injection of antibodies against a specific microbe from donated blood plasma from a person already exposed, to give protection against a disease for up to about three months.

immunocompromised   A condition in which a person's immune system can't respond adequately to an invading organism. Such an impaired immune system makes a patient vulnerable to infection.

immunosuppression   Impairment of a person's immune system by using certain drugs, in order to treat cancer or stop the rejection of transplanted organs.

incubation period   The time between exposure to an infection and the first appearance of symptoms.

infection   The establishment of a colony of disease-causing microorganisms such as bacteria, viruses, or fungi in the body. The organisms reproduce rapidly and cause disease by damaging cells or producing damaging toxins. Infection usually triggers a response from the immune system, which causes many of the symptoms commonly seen in infections.

infestation Colonization by parasites such as mites, ticks, or lice in the skin or by worms (such as tapeworms) in the body.

latency A quiescent period during which a pathogen either does not reproduce or reproduces very slowly. During this time, symptoms of the disease may not appear.

lymphocyte A category of white blood cells with specialized functions in the immune system. B lymphocytes create antibody-producing cells; T lymphocytes activate other white blood cells (such as B lymphocytes) or kill infected cells directly.

mutation A change in the genetic material within a living cell (the DNA).

nef An HIV-encoded protein, some of which suppress HIV replication, others of which enhance replication, and others that have no discernable effect.

pandemic A disease that occurs over a large geographical area (sometimes the entire world) and affects a high proportion of the population (a widespread epidemic).

parasite Any organism living in or on any other living creature, deriving advantages from doing so, while causing disadvantage to the host.

pathogen A microorganism that parasitizes an animal or plant and causes disease; they include protozoans, bacteria, and viruses.

plasmid A loop of DNA that occurs in bacteria that contain genes coding for toxin production, antibiotic resistance, and ability to invade host cells. Plasmids can be transferred between bacteria.

Plasmodium A genus of protozoans (single-celled organisms) that live as parasites within the red blood cells and liver cells of man. The parasite completes the sexual phase of its development in the stomach and digestive glands of a bloodsucking *Anopheles* mosquito; four species cause malaria in man (*P. vivax, P. ovale, P. falciparum, P. malariae*).

pus A liquid caused by inflammation. It consists of leukocytes, dead tissue, and fluid.

pyoderma A condition of the skin involving pus-filled lesions.

retrovirus A member of a family of viruses that use RNA as genetic information and transcribes this information into DNA. The family Retroviridae includes HIV and HTLV (human T-cell lymphotropic virus, human T-cell leukemia virus, or human T-cell leukemia/lymphoma virus).

spleen An organ that removes and destroys worn-out red blood cells and helps fight infection. It fights infection by producing some of the antibodies, phagocytes, and lymphocytes that destroy invading microorganisms. If it is removed, its duties can be taken over by other parts of the lymphatic system, although this makes the patient more susceptible to infection.

T cells One of the two main classes of lymphocytes (a type of white blood cell). T cells play an important part in the body's immune system defenses against infection.

thymus A gland that makes up part of the immune system, by making lymphocytes become T cells. These T cells play an important part in the body's defense against viruses and other infections.

toxin A poisonous protein produced by disease-causing bacteria such as *Clostridium tetani* (which causes tetanus). Bacterial toxins are sometimes subdivided into endotoxins (released from inside dead bacteria), exotoxins (released from the surface of live bacteria), and enterotoxins (which inflame the intestine).

trematodes Parasitic flatworms in the class Trematoda, commonly called "flukes."

trypanosomes Protozoal (single-celled) parasites that cause diseases such as sleeping sickness.

vector Any animal that transmits a particular infectious disease. A vector picks up an organism from a source of infection, carries them within the body, and later deposits them where they infect a new host. Mosquitoes, fleas, lice, ticks, and flies are the most important vectors of disease to humans.

virus   The smallest known type of infectious agent, causing diseases that range from mild (warts and the common cold) to extremely serious (rabies, AIDS, and probably some types of cancer).

white blood cells   Also known as leukocytes, their principal role is to protect the body against infection. There are three main types of white blood cells: granulocytes, monocytes, and lymphocytes. These cells circulate in blood, lymph, and body tissues and either directly or indirectly destroy invading organisms and infected or damaged cells.

zoonosis   Any infectious or parasitic disease of animals that can be transmitted to humans. Many disease organisms can infect only humans or particular animals, but zoonotic organisms are more flexible. They can adapt themselves to many different species. Zoonoses are usually caught from animals closely associated with humans (dogs, cats, parrots, pigs, cattle, rats). Examples include cat-scratch disease, fungal infections, psittacosis, brucellosis, trichinosis, leptospirosis.

APPENDICES

acetaminophen (Trade names: Tylenol, Datril, Temora, Volatile) Over-the-counter pain-killer and fever reducer used in many nonprescription pain relievers. Often prescribed for mild to moderate pain or fever, it cannot treat inflammation. It is given by mouth and may cause stomach upsets.

Side Effects Allergic reactions. Overdose can cause fatal liver problems.

acyclovir (Trade name: Zovirax) An antiviral drug prescribed for the treatment of herpes simplex, shingles, and chicken pox that is available in oral or topical form. Acyclovir works by inhibiting the synthesis of DNA in cells infected by herpes viruses. The drug also has been helpful to patients receiving bone marrow transplants to prevent the subsequent development of herpes simplex infection.

Oral acyclovir Acyclovir is effective in managing both initial and recurrent infections of herpes and localized shingles. It can prevent subsequent viral attacks if taken continuously soon after infection. However, in cases of recurrent genital herpes, acyclovir therapy doesn't make the lesions heal quicker or ease symptoms.

Topical acyclovir The topical form does not prevent new lesions from forming during the course of the disease. When applied to an existing blister, however, it may relieve symptoms, speed healing, and shorten the duration of the infection and the contagious period.

Adverse Effects Adverse effects are rare. The ointment may cause skin irritation or rash. Taken by mouth, the drug may cause headache, dizziness, nausea/vomiting. Rarely, acyclovir injections may cause kidney damage.

adenosine monophosphate (AMP) A compound containing Adenine, Ribose, and one Phosphate group (AMP), this metabolism byproduct seems to help ease the pain of shingles. In one study, 15 of 17 shingles patients who took the drug reportedly felt no pain within two weeks, and were still pain free two years later. The treatment has no side effects and works best within the first few months of pain, when the nerve endings have experienced minimal damage.

amantadine hydrochloride (Trade names: Symmetrel, Symadine) An antiviral drug that is prescribed to prevent and (in the early stages) to treat type-A influenza virus. It is believed to act by preventing a virus from penetrating into the host's cells.

Side Effects Among the most serious adverse effects are central nervous system effects; nervousness, blurred vision, and slurred speech may also occur. The drug should be used with caution in patients with congestive heart failure or during pregnancy and breast-feeding.

amoxicillin (Trade names: Amoxil, Moxilin, Wymox) A semisynthetic oral penicillin antibiotic, similar to ampicillin. This broad-spectrum antibiotic is prescribed in the treatment of several infections caused by gram-positive and gram-negative bacteria, including bronchitis, cystitis, gonorrhea, and ear and skin infections.

Side Effects Nausea and diarrhea; various allergic reactions include rash, fever, swelling of the mouth, itching, and breathing problems.

amphotericin B (Trade name: Fungizone) An antibiotic drug used to treat deep fungal infections of the skin, available as drops, lotion, or cream. It is inactive against both bacteria and viruses. While it can be given by mouth, it is given by intravenous injection to treat serious systemic infections such as cryptococcosis and histoplasmosis. This drug is usually administered in a hospital setting.

Side Effects Adverse effects are likely only when given as injection; these side effects may include muscle pains, vomiting, fever, headache, or (rarely) seizures. There is also a risk of kidney damage.

ampicillin (Trades names: Amcill, Omnipen, Polycillin, Principen) A penicillin-type semi-synthetic antibiotic used to treat conditions caused by a broad spectrum of gram-negative and gram-positive organisms in the urinary, respiratory, biliary, and intestinal tracts. Some of these conditions include cystitis, bronchitis, gonorrhea, typhoid fever, and ear and eye infections. It is inactivated by penicillinase, and therefore cannot be used against organisms that produce this enzyme.

Adverse Effects Nausea, vomiting, fever, or diarrhea. Allergic reactions may include symptoms of rash, diarrhea, and (rarely) fever; swelling of the mouth and tongue; itching; and breathing problems.

azidothymidine (AZT) See ZIDOVUDINE.

AZT See ZIDOVUDINE.

benethamine penicillin An antibiotic that is effective against most gram-positive bacteria, such as streptococci, staphylococci, and pneumococci. This drug is a derivative of benzylpenicillin and can be administered by mouth, although it is usually given as an intramuscular injection.

Side Effects As with all penicillins, allergic reactions are common.

benzathine penicillin G (Trade names: Bicillin, Permapen) Long-acting antibiotic given by mouth or injection that is slowly absorbed and effective against most gram-pos-

itive bacteria, including streptococci, staphylococci, and pneumococci. (See also PENICILLIN.)

Side Effects As with all penicillins, allergic reactions are fairly common.

benzoyl peroxide An antibacterial agent that is extremely effective in suppressing the bacterium *Propionibacterium acnes,* associated with acne. Probably the most popular of the over-the-counter products, it draws the peroxide into the pore where it releases oxygen, killing the bacteria that can aggravate acne. Benzoyl also suppresses fatty acid cells that irritate pores. It is most effective for patients with inflammatory acne; by inhibiting bacteria, it decreases the inflammatory components in the skin. Benzoyl peroxide is sold in strengths ranging between 5 to 10 percent, but the lower concentration is just as effective and less likely to cause irritation. Most over-the-counter products contain benzoyl peroxide in a lotion base; prescription products contain the chemical in a gel base. A fairly new preparation combining 3 percent erythromycin with 5 percent benzoyl peroxide in a gel base may be more effective than either component by itself.

Adverse Effects Some irritation may follow use with benzoyl peroxide, and allergic sensitization has occasionally occurred. *Benzoyl peroxide is closely related to products containing vitamin A (such as Retin-A and Accutane) and they shouldn't be used together.*

bleomycin (Trade name: Blenoxane) An antibiotic obtained from a soil fungus, bleomycin is effective in treating warts that have not responded to other treatment. It is administered by injection.

Adverse Effects Bleomycin can cause toxic side effects in skin and lungs and should not be used with patients who have problems with kidney function or lung disease. Other side effects include localized swelling and the development of pneumonitis or rash.

butoconazole nitrate (Trade name: Femstat) An antifungal drug that is derived from imidazole, used to treat vaginal mycotic infections caused by *Candida* species. Pregnant women should use the drug only in the second and third trimesters.

Side Effects Rarely, side effects include burning or itching.

capsaicin (Trade name: Zostrix) An ointment used to ease the pain of shingles. Its active ingredient is capsaicin, a red pepper derivative used to make chili powder. *Zostrix should be used only after all blisters have disappeared.* Capsaicin blocks the production of a chemical necessary for pain impulse transmission between nerve cells. Zostrix also has been tested as a treatment for psoriasis; however, it has been approved so far by the Food and Drug Administration only for use with shingles.

Side Effects As a counter-irritant, Zostrix should be used only on patients with unbroken healed skin still experiencing pain from shingles, not for those with open, oozing infections. Zostrix does burn, and it won't be effective unless used often and continuously for three weeks. However, the burning lessens or vanishes if treatments are continued.

cefaclor (Trade name: Ceclor) A common cephalosporin-type antibiotic used to treat ear infections, upper and lower respiratory-tract infections, urinary tract infections, skin infections, pharyngitis (sore throat), and tonsillitis. Given by mouth, the drug should be used with caution in patients who are allergic to penicillin.

Side Effects Severe diarrhea, nausea and vomiting, or skin eruptions.

cefadroxil monohydrate (Trade names: Duricef, Ultracef) A cephalosporin antibiotic used to treat certain bacterial infections, including urinary tract infections, skin infections, pharyngitis, and tonsillitis. Given by mouth, it is administered with caution to patients who have a history of allergy to penicillin.

Side Effects Allergic reactions, generalized itching, severe diarrhea, and nausea and vomiting.

cefazolin sodium (Trade name: Ancef; Kefzol) A cephalosporin antibiotic used to treat certain bacterial infections, including respiratory, urinary tract, skin, biliary, bone, joint, genital infections, and septicemia ("blood poisoning"). It is administered with caution to patients with a history of allergy to penicillin.

Side Effects Hypersensitivity reactions and severe diarrhea, nausea, and vomiting.

cefotaxime sodium (Trade name: Claforan) A cephalosporin antibiotic used to treat lower respiratory tract, genitourinary, gynecologic, intra-abdominal, skin, bone, and joint infections and septicemia. Intravenous route only.

Side Effects Itching, colitis, and fungal infections.

cefoxitin sodium (Trade name: Mefoxin) A cephalosporin antibiotic used to treat certain bacterial infections. It should be administered with caution to patients allergic to penicillin or other cephalosporins. Intravenous route only.

Side Effects Allergic reactions, phlebitis, and pain at the injection site.

ceftazidime (Trade names: Ceptaz, Fortaz, Pentacef, Tazicef, Tazidime) A cephalosporin-type of antibiotic used to treat infections of the lower respiratory tract, urinary tract, skin, abdomen, blood, bones and joints, and central nervous system. It should not be used for anyone allergic to cephalosporin antibiotics and with caution in those allergic to penicillin.

Side Effects Itching, fever, skin rash, diarrhea, phlebitis.

ceftriaxone (Trade name: Rocephin) A cephalosporin-type broad-spectrum antibiotic prescribed for infections of the lower respiratory tract, urinary tract, skin, abdomen, bones, joints, and central nervous system. It is used to treat gonorrhea, septicemia, and meningitis.

It is administered as an IV or intramuscular injection.

Side Effects   This drug is usually well tolerated. Occasionally, side effects may include local pain at the injection site, allergic reaction (rash, itching, fever, or chills), blood problems, gastrointestinal problems, headache, or dizziness.

cephalexin (Trade names: Keflex, Biocef, Cephalexin)   A cephalosporin antibacterial prescribed orally to treat certain infections, including respiratory tract, skin, bone, and ear infections. Only available orally.

Side Effects   Nausea, diarrhea, and allergic reactions.

chloramphenicol (Trade names: Chloromycetin, Chloroptic)   An antibiotic and antirickettsial drug derived from the bacterium *Streptomyces venezuelae* (and also produced synthetically) that is effective against a wide variety of microorganisms. Because of its severe side effects, it is usually reserved for serious infections (such as typhoid fever) when less toxic drugs are not effective. It should not be given to pregnant or breastfeeding women or to anyone with a mild infection.

Side Effects   The most serious side effect of this medication is the potential damage to bone marrow.

chlorhexidine (Trade name: Hibiclens)   An antimicrobial agent used as a surgical scrub, hand rinse, and topical antiseptic. It is used in solution, creams, gels, and lozenges and in some preparations combined with cetrimide. In very dilute solutions, it can be used as a mouthwash to control mouth infections.

Side Effects   Rarely, a skin sensitivity to this product can develop.

chloroproguanil   A drug administered by mouth to prevent or treat malaria.

Side Effects   Rarely, large doses may cause stomach discomfort and vomiting.

chloroquine (Trade name: Aralen)   An antimalarial drug prescribed to treat malaria and amebiasis and certain skin conditions (such as lupus erythematosus). It is administered by mouth or injection.

Side Effects   Gastrointestinal problems, headache, visual disturbances, and itching. Those with retina or visual problems or porphyria should not use this drug. Long-term use can lead to eye damage.

ciclopirox olamine (Trade name: Loprox)   A broad-spectrum, topical agent used to treat fungus infections (such as ringworm or tinea) by inhibiting the growth of dermatophytes and *Candida albicans*.

Side Effects   The incidence of adverse reactions with this medication is low. A few patients may notice itching at the application site.

cimetidine (Trade name: Tagamet)   An antihistamine and antiulcer drug that may be a possible drug treatment for chronic hives and for multiple warts in children. According to research at Children's Memorial Hospital in Chicago and New York University, youngsters whose warts did not respond to more traditional treatment received three daily doses of the drug. Within seven weeks, many of the warts had become flatter and less visible; within two months, the warts disappeared completely in 80 percent of the children.

Adverse Effects   Diarrhea, dizziness, and rash.

ciprofloxacin (Trade name: Cipro)   An antimicrobial used to treat lower respiratory and urinary tract infection, infections of skin, bone and joints, and gastrointestinal disease. It is administered by mouth or IV.

Side Effects   Nausea and vomiting, diarrhea, abdominal pain, and headache.

clavulanate potassium (Trade name: Augmentin)   An oral antibacterial combination of the antibiotic amoxicillin and clavulanate potassium (a potassium salt of clavulanic acid, which is produced by the fermentation of *Streptomyces clavuligerus*). It is used to treat infections caused by susceptible strains of a variety of organisms that may be resistant to other antibiotics. Some of the conditions it may treat include lower respiratory tract infections, ear infections, sinusitis, skin infections, urinary tract infections, and bite wounds.

Side Effects This drug is usually well tolerated; most side effects (when they occur) are mild and may include diarrhea, skin rash and itching, vomiting, and vaginitis.

clindamycin (Trade name: Cleocin) An antibacterial drug used to treat acne and serious anaerobic infections that haven't responded, or are resistant, to other antibiotics. Clindamycin is especially effective against most anaerobic bacteria, including *Propionibacterium acnes*. It is also an excellent agent against *Staphylococcus aureus* and streptococcal species.

Adverse Effects Colitis and severe gastrointestinal problems.

clofazimine (Trade name: Lamprene) A dye used primarily in the treatment of leprosy. This drug has a remarkable lack of toxicity, and although there is no evidence of birth defects, it does cross the placenta and cause pigmentation in offspring. Administered by mouth, it should be taken with meals or milk. For most skin conditions, the drug needs to be taken for at least two months before benefit is seen. The drug should not be taken by women during the first three months of pregnancy, by patients prone to diarrhea or recurrent abdominal pain, or by those with kidney or liver disease.

Adverse Effects The most obvious side effect is a pink, red, or brownish-black discoloration of the skin, especially in areas exposed to sunlight. Hair, sweat, sputum, urine, and feces may also be discolored. These pigmentation side effects are related to dosage, however, and begin to fade when therapy is stopped. Other side effects include itching, sensitivity to sunlight, and acnelike skin eruptions. There may also be nausea and vomiting, abdominal pain, and diarrhea.

clotrimazole (Trade names: Gyne-Lotrimin, Lotrimin, Mycelex) A broad-spectrum antifungal drug used in topical applications to treat fungal and yeast infections including ringworm and infections of the genital organs. It is applied as a cream or solution or as vaginal pessaries. It is not prescribed for use in the eyes; contact with eyes should be avoided.

Side Effects Severe skin allergic reactions may occur, as can mild burning or irritation.

cloxacillin (Trade names: Cloxapen, Tegopen) A penicillin-type antibiotic used to treat staphylococcal infections that are resistant to penicillin. Administered by mouth or injection, it should not be taken with acidic fruits or juices or aged cheese. Taken with alcohol, this drug could cause stomach irritation. Use with birth control pills may impair the efficacy of the contraceptive.

Adverse Effects Stomach discomfort and rash, diarrhea or allergic reactions in those sensitive to penicillin.

dapsone (4,4'-diaminodiphenyl-sulfone) An antibacterial drug and a derivative of sulfone used to treat leprosy and dermatitis herpetiformis. Results with this drug (the most often-used of the sulfones) have been variable, but in some cases there have been excellent results. Its mechanism of action is unknown. The introduction of the sulfones in the 1950s had a dramatic impact on the treatment of leprosy, since dapsone was the first safe and effective drug available that stopped the disease and eliminated the need for patient isolation. Although bacterial resistance to dapsone is becoming widespread, it remains the drug of choice in the treatment of leprosy in conjunction with other medication. According to reports, millions of patients have been successfully treated with dapsone for years with a relatively low rate of toxic side effects. Pregnant women should not use dapsone.

Adverse Effects   The adverse effects of this drug tend to be dose related and are uncommon on low doses. Concerns over the safety may have been exaggerated by the high doses in some early studies. Severe allergic reactions may occur. Other side effects may include nausea, vomiting, and, rarely, damage to the liver, red blood cells, and nerves. During long-term treatment, blood tests are conducted to monitor liver function and the red blood cell level. Neurological symptoms (such as psychosis) are believed to be dose related; those with a history of psychiatric problems may be more likely to develop mental problems on this drug.

dideoxyinosine   An antiretroviral drug used to treat HIV infections, restricting the viral replication activity.

doxycycline (Trade name: Vibramycin)   A tetracycline antibacterial drug used to treat a variety of infections caused by bacteria and other microorganisms. It is administered by mouth.

Side Effects   The same as other tetracyclines: Gastrointestinal disturbances, phototoxicity, and discoloration of teeth of children under age eight or in utero. It should not be used in patients with kidney or liver problems or to sensitivity to other tetracyclines, nor should it be prescribed for pregnant women or children under age eight.

econazole (Trade name: Spectrazole)   An antifungal drug used to treat ringworm of the scalp, athlete's foot, jock itch, "sun fungus," nail fungus, candidiasis, and others. Available in powder, cream, lotion, ointment, or vaginal tablet, the medication acts quickly (often within two days), killing fungi by damaging the fungal cell wall. The drug may take up to eight weeks to cure the infection.

Adverse Effects   Rarely, the drug may cause skin irritation.

erythromycin (Trade names: E-mycin, Ery-thro, Erythrocin, Robimycin, Ery-Tab, Erycette)   An antibacterial antibiotic used to treat many bacterial and mycoplasmic infections, especially those that can't be treated with penicillin. In children under age eight, it is the alternative to tetracycline (an antibiotic that can permanently stain developing teeth). Because erythromycin is destroyed by acid in the stomach, the drug should be taken in coated forms or as a compound. Patients with liver disease should not use this drug.

Adverse Effects   Possible side effects include nausea and vomiting, abdominal pain, diarrhea, and an itchy rash. To reduce side effects, *certain brands* of erythromycin may be taken with food to reduce the chance of irritating the stomach. Check with your physician or pharmacist regarding the proper method of taking this medication.

ethambutol (Trade name: Myambutol)   An antibiotic drug used to treat pulmonary tuberculosis in conjunction with other drugs. It is not recommended for small children or for those with optic neuritis.

Side Effects   Diminished visual acuity and allergic reactions (such as rashes). It may sometimes cause visual problems that ease when the drug is withdrawn.

ethionamide (Trade name: Trecator-SC)   An antibacterial drug used to treat tuberculosis, usually in conjunction with other drugs. It is administered by mouth or as a suppository. Patients with liver damage should not use this drug.

Side Effects   Loss of appetite, nausea, and vomiting are common. Other side effects include skin rash, jaundice, mental depression, or gastrointestinal problems.

foscarnet (phosphonoformic acid, trisodium salt)   An antiviral that acts directly on the viral DNA of herpes simplex viruses and cytomegalovirus, and on retroviruses. The major use of foscarnet has been to treat severe infections caused by acyclovir-resistant herpes simplex viruses.

furazolidone (Trade name: Furoxone) An antiinfective and antiprotozoal drug prescribed for certain bacterial or protozoal infections of the gastrointestinal tract. This drug is not prescribed for infants under age one.

Side Effects This drug is not used with drugs that should not be taken with monoamine oxidase (MAO) inhibitors (a class of drugs used primarily to treat depression). Among the more serious reactions are fever and hemolytic anemia (destruction of red blood cells). Skin rash and stomach pain may occur.

gamma benzene hexachloride (lindane) (Trade name: Scabene)   A medication used to treat lice and that is no longer recommended by the National Pediculosis Association because of its potential toxicity. Other products, according to the association, work equally well with less risk. It is not usually given to infants or pregnant women and should not be applied to the face.

Side Effects Among the most serious reactions are neurologic damage and aplastic anemia (a deficiency of the elements of the blood). Eyes or skin may be irritated by topical use. Lindane also may irritate the skin and scalp, or cause itching.

ganciclovir sodium (Trade name: Cytovene) A drug related to acyclovir used to prevent cytomegalovirus infection after bone marrow transplantation and in AIDS patients. It is administered intravenously, orally, and via ocular implants.

Side Effects During clinical trails, this drug was withdrawn in about 32 percent of patients because of adverse reactions, including most frequently liver and kidney problems and fever, rash, and malaise. Other side effects include headache, confusion, sepsis,

swelling, high or low blood pressure, disturbing and intrusive thoughts and dreams, nausea and vomiting, loss of appetite, diarrhea, abdominal pain.

gentamicin (Trade names: Gentacidin, Bristagen, Garamycin, Genoptic Liquifilm) An aminoglycoside antibiotic prescribed to ease the effects of a wide variety of severe bacterial infections. It can be administered by injection or applied as a cream, or as drops to the ears and eyes. It should not be used together with other drugs that may be potentially harmful to the kidneys or hearing. It should be used cautiously with patients who have kidney problems. Blood tests may be given during treatment to monitor kidney function.

Side Effects The more serious adverse reactions (especially at high doses) include kidney, hearing, or balance problems and problems along the pathways between brain and muscles.

griseofulvin (Trade names: Griseofulvin, Fulvicin, Grisactin)   One of the oldest antifungal drugs available in America, it is used to treat infections of the skin, nails, or hair. It is particularly effective against superficial dermatophytes infections of the scalp, beard, palms, soles, and nails, including ringworm of the scalp (tinea capitis), ringworm of the body (tinea corporis), and athlete's foot. It is not effective against bacteria, deep fungi, or *Candida albicans*. Even with prolonged treatment, many nail infections do not respond completely or else they recur. Resistance may develop to this drug. When griseofulvin is taken with a high-fat meal, it is better absorbed and tolerated. Griseofulvin should not be taken by patients suffering with acute intermittent porphyria, since it may cause an acute abdominal attack. The drug may also interact with birth control pills, producing breakthrough bleeding or pregnancy.

Adverse Effects The most common side effects are headache and gastrointestinal problems; others include loss of taste, rashes, and increased sun sensitivity. Long-term treatment may cause liver or bone marrow damage. The most serious problems include abnormal blood conditions.

hydrogen peroxide   A colorless topical antiseptic used to treat skin infections, to cleanse open wounds, or as a deodorant mouthwash. The solution combines with catalase (an enzyme present in the skin) to release oxygen, which kills bacteria and cleanses the infected areas.

Adverse Effects   Strong solutions sometimes irritate the skin.

idoxuridine (IDU)   An antiviral that apparently acts by being incorporated into newly synthesized DNA; this drug is highly toxic to host cells. Thus, clinical use has been limited to topical therapy of herpes simplex infections of the eye because of its high systemic toxicity.

Side Effects   When used in the eye, it may cause irritation, pain, itching, and inflammation or swelling of the eyelids; rare allergic reactions and light sensitivity have been reported.

interferons   Natural cellular products released from infected host cells in response to viral (or other foreign) nucleic acids. While scientists don't fully understand how they act, they know that interferon selectively blocks translation and transcription of viral RNA, stopping viral replication without interfering with normal host cell functions. Interferon may be active against many viruses, but it can only be used in the same species that initially produced it.

Interferon-alpha is approved for use in some patients with hairy cell leukemia, Kaposi's sarcoma, or condylomata acuminata. Studies have shown that interferon-alpha2 nasal spray can prevent upper respiratory infections caused by rhinoviruses. Interferon is also effective against shingles in patients with impaired immune systems.

Combining interferon with either acyclovir or vidarabine is useful in treating various versions of hepatitis. Thanks to recombinant DNA technology, interferon is now available in large enough quantities from bacterial cells and many studies around the country are currently under way.

isoniazid (isonicotinic acid hydrazide, INH)   (Trade names: Cotinazin, INH, Nydrazid) An antibacterial used to prevent and treat tuberculosis, usually given by mouth. Isoniazid may be given to close contacts of patients who have TB to prevent the spread of the disease. Becase TB bacteria soon become resistant to isoniazid, it is usually given in combination with streptomycin or other antibacterial drugs. Since the drug may hasten the depletion of pyridoxine (vitamin B_6) in the body, vitamin B_6 supplements are usually given to prevent nerve damage.

Side Effects   Because long-term treatment may be associated with liver problems, isoniazid should not be used by patients with liver disease. High doses or prolonged treatment has been associated with problems with the peripheral nervous system (the motor and sensory nerves outside the brain and spinal cord). Other side effects that commonly occur are rash and fever; occasionally, patients may experience dry mouth and digestive problems.

kanamycin   (Trade names: Kantrex, Kantrim, Klebcil)   An aminoglycoside antibiotic used to treat certain severe bacterial infections, especially those resistant to other antibiotics. It should not be used at the same time as other ototoxic drugs (medicines potentially harmful to hearing). It is given mainly by injection, but it is administered by mouth for infections of the intestines and by inhalation for respiratory infections.

Side Effects   Mild side effects occasionally occur, including skin rash, fever, headache, nausea and vomiting, and tingling sensations. Others include renal failure and deafness.

ketoconazole (Trade name: Nizoral) An antifungal agent prescribed to treat fungal diseases, including tinea versicolor, candidiasis, coccidiomycosis, and histoplasmosis when other antifungal preparations have not been effective. It should not be used to treat fungal meningitis.

Side Effects The most serious—but rare—adverse reactions are liver disorders. Ketoconazole may also cause nausea, but this may be avoided by taking the drug with food; it should not be taken at the same time as antacids. Other side effects include itching, headache, dizziness, abdominal pain, constipation, diarrhea, nervousness, or rash. Occasionally, patients may experience hives and allergic reactions with the first dose. Drug interactions with ketoconazole can be serious; this drug should not be taken with rifampin, isoniazid, warfarin, cyclosporine, or phenytoin.

lindane See GAMMA BENZENE HEXACHLORIDE.

mebendazole (Trade name: Vermox) An anthelminthic used to treat infestations of pinworms, whipworms, roundworms, and hookworms. Pregnant women should not use this drug.

Side Effects Abdominal pain and diarrhea are among the most serious side effects.

mefloquine (Trade name: Lariam) An antimalarial drug that is effective in preventing and treating chloroquine-resistant falciparum and vivax malaria.

Side Effects Vomiting, dizziness, nausea and fever, chills, diarrhea, fatigue.

metronidazole (Trade names: Flagyl, Metro I.V., Metryl, Protostat, Satric) An antibiotic particularly useful in fighting infections caused by anaerobic bacteria. This antimicrobial drug is used to treat infections of the genital, urinary, and digestive systems, such as amebiasis, trichomonas, and giardiasis. It is administered by mouth or in suppositories. It should not be used by pregnant women in the first trimester or by patients with organic disease, central nervous system disorders, or blood conditions.

Side Effects Possible effects include severe nausea and vomiting, appetite loss, abdominal pain, dark-colored urine, dizziness, neurological disturbances, or decrease in certain white blood cells (neutropenia). Many patients report that this drug creates a metallic taste in the mouth. Drinking alcohol during treatment with this drug can trigger particularly unpleasant reactions such as nausea, vomiting, hot flashes, and headache.

miconazole (Trade names: Micatin, Monistat) An antifungal medicine used on the skin to treat certain fungal infections of the skin and vagina, such as ringworm of the scalp, body, and feet, fungal meningitis, coccidioidomycosis, and candidiasis. It is given intravenously or by injection to treat systemic fungal infections, as well as topically or intravaginally.

Side Effects Among the more serious reactions following application to the skin are irritation and burning. When used systemically, the drug may trigger nausea, itching, phlebitis, and anemia.

neomycin (Trade names: Mycifradin, Myciguent, Neobiotic) An aminoglycoside antibiotic used to treat infections of the intestine, eyes, and (topically) of the skin caused by a wide range of bacteria. It is usually applied in creams or drops with other antibiotics, but it can also be given by mouth. Neomycin should not be used by anyone with kidney problems or an intestinal obstruction.

Side Effects Possible adverse effects include nausea and vomiting, rash, itching, diarrhea, hearing loss, dizziness, and tinnitus (ringing in the ears). Application of this medication to the skin may lead to allergic reactions.

niclosamide (Trade name: Niclocide) An anthelminthic prescribed to treat beef or fish tapeworm infestation. Its safety for small children, pregnant women, or nursing mothers has not been established.

Side Effects Rectal bleeding, palpitations, hearing loss, swelling, nausea, and vomiting.

norfloxacin (Trade name: Chibroxin, Noroxin) An oral antibacterial drug prescribed for the treatment of urinary tract infections. It is not recommended for children or pregnant women. Nitrofurantoin drugs should not be used together with this medicine.

Side Effects Nausea, dizziness, and headache have been reported.

nystatin (Trade names: Mycostatin, Nilstat, Nystex, O-U Statin) An antifungal antibiotic for the treatment of fungal infections of the gastrointestinal tract, vagina, and skin. It is applied as a cream for skin infections, by mouth for oral and intestinal infections, as pessaries or suppositories for vaginal and anal infections, or as eye drops for eye infections.

Side Effects There are no known serious side effects; some patients may experience mild gastrointestinal irritation or mild skin reactions.

ofloxacin (Trade name: Floxin) A broad-spectrum injectable and oral antimicrobial used to treat adults with mild to moderate infections caused by susceptible strains of certain microorganisms in a variety of infections involving the lower respiratory tract, skin, urinary tract, and prostate. It is also used to treat a variety of sexually transmitted diseases. It should not be given to anyone allergic to drugs in the quinolone group.

Side Effects Nausea, insomnia, headache, dizziness, diarrhea, vomiting, rash, itching, vaginitis, tendonitis, and tendon rupture.

oxytetracycline (Trade name: Terramycin) One of the tetracyclines, this antibiotic is used to treat a wide variety of bacterial and rickettsial infections, including chlamydia, syphilis, Rocky Mountain spotted fever, and cholera. It is administered by mouth or injec-

tion, or applied to the skin as a cream. Oxytetracycline should be used with caution in patients with kidney or liver problems.

Adverse Effects Possible side effects include rash, increased skin sensitivity to the sun, nausea, and vomiting. Because it may discolor developing teeth, it is not prescribed for pregnant women or children under age eight.

para-aminosalicylic acid (PAS) A drug that is chemically related to aspirin that is used (together with isoniazid or streptomycin) to treat various types of tuberculosis. It is administered by mouth.

Side Effects Nausea and vomiting, diarrhea and abdominal pain, fever, rash, goiter, hypokalemia (loss of potassium in the blood), and acid-base imbalance.

penicillin (penicillin G [benzylpenicillin]) (Trade names: Bicillin, Cilloral, Crystapen, Falapen, Liquapen, Pentids, Permapen, Pfizerpen) An antibiotic derived from cultures of species of the mold *Penicillium notatum* used to treat a wide variety of bacterial infections, such as meningococcal, pneumococcal, and streptococcal infections, syphilis and many other diseases. It is rapidly absorbed when injected, but it is inactivated by stomach acid. It is often not effective against staphylococcus aureus. There are several similar drugs prepared from *P. notatum* (benethamine penicillin and benzathine penicillin) and a group of antibiotics derived from the penicillins, known as semisynthetic penicillins (including ampicillin and cloxacillin).

Side Effects Allergic reactions are common, and include skin rash, hives, and anaphylaxis. Any patient who has had an allergic reaction to one type of penicillin should not be given any other. Other side effects include vomiting and diarrhea.

penicillin V (phenethicillin) An antibiotic similar to penicillin that is active against gram-positive bacteria (except certain strains of staphylococci). It can be administered by mouth.

Side Effects Diarrhea and allergic reactions.

permethrin (Trade names: Elimite, Rid) A drug used on the skin to treat head lice and their nits. It should not be used by anyone allergic to pyrethrine, pyrethroids, or chrysanthemum flowers.

Side Effects Reported reactions include itching, mild burning or stinging, numbness, discomfort, mild redness, or scalp rash.

piperazine (Trade names: Antepar, Bryrel) A drug used to treat infestations by roundworms and thread worms. It is administered by mouth.

Side Effects Rarely, side effects (nausea and vomiting, headache, tingling, and rashes) may follow high doses.

podofilox (Trade name: Condylox) An antimitotic drug synthesized from plants used to treat external genital warts (condyloma acuminatum). It is not used to treat perianal or mucous membrane warts. Correct diagnosis of the lesions is essential.

Side Effects There is a likelihood of side effects, including burning, pain, inflammation, erosion, and itching; burning and itching occur more often among women. Other, more rare side effects include pain with intercourse, insomnia, tingling, bleeding, tenderness, chafing, bad odor, dizziness, scarring, blisters, crusting, and swelling.

polymyxin B (Trade name: Aerosporin) An antibiotic prescribed for infections caused by *Pseudomonas,* such as urinary tract infections, septicemia ("blood poisoning"), and eye infections.

Side Effects It should be used with extreme caution in patients with kidney problems. Drug fever, kidney, and liver problems may be caused by this drug. Mild dizziness may also occur.

polymyxins A group of antibiotics derived from the bacterium *Bacillus polymyxa* used to treat gram-negative bacterial infections that cause a variety of conditions such as meningitis, corneal ulcers, and ear infections. The polymyxins include colistin and polymyxin B.

Side Effects Taken orally, colistin is associated with pseudomembranous enterocolitis—a severe, life-threatening type of diarrhea sometimes caused by antibiotics. It may also cause liver problems and various neurologic changes when taken internally. When applied on the skin, irritation and allergic reactions may occur.

praziquantel (Trade name: Biltricide) A drug used to treat schistosome infections and infections of liver fluke.

Side Effects Praziquantel is usually well tolerated; side effects are usually mild and don't last long. They include headache, dizziness, abdominal discomfort, fever, hives.

pyrantel pamoate An anthelminthic used to treat infestation of roundworms or pinworms. It should be used with caution in patients with anemia or severe malnutrition.

Side Effects Nausea, abdominal cramps, diarrhea, dizziness, and skin rash.

pyrazinamide An antimycobacterial drug prescribed in combination drug therapy to treat hospitalized patients with tuberculosis who don't respond to other drugs. Patients with severe liver damage should not use this drug.

Side Effects Joint pain, fever, and rash. At high doses, the drug may cause toxic effects on the liver.

pyrethrin (Trade name: A-200 shampoo) Used together with piperonyl butoxide, this is a fixed-combination medication used to treat head, body, and pubic lice and scabies. Patients with a sensitivity to ragweed should not use this medication.

Side Effects Irritation of skin and mucous membranes.

pyrimethamine (Trade names: Daraprim, Fansidar) An antimalarial prescribed in the treatment of malaria and toxoplasmosis. It should not be used to treat chloroguanide-resistant malaria, and it is prescribed cautiously in patients with toxoplasmosis because the dosage needed may be near toxic levels. It also may be used together with sulfadozine to treat malaria. This combination should not be used to treat pregnant women at term or while nursing, infants under age two months, or patients with the blood disorder megaloblastic anemia.

Side Effects   Adverse reactions occur especially with large doses, and may include blood disorders, very sore tongue (atrophic glossitis), low levels of some types of white blood cells (leukopenia), and convulsions. Side effects to the pyrimethamine and sulfadoxine combination may include pancreatitis, depression, convulsions, hallucinations, and several types of blood disorders.

quinacrine (Trade name: Atabrine)   A drug used since World War II to suppress malaria; it is now used to treat the intestinal infections, giardiasis, or cestodiasis. It should not be used during pregnancy or together with the drug primaquine, and it should be administered with caution to patients over age 60 or anyone with a history of psychosis.

Side Effects   Possible adverse effects include nausea and vomiting and yellow discoloration of the skin and urine. Prolonged use can cause blood disorders or psychological problems. Other side effects include severe psoriasis, aplastic anemia, acute kidney problems.

quinine (Trade name: Quinamm, Quinine) The oldest drug treatment for malaria. Quinine had been abandoned and replaced by more effective, less toxic drugs, but in the wake of resistant forms of malaria it is being reintroduced as a potential malaria treatment. Today, it is used mainly to treat strains of the disease that are resistant to other antimalarial drugs (especially in malaria caused by *Plasmodium falciparum*). Patients with certain types of heart problems should not use this drug.

Side Effects   Large doses of this drug are needed, and therefore there is a high risk of adverse effects due to severe poisoning: headache, fever, nausea and vomiting, confusion, hearing loss, ringing in the ears, and blurred vision.

ribavirin (Trade name: Virazole)   An aerosol antiviral drug prescribed to treat respiratory syncytial virus (RSV) infections of the lower respiratory tract in infants and small children and other RNA and DNA viruses. It is not recommended for infants who need help in breathing, and its role in healthy children remains to be defined. It also appears to have some effectiveness against influenza A and B, but its role in treating these diseases is not defined. It has also been used successfully against lassa fever.

Side Effects   Reported side effects include bacterial pneumonia, pneumothorax, breathing cessation (apnea), low blood pressure, and cardiac arrest (these reported conditions could have been caused by the underlying disease and not the medication). Other side effects may include eye infection, impaired breathing function, and an increase in immature red blood cells (reticulocytosis).

rifampin (Trade names: Rifadin, Rimactane) An antibacterial drug prescribed to treat various infections, particularly tuberculosis. It is also used to prevent meningococcal meningitis in people who are exposed to someone with the disease. It is usually prescribed with other antibacterials because some strains of bacteria quickly develop resistance to rifampin alone. The drug should not be used by pregnant women or anyone with liver problems.

Side Effects   Liver toxicity and a syndrome that resembles influenza. Other side effects include a harmless, orange-red discoloration of urine, saliva, and other body secretions; gastrointestinal distress; aches and cramps; jaundice; rash; or itching.

rimantadine   An analog of amantadine that shares the same effectiveness, but appears to produce fewer side effects.

silver sulfadiazine (Trade name: Silvadene) A topical antibacterial cream used to prevent infections in skin grafts or second- and third-degree burns. It is especially helpful in keeping burn sites sterile, reducing the chance of secondary infection.

Adverse Effects   Possible side effects include allergic reactions (with rash, itching, or burning). Long-term use may rarely produce serious blood disorders or kidney damage. It is not recommended for patients who are sensitive to sulfonamide drugs, nor should it be used for newborns or premature infants.

streptomycin   An aminoglycoside antibiotic derived from *Streptomyces griseus* that is used to treat a wide variety of bacterial infections, including tularemia, plague, brucellosis, and glanders. It is administered by injection and is sometimes given together with a penicillin drug to treat endocarditis (inflammation of the lining of the heart and its valves). Streptomycin was once used to treat a variety of other infections, but it has now been surpassed by newer more effective drugs with less serious side effects. When it was discovered, it was the first effective drug treatment for tuberculosis; it is still sometimes used (together with isoniazid) to treat a resistant strain of bacteria. Streptomycin should be used with caution by the elderly and those with kidney problems.

Side Effects   Its most serious adverse affect is the possibility of damage to the inner ear, disturbing balance and causing dizziness, ringing in the ears and deafness. For this reason, patients with labyrinthine disease should not take this drug. It must also be used with caution with those with kidney problems and the elderly. Other possible problems include facial numbness, tingling in the hands, headache, malaise, nausea, and vomiting.

sulfacetamide   (Trade names: Bleph-10, Cetamide, Sebizon, Sulamyd, Sulf-10, Sulfacet-R)   A topical sulfonamide-type of antibacterial drug used to treat conjunctivitis (pinkeye) and sometimes given to treat blepharitis (inflammation of the eyelids). It may also be used to prevent infection after an eye injury or the removal of a foreign object. Those with impaired kidney function should not use this drug.

Adverse Effects   Stinging and possible allergic reactions such as itching, redness, and swelling of the eyelids.

Sulfacet-R   Brand name drug for a topical combination medicine containing a scabicide (sulfur), an antibacterial (sulfacetamide sodium), and an antiseptic and astringent (zinc oxide).

sulfachlorpyridazine   A sulfonamide-type of antibacterial drug used to treat infection (especially of the urinary tract). It should not be used if the urinary tract is blocked.

Adverse Effects   Among the more serious reactions are photosensitivity and severe allergic reactions.

sulfacytine   A sulfonamide antibacterial used to treat infection, especially pyelonephritis and cystitis. It should not be used in patients who have porphyria or an obstructed urinary tract.

Side Effects   Photosensitivity, severe allergic reactions, a variety of blood conditions, or crystals in the urine (crystalluria).

sulfadiazine   Sulfonamide antibacterial prescribed to treat infection (especially of the urinary tract) and to prevent the development of rheumatic fever. They should not be used in patients who have porphyria or an obstructed urinary tract.

Side Effects   Photosensitivity, severe allergic reactions, a variety of blood conditions, or crystals in the urine (crystalluria).

sulfamethoxazole (Trade name: Gantanol) A sulfonamide-type antibacterial used to treat ear infection (otitis media), pinkeye, skin infections, and certain urinary tract infections. When combined with the antibacterial drug trimethoprim (as Bactrim or Septra), the two are given to treat a variety of respiratory tract infections, including pneumocystic pneumonia. It should not be given during the last trimester of pregnancy, during breast-feeding, or to children under age two months.

Adverse Effects Rash, fever, nausea, vomiting, diarrhea, headache, dizziness, muscle or joint pain, or crystals in the urine.

sulfonamides (sulfa drugs) A large group of synthetic antibacterial agents that are effective in treating infections caused by many gram-negative and gram-positive microorganisms responsible for urinary tract infections, some types of pneumonia, and middle-ear infections, among other diseases. The sulfonamides are derived from a red dye known as sulfanilamide. Before the development of penicillin drugs, the sulfonamides were widely used to treat infections. Most sulfonamides are given by mouth and are available in a range of effectiveness from short- to long-acting, depending on the speed with which they are excreted from the patient's body. Most (including sulfamethoxazole and sulfaphenazole) are quickly absorbed from the stomach and small intestine and should be taken at frequent intervals. Some (such as sulfadoxine) are used for leprosy and malaria; sulfalene is a long-acting drug that need only be taken once a day. Others (such as sulfaguanidine) are poorly absorbed and are used to treat infections of the gastrointestinal tract, such as bacillary dysentery and gastroenteritis.

Side Effects Hemolytic anemia, agranulocytosis, thrombocytopenia or aplastic anemia, drug fever or jaundice, or allergic reactions. Adverse effects are more common with the long-acting sulfonamides that are given for more than 10 days. Sulfonamides are also given cautiously to people with impaired liver or kidney function. They are not given in the last three months of pregnancy or to infants because of the risk of mental retardation. In general, patients should avoid exposure to direct sunlight when taking these drugs. Prolonged use of these drugs leads to the development of resistant strains of microorganisms in the gut.

sulfones One of a group of drugs closely related to the sulfa drugs in their structure and the way they act. Sulfones are powerful agents in the fight against the bacteria that cause leprosy and tuberculosis. Patients who take these drugs require frequent evaluation, including complete blood counts, a chemistry profile (including liver and kidney tests), and urine tests.

sulfisoxazole (Trade name: Gantrisin) A sulfonamide-type of antibacterial drug used to treat urinary tract infections (including vaginitis, cystitis, and pyelonephritis) and eye infections (pinkeye).

Adverse Effects Nausea, vomiting, appetite loss, diarrhea, headache, dizziness, or rash. There may be a severe hypersensitivity reaction. The drug is not given during the last trimester of pregnancy, or to children under age two months.

tetracycline (Trade names: Achromycin, Cyclopar, Panmycin, Polycycline, Sumycin, Tetracyn, Tetrex, Topicycline) Any one of a group of broad-spectrum antibiotics derived from cultures of *Streptomyces* bacteria (chlortetracycline, doxycycline, oxytetracycline, and tetracycline). They are prescribed for the treatment of many bacterial and rickettsial infections, including respiratory-tract infections, syphilis, and acne. Because tetracycline may cause permanent discoloration of the teeth, it is not used during the last half of pregnancy or during a child's first eight years of life. Patients with significant liver or kidney problems should not use this drug.

Side Effects Nausea and vomiting and

diarrhea are fairly common side effects. Others include more severe gastrointestinal disturbances, kidney and liver damage, inflammatory lesions in the anal-genital area, hemolytic anemia, and rash. Patients may also be susceptible to infection with tetracycline-resistant organisms.

thiabendazole (Trade name: Mintezol) An anthelmintic used to treat a variety of worm infestations, including roundworms, pinworms, and hookworms. People with erythema multiforme (an allergic syndrome associated with some drugs) or Stevens-Johnson syndrome (a severe form of erythema multiforme) should not use this medication.

Side Effects Loss of appetite, central nervous system effects, severe gastrointestinal problems, dizziness, and low blood pressure.

tolnaftate (Trade names: Aftate, Tinactin) An antifungal drug used to treat superficial fungus infections of the skin, including some types of ringworm (including athlete's foot, ringworm of the body, and tinea versicolor). It is available without a prescription as a cream, powder, or aerosol. Tolnaftate is not effective in candidiasis.

Side Effects In rare cases, it may cause skin irritation or rash.

trifluridine (trifluorothymidine) This antiviral drug interferes with DNA synthesis and is effective in treating eye infections caused by herpes simplex 1 and 2.

Side Effects Burning or stinging in the eye.

trimethoprim (Trade names: Proloprim, Trimpex) An antibacterial drug used to treat various infections such as malaria, chronic infections of the urinary tract, and infections of the middle ear and bronchi. It should not be used to treat streptococcal pharyngitis (strep throat). It is often administered by mouth in a combined preparation with sulfamethoxazole (Bactrim, Septra).

Side Effects A range of blood abnormalities, allergies, gastrointestinal problems, and central nervous system problems. Long-term treatment may cause an impairment of bone marrow production.

trimethoprim and sulfamethoxazole (Trade names: Bactrim, Septra) A fixed-combination antibacterial drug used to treat urinary tract infections, ear infections, and shigellosis. It is not recommended for use in infants under age two months, or in the last three months of pregnancy. It should be used with caution by patients with kidney or liver problems, or who have a possible folate deficiency.

Side Effects Crystals in the urine, rash, fever, and allergic reactions.

undecylenic acid (Trade names: Breezee Mist Foot Powder; Fungi-Nail Solution, Gordochom solution) An antifungal agent used to treat athlete's foot and ringworm. It is applied to the skin as a powder, ointment, lotion, or aerosol spray, but should not be used in the eyes or on mucous membranes. Diabetic patients should use this drug with caution.

Side Effects Skin irritation and allergic reactions.

vidarabine An antiviral that interferes with viral DNA synthesis. It is used to treat herpes simplex infections and appears to be less susceptible to development of drug-resistant viral strains than idoxuridine (used to treat herpes simplex infections of the eye).

When used against herpes simplex encephalitis, it has cut mortality from 70 percent to 28 percent; therapy is most effective when started early, and is least effective when begun once the patient is comatose. It is also effective in treating shingles infections in those with an impaired immune system, shortening the period of viral shedding and lessening the incidence of postherpetic neuralgia.

While effective, however, studies have shown that acyclovir is more effective than vidarabine against both shingles and herpes simplex encephalitis.

Side Effects   Possible effects for treatments in the eye include tearing, irritation, pain, and sensitivity to light. Systemic use may cause nausea, vomiting, tremor, and phlebitis at the infusion site. This drug may be toxic to bone marrow and liver when given in high doses.

Zostrix   See CAPSAICIN.

zalcitabine (Trade name: Hivid)   A new antiretroviral drug used in combination with AZT (zidovudine) to treat adult patients with advanced HIV infection whose condition is deteriorating.

Side Effects   Only limited data on safety are available, but side effects that have been reported include oral ulcers, nausea, loss of appetite, abdominal pain, vomiting, rash and itching, dizziness, headache, fatigue, and sore throat.

zidovudine (Trade name: Retrovir)   An antiviral drug formerly known as azidothymidine (AZT) that is used in the treatment of AIDS and severe AIDS-related complex. The drug slows the growth of HIV infection in the body but cannot cure the infection; it works by interfering with DNA synthesis. It is used in conjunction with other drugs that help eradicate HIV.

Side Effects   Nausea, headache, and insomnia.

Appendix II
Home Disinfection

Most of the items needed to keep infections from spreading at home are readily available:

- sanitary running (hot and cold) water
- separate eating, bathing, and sleeping areas
- towels
- soap
- paper towels
- washing machine/dryers

Disinfection means the elimination of most germs on household surfaces. They include the following products:

Antiseptic: a germicide used for human skin (not inanimate objects), such as

- alcohol
- iodine
- povidone-iodine (Betadine)
- hydrogen peroxide
- chlorhexidine

Disinfectant: A chemical germicide used to disinfect surfaces; most must not be used on human skin. All common disinfectants kill HIV, other viruses, and bacteria if used properly. Any household product called a "disinfectant" contains either ethyl alcohol (ethanol), isopropyl alcohol (isopropanol), a chlorine compound, ammonia, phosphoric acid, or pine oil.

- alcohol (also an antiseptic); can be used to wipe off thermometers
- ammonium (quaternary ammonium compounds are used in hospitals to wipe down floors, walls, and furniture)
- chlorine (household bleach) usually found in a liquid called sodium hypochlorite; can be used to wipe down bathroom, diaper changing table and pail, toys, and cutting boards (to use, mix ¼ cup bleach in 1 gallon of cool water or 1 tbs. bleach in 1 quart of water in a spray bottle; make a fresh mixture every few days)

Bathroom Cleaning

Colds, flu, and diarrhea can be spread from contaminated surfaces and cloth towels. To limit infection, use any household disinfectant and

- wipe bathroom faucets, toilets, and light switches regularly when family members are sick
- wash hands after using the toilet
- wash hands after changing a baby's diaper

Kitchen Cleaning

- wipe countertops with hot soapy water and let dry thoroughly
- wipe cutting boards with hot soapy water; clean in dishwasher if possible
- thoroughly wash hands before preparing food and after handling raw meat

Appendix III
Health Organizations

International

World Health Organization
Avenue Appia
CH 1211 Geneva 27, Switzerland

Governmental

Centers for Disease Control
  Center for Prevention Services
  Center for Environmental Health
  Center for Health Promotion and
    Education
  Center for Infectious Diseases
  Division of Tuberculosis Control
1600 Clifton Road, NE
Atlanta, GA 30333
(404) 639-3311 (general number)
(404) 639-3534 (public inquiries)

*National Institute of Allergy and Infectious
Diseases*
National Institutes of Health
9000 Rockville Pike
Bldg. 31, Rm. 7A32
Bethesda, MD 20892
(301) 496-5717

U.S. Dept. of Health and Human Services
Public Health Service
200 Independence Avenue, SW
Washington, DC 20201

U.S. Department of Agriculture

U.S. Food and Drug Administration
hfi-40
5600 Fishers Lane
Rockville, MD 20857
(301) 472-4750

AIDS

*World Health Organization Collaborating Center
on AIDS*
c/o Centers for Disease Control
1600 Clifton Road, NE
Atlanta, GA 30333

National Association of People with AIDS
Ste. 700
1413 K Street, NW
Washington, DC 20005
(202) 898-0414

AIDS Education Office of the American Red Cross
8111 Gatehealth Road
Falls Church, VA 22042
(703) 206-7130

Women and AIDS Resource Network
Ste. 513
30 Third Avenue
Brooklyn, NY 11217
(718) 596-6007

Chronic Fatigue Syndrome

*Chronic Fatigue and Immune Dysfunction Syn-
drome Association of America*
P.O. Box 220398
Charlotte, NC 28222
(800) 442-3437

National Chronic Fatigue Syndrome Association
Ste. 222
3521 Broadway
Kansas City, MO 64111
(816) 931-4777

Food Safety

Food Safety and Inspection Service
Rm. 1175—South Building
1400 Independence Avenue, SW
Washington, DC 20250
(202) 720-7943
(202) 720-1843 (fax)

General Information

American Public Health Association
1015 15th Street, NW
Washington, DC 20005
(202) 789-5600

Canadian Public Health Association
(613) 725-3769

National Foundation for Infectious Diseases
P.O. Box 42022
Washington, DC 20015

Helicobacter Pylori

International Research Foundation for Helicobacter and Intestinal Immunology
P.O. Box 7965
Charlottesville, VA 22906
(804) 977-1594 (unattended voice mail and faxback line)
(804) 977-8760 (office fax)
website: http://www.helico.com/

Hepatitis

American Liver Foundation
1425 Pompton Avenue
Cedar Grove, NJ 07009
(201) 256-2550

International Travel

International Association for Medical Assistance to Travelers
417 Center Street
Lewiston, NY 14092
(716) 725-9826

IAMAT
40 Regal Road

Guelph, Ontario, N1K 1B5
Canada
(519) 836-0102
(613) 836-3412

Leprosy

American Leprosy Missions
(800) 223-0179
(201) 794-8650 in New Jersey

Respiratory Diseases

American Lung Association
1740 Broadway
New York, NY 10019

Sexually Transmitted Diseases

American Social Health Association
P.O. Box 13827
Research Triangle Park, NC 27709
(919) 361-8400
(919) 361-8425 (fax)
website: http://sunsite.unc.edu/ASHA/

American Venereal Disease Association
Box 22349
San Diego, CA 92122

Herpes Resource Center
American Social Health Association
P.O. Box 13827
Research Triangle Park, NC 27709

Urinary Tract Infections

National Kidney and Urologic Diseases
Information Clearinghouse
3 Information Way
Bethesda, MD 20892
(301) 654-4415

National Kidney Foundation
Dept. UTI
30 E. 33rd Street
New York, NY 10016
(212) 889-2210

Appendix IV
Disease Hot Lines

AIDS

CDC National AIDS Information Hot Line
(800) 342-2437 (24-hour toll free)
(800) 344-7432 (Spanish line 8 A.M.–2 A.M.,
every day except holidays)
(800) 243-7889 (TDD) (10 A.M.–10 P.M.,
Monday–Friday)
   Provides information to the public on the prevention and spread of HIV/AIDS sponsored by the Centers for Disease Control and Prevention.

CDC Clinical Trials Information Service
(800) 874-2572 (English and Spanish
9 A.M.–7 P.M.)
(800) 243-7012 (TDD)
   Provides current information on federally and privately sponsored clinical trials for AIDS patients and others with HIV infection, and on the drugs used in those trials. Sponsored by the Centers for Disease Control and Prevention, the Food and Drug Administration, the National Institute of Allergy and Infectious Diseases, and the National Library of Medicine. All calls are confidential.

CDC National AIDS Clearinghouse
(800) 458-5231 (English and Spanish
9 A.M.–7 P.M.)
(800) 243-7012 (TDD)
   Collects, classifies, and distributes up-to-date information and educational materials; provides expert assistance to HIV and AIDS prevention professionals. Makes referrals nationally to AIDS organizations for publications and HIV/AIDS-related services. Provides information and publications in English and Spanish.

Immune Deficiency Foundation
(301) 461-3127

National Indian AIDS Hot Line
(800) 283-2437 (8:30 A.M.–12 P.M. and
1 P.M.–5 P.M., Pacific time)
   Provides printed materials and information about AIDS and AIDS prevention in the Indian community.

Project Inform HIV/AIDS Treatment Hot Line
(800) 822-7422 (10 A.M.–4 P.M., Monday–Saturday, Pacific time)
(415) 558-9051 (in California) (10 A.M.–4 P.M.,
Monday–Saturday, Pacific time)
   Provides treatment information and referral for HIV-infected individuals; information on clinical trials. No diagnosis.

National Gay Task Force Crisis Line (for AIDS)
800-221-7044; 212-529-1604 in NY, AK, HI

Other Sexually Transmitted Diseases

*Centers for Disease Control STD
National Hot Line*
(800) 227-8922 (8 A.M.–11 P.M. EST,
Monday–Friday)
   Information about all sexually transmitted diseases; referral to community clinics offering free or low-cost exams and treatment.

Herpes Resource Center
(415) 328-7710

Food Safety
*Food Labeling Hot Line
Meat and Poultry Hot Line*

Turkey Hot Line
(800) 535-4555 (10 A.M.–4 P.M.)

Provides information on safe handling, preparation, and storage of meat, poultry, and eggs and provides tips on buying turkey, holiday food safety, and understanding labels on meat and poultry. Sponsored by the U.S. Department of Agriculture.

Seafood Hot Line
(800) FDA-4010 (24 hours a day, English and Spanish; noon–4 P.M. specialists are available to answer specific questions)
(202) 205-4314 (in Washington, DC; noon–4 P.M.)

Provides information on seafood buying, handling, and storage for home consumption. Also provides seafood publications and prerecorded seafood safety messages. Items and information not related to seafood are available also. To receive publications on food labeling and nutrition, callers can press "1" if using a touch telephone and then "2" for a list of available publications. Sponsored by the Food and Drug Administration.

Hepatitis

Hepatitis/Liver Disease Hot Line
(201) 256-2550

Rabies

CDC Division of Viral and Rickettsial Diseases
(404) 639-1075
(404) 639-2888 (after hours)

Patient or physicians can call if you are bitten and local/state officials are not available.

Tuberculosis

CDC Division of Tuberculosis Control
(404) 639-8120

Vaccine Injury

National Vaccine Compensation Program
(800) 338-2382

Appendix V
Health Publications

Infection Control Standards

Caring for Our Children: National Health and Safety Performance Standards: Guidelines for Out-of-Home Child Care Programs
American Public Health Association
(202) 789-5636

International Travel and Infectious Disease

Health Information for International Travel
    Centers for Disease Control
Offered by most local and state health departments, some public libraries. Also can be ordered (Publication #8280) for $5 from
Superintendent of Documents
Washington, DC 20402-9235
(202) 783-3238

International Health Guide by Stuart Rose, M.D.
Travel Medicine Inc.
351 Pleasant Street
Suite 312
Northhampton, MA 01060
(800) 872-8633
    Updated yearly.

International Travel and Health
    Published by the World Health Organization, this booklet includes vaccine requirements and health advice.

WHO Regional Office for the Americas
49 Sheridan Avenue
Albany, NY 12210
    or
Canadian Public Health Association
Publications Department
400-1565 Carling Avenue
Ottawa, Ontario K1Z 8R1
Canada
(613) 725-3769
(613) 725-9826 (Fax)

Don't Drink the Water: The Complete Traveller's Guide to Staying Healthy in Warm Climates
Canadian Public Health Association
Canadian Society for International Health
(613) 725-3769
(613) 725-9826 (Fax)
    A regularly updated guide by Dr. J. S. Keystone.

Travelling Healthy Newsletter
$29/six issues
108-48 70th Road
Forest Hills, NY 11375

Wilderness Medicine News Letter
$24/six issues
P.O. Box 9
Pitkin, CO 81241

Appendix VI
Infectious Disease–Related Web Sites

AIDS

AIDS & HIV Resource Center
Forums, newsletters, message boards, Internet sites, online support
AMERICA ONLINE keyword: aids

The Body-A Multimedia AIDS and HIV Information Resource
Articles, discussions, medical and legal advice, new treatments
http://www.thebody.com

Center for AIDS Prevention Studies
Fact sheets, forums, articles, programs, bibliography
http://www.epibiostat.ucsf.edu/capsweb

CDC National AIDS Clearinghouse
Transcripts, Quicktime videos, searchable database
http://www.cdcnac.org

European Information Center for HIV and AIDS
Stats, charts, journal archives
http://hiv.net

Gay Men's Health Crisis on the Web
Information of all kinds
http://www.gmhc.org

Gay Men's Health Crisis: I Can't Cope with My Fear of AIDS
http://www.gmhc.org/stopping/fear.html

JAMA HIV/AIDS Information Center
JAMA articles, guidelines, fact sheets, links, hot lines, groups
http://www.ama-assn.org/special/hiv/
   hivhome.htm

National Commissions on AIDS
Articles, information
gopher://odie.niaid.nih.gov:70/11/aids/nca

Positively HIV, Inc. & The HIV-ALIVE Nutritional Project
Information, projects, resources, CyberQuilt
http://www.hivalive.org

Red Ribbon Net
coffeehouse, classifieds, online AIDS charity contributions
http://www.redribbon.com

ACT-UP New York
AIDS Coalition to Unleash Power site
http://www.actupny.org

Estate Project for Artists with AIDS
Help in finding financial support and grants, artists profiles
http://www.artistswith aids.org

Pets Are Wonderful Support
Pets and AIDS patients
http://www.pawssf.org

United in Anger
Photo documentary, poetry
http://www.panix.com/~bytsura.uia.shtml

AIDS News Clips
Clipping service
COMPUSERVE *go* aidsnews

AIDS Related Information
Hundreds of articles, reports
gopher://odie.niaid.nih.gov/11/aids

Berkeley AIDS Gopher
Onsite articles, links
gopher//uclink.berkeley.edu:1901/11/
    other/aids

CDC Gopher
Articles, reports, public service announce-
ments
gopher://cdcnac.aspensys.com:72/11

New York Times AIDS
Current articles on HIV/AIDS
http://nytsyn.com/live/Aids

AIDS Virtual Library
Index of Net resources, including FAQs,
gophers, organizations
http://pknetq.com/aidsvl/index.html

AIDS Patent Project
Abstracts, copies of patents relating to AIDS
http://patents.cnidr.org

AIDS Treatment Data Network
Comprehensive treatment resource
http://www.aidsnyc.org/network/index.
    html

Calypte Biomedical
Articles, weekly column on urine HIV tests
http://www.calypte.com/AIDS

Medscape-AIDS
Technical articles, columns, clinical news
http://www.medscape.com/Home/Topics/
    AIDS/AIDS.html

Bacterial and Fungal Diseases

The Swedish Karolinska Institute
http://www.mic.ki.se/Diseases/index.html

The E. coli index
Links to microbiological research sites, companies, publishers, and journals
http://sun1.bham.ac.uk/bcm4ght6/res.html

Communicable Disease Surveillance Centre

United Kingdom–based web site with links to
research institutions and disease-monitoring
organizations
http://www.open.gov.uk/cdsc

Ebola

An Interview with Dr. Frederick A. Murphy
Discussion with former director of the CDC's
National Center for Infectious Diseases
http://outcast.gene.com/ae/WN/NM/
    interview_murphy.html

Ebola Information
Media reports, links to CDC and WHO
http://www.geocities.com/Cape
    Canaveral/Lab/5738

Ebola Page
Medical newsgroups, mailing lists, associations
http://www.uct.ac.za/microbiology/
    ebopage.html

Ebola Reading List
Bibliography on Ebola and hemorrhagic fever
http://www.bocklabs.wisc.edu/ebola.html

Outbreak: Ebola on the Net
Chronology of Ebola outbreak, with general
information and WHO fact sheets
http://www.outbreak.org

Outbreak Updates
University of Wisconsin web clipping service,
links to basic tutorial
http://www.bocklabs.wisc.edu/outbreak.
    html

E. Coli

The E. coli Index
Links to microbiological research sites, companies, publishers, and journals
http://sun1.bham.ac.uk/bcm4ght6/res.html

Emerging Diseases

Emerging and Re-Emerging Viruses
Scholarly information
http://www.uct.ac.za/microbiology/ebola.
  html

Emerging Infections Information Network
Yale's School of Public Health information
center, with seminars (including lectures,
slides, and audio clips) and live chat sessions;
e-mail questions answered
http://info.med.yale.edu/EIINet.html

Emerging Infectious Diseases Journal
CDC's quarterly journal
http://www.cdc.gov/ncidod/EID/eid.htm

Emerging Infectious Diseases Resource Links
CDC site with links to health journals,
resources, agencies
http://www.cdc.gov/ncidod/id_links.htm

Emerging Viruses
Department of Microbiology at the University
of Cape Town site
http://www.uct.ac.za/microbiology

The Hot Zone
Web page by Richard Preston, author of the
best-seller *The Hot Zone*
http://mixer.visi.com/~chris/hotzone

Outbreak Page
Press releases are updated often.
http://www.who.ch/outbreak/
  outbreak_home.html

ProMED
Mailing lists, discussions.
http://www.healthnet.org/programs/
  promed.html

WHO Division of Control of Tropical Diseases
Information, links to virology and schistosomiasis newsgroups
http://www.who.ch/ctd

*WHO: Emerging and Other Communicable Dis-
eases Surveillance and Control*
Weekly Epidemiological Record, updated
new briefs
http://www.who.ch/emc/emc_home.htm

Food-borne Diseases

The E. coli Index
Links to microbiological research sites, companies, publishers, and journals
http://sun 1.bham.ac.uk/bcm4ght6/res.html

Herpes

The Herpes Zone
http://www.herpeszone.com

Herpes
http://www.azstarnet.com

Herpes Home Page
http://www.racoon.com/herpes

Infectious, Contagious Diseases

General information, with latest news on out-
breaks
AMERICA ONLINE keyword: Infectious,
Contagious Diseases

Infectious Disease Weekly
Abstracts of the week's news in infectious disease (full stories available only through subscription); e-mail service available
http://www.newsfile.com/li.htm

National Center for Infectious Diseases
http://www.cdc.gov/ncidod/ncid.htm

Leprosy

*WHO Action Programme for the Elimination of
Leprosy*
General information
http://www.who.ch/programmes/lep/
  lep_home.htm

Medical Microbiology Home
Singapore General Hospital information
http://biomed.nus.sg

Medscape: Infectious Diseases
Aimed at medical community (requires registration)
http://www.medscape.com

Microbial Underground
St. Bartholomew's Hospital in London site
http://www.Isumc.edu/campus/micr/
   mirror/public_html/index.html

National Center for Infectious Diseases
General information on travel health, disease, prevention
http://www.cdc.gov/nicidod/ncid.htm

National Foundation for Infectious Diseases
Links to WWW sources on many infectious diseases
http://www.scp.com/NFID

Parasitic Diseases
Karolinska Institute site for general information
http://www.mic.ki.se/Diseases/index.html

Plague Links
Links to information clearinghouses
http://ccme-mac4.bsd.uchicago.edu/
   CCMEDocs/Plague

University of Rochester Infectious Diseases Unit
http://www.urmc.rochester.edu/SMD/
   InfDis/id.htm

Virtual Library: Epidemiology
Agencies, research sites, mailing lists
http://www.epibiostat.ucsf.edu/epidem/
   epidem.html

Plagues

The Black Death
History of the plague
http://jefferson.village.virginia.edu/osheim/
   intro.html

Plagues
Lecture series
http://www.ento.vt.edu

People's Plague Interactive Quiz
http://www.pbs.org/ppol/quiz.html

Lyme Disease

American Lyme Disease Foundation
Homeowners guide, support link for sufferers
http://www.w2.com/docs2/d5/lyme.html

Lyme Disease Information Resource
Senate bills on insurance, new drugs, support guide, discussion, general health links
http://www.sky.net

Lyme Disease Network
Newsletter, discussion groups, diagnosis/treatment manual, court cases, national support groups
http://www.lymenet.org

LYMENET-L
Bimonthly newsletter tracking research, treatment, politics
E-mail listserv@legigh.edu (type in message
   body: subscribe lymenet-1<your full name>)

sci.med.diseases.lyme
Discussions of new treatments, insurance advice, information
USENET sci.med.diseases.lyme

Malaria

Malaria Weekly
Weekly abstracts on news, research, official releases (by subscription)
http://www.newsfile.com/1m.htm

Papillomavirus

Papovaviruses
http://www-micro.msb.le.ac.uk

Sexually Transmitted Diseases (Other Than AIDS)

American Social Health Association
A complete directory of telephone hot lines, plus news releases and the ABCs of STDs, from antigens to urethritis
http://sunsite.unc.edu/ASHA

Travel-related Diseases

Travel Health
Detailed information and links to CDC sites and the state department travel advisories
http://www.travelhealth.com

Tuberculosis

Brown University TB/HIV Laboratory
Scientific articles, online history
http://www.brown.edu

Centers for Disease Control Tuberculosis Page
Basic information
http://www.cdc.gov

Multidrug-resistant Tuberculosis—Annotated Bibliography
Brief descriptions of the latest literature; hypertext links to Medline article subscription service
http://uhs.bsd.uchicago.edu/uhs/topics/
    resist.tb.bib.html

The People's Plague Online
Educational site on TB
http://www.pbs.org/ppol

TB Weekly
News abstracts, research, journal articles; subscription-only access to full text
http://www.newsfile.com/1t.htm

Tuberculosis Resources
Columbia Presbyterian Hospital and the New York City Health Department presents series of pamphlets on TB in English and Spanish, with protocols for health care providers
http://www.cpmc.columbia.edu/tbcpp

WHO Global Tuberculosis Programme
New report on TB epidemic; e-mail links
http://www.who.ch

Vaccines

Adult Vaccinations
Mass. public health department text file
http://vh.radiology.uiowa.edu

CDC Immunization Information Page
Hypertext file details disease, treatment
http://www.cdc.gov

Vaccines & Diseases News
Journal abstracts
http://www.biol.tsukuba.ac.jp

Virology

Virus Diseases
Karolinska Institute's informational site
http://www.mic.ki.se/Diseases/index.html

BIBLIOGRAPHY

Adler, Stuart. "Risk of Human Parvovirus B19 Infections," *The Journal of Infectious Diseases* 168(1993):361–68.

Adler, Tina. "Mauling mosquitoes naturally: new ways to silence the buzz," *Science News* 149(April 27, 1996):270–71.

Akue, J. P., T. G. Egwant, E. Devaney. "High levels of parasite-specific IgG4 in the absence of microfilaremia in Loa loa infection," *Tropical Medical Parasitology* 45(1994): 246–48.

Almond, J. W., et al. "Will bovine spongiform encephalopathy transmit to humans?" *British Medical Journal* 311(Nov. 25, 1995): 1415–21.

Anasari, A., et al. "Comparison of Cloth, Paper and Warm Air Drying in Eliminating Viruses and Bacteria from Washed Hands," *American Journal of Infection Control* 19:5(1991):243–49.

Anderson, Kenneth N., ed. *Mosby's Medical, Nursing and Allied Health Dictionary.* 4th ed. Boston: Mosby, 1994.

Associated Press. "Abuse of antibiotics produces superbugs," *Associated Press wire* (Nov. 25, 1995).

———. "Herb-based drug is effective in preventing malaria deaths," *Associated Press wire story* (July 11, 1996).

———. "Aviron's cold adapted influenza vaccine." Mountain View, Calif.: Aviron. Nov. 5, 1996, pp. 33–34.

———. "Parainfluenza virus type 3." Mountain View, Calif.: Aviron. Nov. 5, 1996, p. 35.

———. "Epstein-Barr virus." Mountain View, Calif.: Aviron. Nov. 5, 1996, pp. 35–36.

———. "Cytomegalovirus." Mountain View, Calif.: Aviron. Nov. 5, 1996, p. 36.

———. "Herpes simplex type 2." Mountain View, Calif.: Aviron. Nov. 5, 1996, pp. 36–37.

———. "Respiratory syncytial virus." Mountain View, Calif.: Aviron. Nov. 5, 1996, p. 37.

———. "FDA first once-daily anti-infective for three respiratory diseases," *Associated Press wire* (Dec. 20, 1996).

———. "FDA oks new respiratory drug," *Associated Press wire* (Dec. 21, 1996).

———. "Army to study Gulf War research," *Associated Press wire story* (Dec. 26, 1996).

Barbour, Alan G., and Durland Fish. "The biological and social phenomenon of Lyme disease," *Science* 260(June 11, 1993): 1610–16.

Barthold, S. W. "Antigenic stability of borrelia burgdorferi during chronic infections of immunocompetent mice," *Infection and Immunity* 61:12(Dec. 1993):4955–61.

Beardsley, Tim. "Trends in preventive medicine: Better than a cure," *Scientific American* 272(Jan. 1995):88–95.

Beeler, J., F. Varricchio, and R. Wise. "Thrombocytopenia after immunization with measles vaccines: review of the Vaccine Adverse Events Reporting System (1990 to 1994), *Pediatric Infectious Disease Journal* 15(1996):88–90.

Berenbaum, May R. *Bugs in the System: Insects and Their Impact on Human Affairs.* Boston: Addison-Wesley, 1995.

Berenguer, J., M. Santiago, and F. Laguna. "Tuberculous meningitis in patients infected with the HIV virus," *New England Journal of Medicine* 326(1992):668–72.

Biddle, Wayne. *A Field Guide to Germs.* New York: Doubleday, 1995.

Bishop, Jerry. "Study suggests cause and cure for ulcers," *Wall Street Journal* (May 1, 1992):B-1.

Blake, P. A. "Epidemiology of Cholera in the Americas," *Gastroenterology Clinics of North America* 22(1993):639–60.

Blumenthal, Susan. "Another ear infection?" *Ladies Home Journal* 112(June 1995):118.

Bower, Bruce. "Virus may trigger some mood disorders," *Science News* 147(June 17, 1995):132.

Breiman, R., et al. "Emergence of Drug-Resistant Pneumococcal Infections in the United States," *JAMA* 271:23(1994): 1831–35.

Briseno-Garcia, B., H. Gomez-Dantes, E. Argott-Ramirez. "Potential risk for dengue hemorrhagic fever: The isolation of sero-type dengue-3 in Mexico," *Emerging Infectious Diseases* 2:2(1996):841–44.

Brown, E. E., D. A. Peura. "Diagnosis of *Helicobacter pylori* infection," *Gastroenterology Clinics of North America* 22:1(March 1993):105.

Brown, Kathryn Sergeant. "Skip the flu: it can be done," *Woman's Day* (Oct. 10, 1995):100.

Bulbin, A., and M. S. Simberkoff. "Prevention of pneumonia in the elderly," *Infections in Medicine* 12(8):385, 389–394, 1995.

Bull, J. J. "Virulence," *Evolution* 48(1994): 1423–37.

Carey, R. F., W. A. Herman, et al. "Effectiveness of latex condoms as a barrier to human immunodeficiency virus-sized particles under conditions of simulated use," *Sexually Transmitted Diseases* 19(1992): 230–34.

Centers for Disease Control. "Condoms for prevention of sexually transmitted diseases," *Morbidity and Mortality Weekly Report* 37(1988): 133–37.

———. "Screening for tuberculosis and tuberculosis infection in high-risk populations," *MMWR* 39:RR-8(1990):1–7.

———. "Summary of Notifiable Diseases, United States," *Morbidity and Mortality Weekly Report*. Atlanta: Centers for Disease Control, 1992.

———. "The Management of Acute Diarrhea in Children: Oral Rehydration, Maintenance and Nutritional Therapy," *Morbidity and Mortality Weekly Report* 41(1992):RR–16.

———. "E Coli 0157:H7 Information Package," March 1993. *Morbidity and Mortality Weekly Report* 42(1993):RR–1.

———. "Initial therapy for tuberculosis in the era of multi-drug resistance: Recommendations of the Advisory Council for the elimination of tuberculosis," *MMWR* 42:RR-7(1993):1–8.

———. "Summary of Notifiable Diseases, United States," *Morbidity and Mortality Weekly Report*. Atlanta: Centers for Disease Control, 1993.

———. "Bacteria take new role as cancer vaccine," *Science News* 148(Nov. 25, 1995): 357.

———. "New drug sweeps clean in HIV model," *Science News* 148(Nov. 18, 1995):324.

Centofanti, Marjorie, "Just lookin' for a home: many bacteria sneak into cells via entry routes already in place," *Science News* 149(Jan. 6, 1996):12–13.

Chapnick, Edward K., John Protic, et al. "Congratulations: It's a worm!" *Infections in Medicine* 13:8(1996):653–54.

Clancy, Cornelius J., et al. "Fungemia caused by *Candida lusitaniae*," *Infections in Medicine* 13:11(1996):940, 948–51.

Clemens, J. D., D. A. Sack, and J. R. Harris. "Field trial of oral cholera vaccines in Bangladesh: Results form three-year followup," *Lancet* 335(1990):270–3.

Covacci, A., S. Censini, M. Bugnoli, et al. "Molecular characterization of the 128-kDa immunodominant antigen of Helicobacter pylori associated with cytotoxicity and duodenal ulcer," *Proceeds of the National Academy of Science* 90(1993): 5791–95.

Cover, T. L., M. J. Blaser. "Helicobacter pylori: a bacterial cause of gastritis, peptic ulcer disease and gastric cancer," *American Society of Microbiology newsletter* 61(1995):21–26.

Crabtree, J. E., et al. "Expression of 120 kilodalton protein and cytotoxicity in Helicobacter pylori," *Journal of Clinical Pathology* 45(1992):733–4.

Crosby, Alfred W. *America's Forgotten Pandemic: The Influenza of 1918.* New York: Cambridge University Press, 1990.

Custer, Joseph. "Croup and Related Disorders," *Pediatrics in Review* 14:1(1993): 17–28.

Dealler, S. F. and R. W. Lacey. "Transmissible spongiform encephalopathies: the therat of BSE to man," *Food Microbiology* 7(1990): 253–79.

Dobkin, Jay F. "Influenza and HIV in '97: The big one?" *Infections in Medicine* 14:1(1997): 10.

Ebert, D. "Virulence and local adaptation of a horizontally transmitted parasite," *Science* 265(1994):1084–86.

Ewald, P. W. *The Evolution of Infectious Disease.* Oxford, U.K.: Oxford University Press, 1994.

———. "Guarding against the most dangerous emerging pathogens: insights from evolutionary biology," *Emerging Infectious Diseases* 2:4(1996):245–57.

———. "The hepatitis G enigma: researchers corner new viruses associated with hepatitis," *Science News* 149(April 13, 1996): 238–39.

Farci, P. "Lack of protective immunity against reinfection with hepatitis C virus," *Science* 258(Oct. 2, 1992): 135–40.

Farley, Dixie. "On the teen scene: TSS—reducing the risk," *FDA Consumer* (Oct. 1991):24.

——— "Help for cuts, scrapes and burns: OTC options," *FDA Consumer* (May 1996):13–15.

———. "Fighting Fleas and Ticks," *FDA Consumer* (July–August 1996):23–29.

———. Treating Tropical diseases," *FDA Consumer* (Jan.–Feb. 1997):26–30.

Farrington, P., et al. "A new method for active surveillance of adverse events from DTP and MMR vaccines," *Lancet* 345(1995): 567–69.

Fauci, A. S. "Multifactorial nature of human immunodeficiency virus disease: implications for therapy," *Science* 262(1993): 1008–11.

FDA Consumer. "Penicillins," *FDA Consumer* (July–August 1990):29–30.

———. "Report on rotavirus vaccine," *FDA Consumer* (July–Aug. 1995):3.

———. "HIV-Related use of antibiotic," *FDA Consumer* (November 1996): 3.

———. "First drug for rare parasitic diseases," *FDA Consumer* (September 1996):4.

———. "New pertussis vaccine safer for infants," *FDA Consumer* (October 1996):2.

———. "New drug for AIDS-related eye infection, *FDA Consumer* (October 1996): 4.

———. "First urine test for HIV," *FDA Consumer* (October 1996):5.

———. "AIDs drug approved in 119 days," *FDA Consumer* (October 1996):5.

———. "Drug for testing HIV wasting gets early approval," *FDA Consumer* (November 1996):2.

———. "FDA Warning concerning certain Italian cheese," *FDA Consumer* (Nov. 1996):3–4.

———. "Breath Test for Ulcer Bacterium," *FDA Consumer* 31:1(Jan.–Feb. 1997):3.

———. "Certain antimicrobial drugs related to tendon problems," *FDA Consumer* 31:1(Jan.–Feb. 1997):4.

Feng, P. "Escherichia coli Serotype 0157:H7: Novel vehicles of infection and emergence of phenotypic variants," *Emerging Infectious Diseases* 1:2(1995):47–52.

Fikrig, E. Barthold, et al. "Protection of mice against the Lyme disease agent by immunizing with recombinant OSPA," *Science* 250(Oct. 26, 1990):553–56.

Franco, Eduardo. "Human Papillomavirus and the National History of Cervical Cancer," *Infections in Medicine* (January 1993): 57–64.

Furley, Dixie. "Treating tropical diseases," *FDA Consumer* 31:1(Jan.–Feb. 1997):26–30.

Gale, J. L. et al. "Risk of serious acute neurological illness after immunization with diphtheria-tetanus-pertussis vaccine," *JAMA* 271 (1994):37–41.

Gantz, Nelson, et al., eds. *Manual of Clinical Problems in Infectious Disease*. Boston: Little, Brown, 1994.

Garraud O., et al. "Identification of recombinant filarial proteins capable of inducing polyclonal and antigen-specific IgE and IgG4 antibodies," *Journal of Immunology* 155(1316–25):1995.

Garrett, Laurie. *The Coming Plague*. New York: Farrar, Straus and Giroux, 1994.

Girgis, N., et al. "Dexamethasone adjunctive treatment for TB meningitis," *Journal of Pediatric Infectious Disease* 10(1991):179–83.

Goddard, Jerome. "Viruses transmitted by mosquitoes: dengue fever," *Infections in Medicine* 13:11(1996):933–34.

Gottfried, Robert S. *The Black Death*. New York: Free Press, 1983.

Griffin, M. R., et al. "Risk of seizures and encephalopathy after immunization with the DTP vaccine," *JAMA* 263(1990): 1641–45.

Gubler, D. J., and G. G. Clark. "Dengue/dengue hemorrhagic fever: The emergence of a global health problem," *Emerging Infectious Diseases* 1:2(1995): 55–57.

Guinee, Vincent F. "Epidemic," *Colliers Encyclopedia CD-Rom (vol 9) online*. Released Feb. 28, 1996.

Gutman, L. T., J. Moye, and B. Zimmer. "Tuberculosis in HIV-exposed or infected U.S. children," *Journal of Pediatric Infectious Disease* 13(1994):963–68.

Haney, Daniel Q. "Kid Diarrhea vaccine effective," *Associated Press* (Sept. 18, 1996).

———. "Drug-resistant fungi emerging," *Associated Press* (Sept. 17, 1996).

Harden, Virginia. *Rocky Mountain Spotted Fever*. Baltimore: Johns Hopkins University Press, 1990.

Harvard Women's Health Watch, "New clue to CFS," *Harvard Women's Health Watch* (Nov. 1995):6.

Haslam, R. H. "Role of computed tomography in the early management of bacterial meningitis," *Journal of Pediatrics* 119(1991): 152–59.

Hill, A. V. S., et al. "Common West African HLA antigens are associated with protection from severe malaria," *Nature* 252(1991):595–600.

Hingley, Audrey. "Rabies on the Rise," *FDA Consumer* (November 1996):25–29.

Hobby, Gladys. *Penicillin: Meeting the Challenge*. New Haven, Conn.: Yale University Press, 1985.

Hoeprich, Paul D., et al., eds. *Infectious Diseases* (5th ed). Philadelphia: Lippincott, 1994.

Hoke, C. H. et al. "Protection against Japanese encephalitis by inactivated vaccines," *New England Journal of Medicine* 319(1988): 608–14.

Holman, R. C., et al. "Epidemiology of Creutzfeldt-Jakob disease in the United States 1979–1990," *Neuroepidemiology* 14(1995):174–81.

Horgan, John. "The no-name virus: questions linger after the four corners outbreak," *Scientific American* 271:6(Dec. 1994):34.

Hotez, Peter J., and David I. Pritchard. "Hookworm Infection," *Scientific American* 272:6(June 1995):68–74.

Hughes, J. M., and F. C. Tenover. "Infectious disease challenges of the 1990s," *Infections in Medicine* 13:9(1996):788, 798–99.

Institute of Medicine, et al., eds.

Institute of Medicine. *Adverse effects of pertussis and rubella vaccines*. Washington, D.C.: National Academy Press, 1991.

Emerging Infections: Microbial Threats to Health in the United States. Washington, D.C.: National Academy Press, 1992.

———. *Vaccines Against Malaria: Hope in a Gathering Storm*. Washington, D.C.: IOM Board on International Health, 1996.

Johnson, Hillary. *Osler's Web: Inside the Labyrinth of the Chronic Fatigue Syndrome Epidemic*. New York: Crown, 1996.

Johnson, Howard, et al. "How interferons fight disease," *Scientific American* 270:5(May 1994):68–75.

Kantor, Fred S. "Disarming Lyme disease," *Scientific American* 271:3(September 1994): 34–39.

Kayhty, Helena, and Juhani Eskola. "New vaccines for the prevention of pneumococcal infections," *Emerging Infectious Diseases* 2:4(1996):289–98.

Khouri, Y., et al. "Mycobacterium TB in children with human HIV type 1 infection," *Journal of Pediatric Infectious Disease* 11(1992):950–55.

King, Linda. "The facts on feline AIDS," *McCall's* (Oct. 1996):166.

Kiple, Kenneth, ed. *The Cambridge World History of Human Disease.* Cambridge, England: Cambridge University Press, 1993.

Klion, A. D., et al. "Loiasis in endemic and nonendemic populations: immunologically mediated differences in clinical presentation," *Journal of Infectious Diseases* 163(1991):1318–25.

Knight-Ridder Newspapers. "Public at risk from old, new diseases," *Knight-Ridder News Services* (Jan. 17, 1996).

Kraut, Alan M. *Silent Travelers.* New York: Basic Books, 1994.

Krieg, Joann P. *Epidemics in the Modern World.* New York: Macmillan/Twayne, 1992.

Kubic, Mike. "New Ways to prevent and treat AIDS," *FDA Consumer* 31:1(Jan.–Feb. 1997):7–11.

Lacey, R. W. "Bovine spongiform encephalopathy is being maintained by vertical and horizontal transmission," *British Medical Journal* 312(Jan. 20, 1996): 180–81.

Lederberg, Joshua, et al., eds. *Emerging Infections.* Washington, D.C.: National Academy Press, 1992.

Leigh Brown, A. J., and E. C. Holmes. "Evolutionary biology of the human immunodeficiency virus," *Annual Review of Ecology and Systematics* 25(1994):127–62.

Lemonick, Michael. "Germ Warfare: Infectious diseases can strike anywhere, anytime," *Time* (Sept. 13, 1996):59–62.

Levin, Bruce R. "The evolution and maintenance of virulence in microparasites," *Emerging Infectious Diseases* 2:2(1996): 93–102.

Levin, B. R., and J. J. Bull. "Short-sighted evolution and the virulence of pathogenic microorganisms," *Trends in Microbiology* 2(1994):76–81.

Levine, Arnold J. *Viruses.* New York: Scientific American Library, 1992.

Levy, S. B. *Antibiotic Paradox: How Miracle Drugs Are Destroying the Miracle.* New York: Plenum Press, 1992.

Lin, J. S., et al. "Underdiagnosis of Chlamydia trachomatis infection: diagnostic limitations in patients with low-level infection," *Sexually Transmitted Diseases* 19(1992): 259–65.

Lipkin, R. "New 'design rule' yield novel drugs," *Science News.* 147(June 17, 1995):374.

Lipsitch, M., and M. L. Nowak. "The evolution of virulence in sexually transmitted HIV/AIDS," *Journal of Theoretical Biology* 174(1995):427–40.

Long, Michael. "In the woods, an unspotted fever," *Health* 8(March 1, 1994):17.

Los Angeles News Service. "Researchers: immune system fix possible," *LA News Service* (Jan. 27, 1997).

Lutwick, L. et al. "There is always something small that's too big for some of us," *Infections in Medicine* 13:9(1996):761–62, 767.

Lutwick, L. "Prion's progress: Are you what you eat?" *Infections in Medicine* 13:12(1996):1037, 1041–43.

Marshal, B. J. "Helicobacter pylori," *American Journal of Gastroenterology* 89:81(Aug. supp. 1994):S-116.

Marshall, E. "Hantavirus Outbreak Yields to PCR," *Science* 262(1993):832–36.

Mason, Michael. "Forget stress and spicy foods: the real culprit may be just a kiss away," *Health magazine* (1994).

McCarthy, S. A., et al. "Toxigenic Vibrio cholerae 01 and Cargo Ships Entering Gulf of Mexico," (letter) *Lancet* 339(1992):624–25.

Miller, D. L. et al. "Pertussis immunization and serious acute neurological illnesses in children," *British Medical Journal* 307(1993): 1171–76.

Miller, E., et al. "Risk of aseptic meningitis after measles, mumps and rubella vaccine in UK children," *Lancet* 341(1993):979–95.

Monastersky, Richard. "Health in the hot zone: how would global warming affect humans?" *Science News* 149(April 6, 1996):218–19.

Moore, Patrick S., and Claire V. Broome. "Cerebrospinal meningitis epidemics," 271:5(Nov. 1994):38–45.

Moore, Patrick S. "Meningococcal meningitis in subsaharan Africa: A model for the epidemic process," *Clinical Infectious Diseases* 14:2(Feb. 1992):515–25.

Morbidity and Mortality Weekly Report, "Cholera associated with an international air flight," MMWR 4(1992):134–35.

———. "Importation of cholera from Peru," *MMWR* 4(1991):258–59.

———. "Dengue fever at the U.S.-Mexico border, 1995–1996," *MMWR* 45:39(1996): 841–44.

———. "World Health Organization consultation on public health issues related to bovine spongiform encephalopathy and the emergence of a new variant of Creutzfeldt-Jakob disease," *MMWR* 45:14(1996):295–303.

———. "Surveillance for Creutzfeldt-Jakob disease—United States" *MMWR* 45:31(1996):665–69.

Morrison, D. C., and J. L. Ryan, eds. *Novel Therapeutic Strategies in the Treatment of Sepsis.* New York: Marcel Dekker, 1996.

Morse, Stephen S., ed. *Emerging Viruses.* New York: Oxford University Press, 1993.

Murdoch, Guy. "Swimmer's ear," *Consumer's Research Magazine* 75(Aug. 1, 1992):2.

Musgrove, C., et al. "Campylobacter pylori: clinical, histological and serological studies," *Journal of Clinical Pathology* 41(1988):11316–21.

Newell, D. G., et al. "Estimation of prevalence of Helicobacter pylori infection in an asymptomatic elderly population compar-

ing urea breath test and serology," *Journal of Clinical Pathology* 44(1991):385–87.

Nowak, Rachel. "Cause of fatal outbreak in horses and humans traced," *Science* 268(April 7, 1995):32.

Palumbo, P., et al. "Population-based study of measles and measles immunization in HIV-infected children," *Pediatric Infectious Disease Journal* 11(1992):1008–14.

Parsonnet, J., et al. "*Helicobacter pylori* infection and the risk of gastric carcinoma," *New England Journal of Medicine* 325(1991): 1127–31.

Patchett, S., et al. "Helicobacter pylori and duodenal ulcer recurrence." *American Journal of Gastroenterology* 87(1992):24–27.

Patlak, Margie. "Book reopened on infectious diseases," *FDA Consumer* 30(April 1996): 19–23.

Paul, John R. *A History of Poliomyelitis.* New Haven: Yale University Press, 1971.

Payer, Lynn. *Disease-Mongers.* New York: John Wiley, 1992.

Peeling, R. W. "Chlamydia trachomatis and *Neisseria gonorrhoeae*: pathogens in retreat?" *Current Opinion in Infectious Diseases* 8(1995):26–34.

Peeling, R. W., and Robert C. Brunham. "Chlamydiae as pathogens: New species and new issues," *Emerging Infectious Diseases 2:4* (October–December 1996): 307–319.

Podolsky, Doug. "Kill the bug and you kill the ulcer," *U.S. News & World Report* (May 13, 1991):94.

Prusiner, S. B. "Molecular biology of prion diseases," *Science* 252 (June 14, 1991): 1515–22.

———. "The prion diseases," *Scientific American* 272:1(Jan. 1995):48–57.

Quetel, Claude. *History of Syphilis.* Baltimore: Johns Hopkins University Press, 1992.

Raloff, Janet. "How climate perturbations can plague us," *Science News* 148(Sept. 23, 1995):196–97.

———. "When pertussis is not a whooping cough," *Science News* 148(Nov. 25, 1995).

———. "Oldest Lyme-carrying microbes found," *Science News* 148(Dec. 2, 1995): 373.

———. "Pesticides may challenge human immunity," *Science News* 149(March 9, 1996):149.

———. "Stress undercuts flu shots," *Science News* 149(April 13, 1996):231.

———. "Antibiotics take a bite out of bad gums," *Science News* 149(May 18, 1996): 308.

Ranger, Terence, and Paul Slack. *Epidemics and Ideas*. Cambridge, England: Cambridge University Press, 1992.

Rantala, J., et al. "Epidemiology of Guillain-Barre syndrome in children: relationships of oral polio vaccine administration to occurrence," *Journal of Pediatrics* 124(1994): 220–23.

Sabin, Francene. *Microbes and Bacteria*. Mahwah, N.J.: Troll, 1985.

Saracco, A., et al. "Man-to-woman sexual transmission of HIV: longitudinal study of 343 steady partners of infected men," *Journal of Acquired Immune Deficiency Syndrome* 6(1993):497–502.

Schaechter, M., et al., eds. *Microbial Disease*. Baltimore: Williams & Wilkins, 1993.

Schrag, S., and P. Wiener. "Emerging infectious diseases: what are the relative roles of ecology and evolution?" *Trends in Ecology and Evolution* 10(1995):319–23.

Science News. "Turning DNA into an antibiotic," *Science News* 149(Jan. 20, 1995):47.

———. "Another round in the prion debate," *Science News* 147(June 17, 1995):383.

———. "Tuberculosis gene may explain dormancy," *Science News* 149(April 20, 1996):255.

———. "Nitric oxide at war with homocysteine?" *Science News* 149(April 27, 1996): 269.

———. "Get the infection, not the disease," *Science News* 148(Sept. 2, 1995):153.

Seachrist, Lisa. "The once and future scourge: could common anti-inflammatory drugs allow bacteria to take a deadly turn?" *Science News* 148(Oct. 7, 1995):234–35.

———. "Amount of virus sets cancer risk," *Science News* 148(Sept. 23, 1995):197.

Shen, Chen-Yang, et al. "Cytomegalovirus Transmission in Special Care Centers for Mentally Retarded Children," *Pediatrics* 91:1(1993):517–21.

Shulman, Stanford T., et al., eds. *The Biologic and Clinical Basis of Infectious Diseases*. 4th ed. Philadelphia: Saunders, 1992.

Simone, P. M., and M. D. Iseman. "Drug resistant tuberculosis: A deadly and growing danger," *Journal of Respiratory Disease* 13(1992):960–71.

Singleton, Paul. *Introduction to Bacteria*. 2nd ed. New York: John Wiley, 1992.

Smeltzer, Suzanne, and Brenda Bare, ed. *Brunner and Suddarth's Textbook of Medical and Surgical Nursing*. 7th ed. New York: Lippincott, 1992.

Smith, A., ed. "Antibiotic Update," *Pediatric Annals* 22:3(1993).

Smith, J. D. G., et al. "PCR detection of colonization by Helicobacter pylori in conventional euthymic mice based on the 16S ribosomal gene sequence." *Clinical Diagnostic Lab Immunol.* 3(1996):66–72.

Squires, Sally. "The most misused medicine in America," *Good Housekeeping* (November 1995):90–93.

———. "New treatment helps ease pain of shingles," *Washington Post News Service* (Oct. 24, 1995).

Stanley, S. K., et al. "Effect of immunization with a common recall antigen on viral expression in patients infected with HIV type 1," *New England Journal of Medicine* 334(1996):1222–30.

Starke, J. R., R. F. Jacobs, and J. Jereb. "Resurgence of tuberculosis in children," *Journal of Pediatrics* 120(1992):839–55.

Steffen, R., and R. H. Behrens. "Travelers' malaria," *Parasitology Today* 8(1992):61–66.

Sternberg, Steve. "Human version of mad cow disease?" *Science News* 149(April 13, 1996):228.

———. "Chance reveals deadly rotavirus secret," *Science News* 149(April 6, 1966):213.

Stoffman, Phyllis. *The Family Guide to Preventing and Treating 100 Infectious*

Illnesses. New York: John Wiley & Sons, 1995.

Taylor, Jeffrey, et al. "Amebic meningoencephalitis," *Infections in Medicine* 13:12(1996): 1017, 1021–24.

Tompkins, L. S., and S. Falkow. "The new path to preventing ulcers," *Science* 267(1995):1621–22.

Travis, John. "AIDS update '96: New drugs, new tests, new optimism mark recent AIDS research," *Science News* 149(March 23, 1996):184–86.

———. "Body's proteins suppress AIDS virus," *Science News* 148(Dec. 9, 1995):388.

———. "Swallowing *Shigella*: Can bacteria that cause food poisoning deliver oral DNA vaccines?" *Science News* 149(May 11, 1996):302–3.

———. "Digging into TB's history with genetics," *Science News* 147(June 3, 1995).

———. "Making big mountains out of tiny bacteria," *Science News* 148(Sept. 23, 1995):197.

———. "HIV-2 offers protection against HIV-1," *Science News* 147(June 17, 1995):373.

———. "Body's proteins suppress AIDS virus," *Science News* 148(Dec. 9, 1995):388.

———. "The worm turns: into a source of new drugs," *Science News* 149(March 9, 1996):148.

Velin, Bob. "FDA takes aim at mad cow disease," *USA Today* (Sept. 12, 1996).

Vila, Ileana, et al. "Chronic Q fever in an avian," *Infections in Medicine* 13:11(1996): 977–88.

Vinetz, J. M., et al. "Sporadic urban leptospirosis," *Annals of Internal Medicine* 125(1996):794–98.

Vlacha, V., et al. "Recurrent thrombocytopenic purpura after repeated MMR vaccination," *Pediatrics* 97(1996):73–79.

Vogt, Shelly. "Psittacosis," *Veterinary Technician* 15(Sept. 1, 1994):483.

Walker, D. H., and J. S. Dumler. "Emergence of the erlichioses as human health problems," *Emerging Infectious Diseases* 2:1(1996):18–29.

Walsh, J. H., and W. Peterson. "The treatment of Helicobacter pylori infection in the management of peptic ulcer disease," *The New England Journal of Medicine* 333(15)(Oct. 12, 1995):984.

Watson, D. A., and D. M. Musher. "The pneumococcus: sugar-coated killer," *Infections in Medicine* 13(5):373–76, 379–81, 429–32, 1996.

Whitley, R. J., and D. T. Durack, eds. *Infections of the Central Nervous System.* New York: River Press, 1991.

Will, R. G., et al. "A new variant of Creutzfeldt-Jakob disease in the UK," *Lancet* 347(1996):921–25.

Williams, Gurney. "8 New Health Threats: How to protect your family," *Family Circle* (Oct. 8, 1996):66–76.

Williams, J. D., and J. Burnie, eds. *The Epidemiology of Acute Bacterial Meningitis in Tropical Africa.* New York: Academic Press, 1987.

Wilson, Mary E. *A World Guide to Infections.* New York: Oxford University Press, 1991.

Wotherspoon, A. C., et al. "Helicobacter pylori-associated gastritis and primary B-cell gastric lymphoma." *Lancet* 338(1991): 1175–76.

Yamauchi, T., et al. "Transmission of live, attenuated mumps virus to the human placenta," *New England Journal of Medicine* 290(1974):710–12.

Zamula, Evelyn, "Adults need tetanus shots, too," *FDA Consumer* (July–Aug. 1996): 13–18.

INDEX

Page numbers in **boldface** indicate main articles. Page numbers followed by *d* indicate definition in Glossary.